Psychiatric Issues in Parkinson's Disease

Edited by

Matthew Menza and Laura Marsh

Psychiatric Issues in Parkinson's Disease

Edited by

Matthew Menza

Professor and Vice Chair
Department of Psychiatry
Robert Wood Johnson Medical School
Piscataway, NJ
USA

Laura Marsh

Associate Professor of Psychiatry and Neurology
Department of Psychiatry and Behavioral Sciences
Johns Hopkins University of Medicine
Baltimore, MD
USA

Foreword by
Jeffrey L Cummings

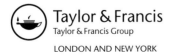

Taylor & Francis
Taylor & Francis Group

LONDON AND NEW YORK

© 2006 Taylor & Francis, an imprint of the Taylor & Francis Group

First published in the United Kingdom in 2006 by Taylor & Francis, an imprint of the Taylor & Francis Group, 2 Park Square, Milton Park, Abingdon, Oxon OX14 4RN

Tel.:   +44 (0)20 7017 6000
Fax.:   +44 (0)20 7017 6699
Website: http://www.tandf.co.uk/medicine
E-mail: info.medicine@tandf.co.uk

Although every effort has been made to ensure that all owners of copyright material have been acknowledged in this publication, we would be glad to acknowledge in subsequent reprints or editions any omissions brought to our attention.

Although every effort has been made to ensure that drug doses and other information are presented accurately in this publication, the ultimate responsibility rests with the prescribing physician. Neither the publishers nor the authors can be held responsible for errors or for any consequences arising from the use of information contained herein. For detailed prescribing information or instructions on the use of any product or procedure discussed herein, please consult the prescribing information or instructional material issued by the manufacturer.

A CIP record for this book is available from the British Library.
Library of Congress Cataloging-in-Publication Data
Data available on application

ISBN 1-84184-491-8
ISBN 978-1-84184-491-6

Distributed in North and South America by
Taylor & Francis
2000 NW Corporate Blvd
Boca Raton, FL 33431, USA
Within Continental USA
Tel: 800 272 7737; Fax: 800 374 3401
Outside Continental USA
Tel: 561 994 0555; Fax: 561 361 6018
E-mail: orders@crcpress.com

Distributed in the rest of the world by
Thomson Publishing Services
Cheriton House
North Way
Andover, Hampshire SP10 5BE, UK
Tel.: +44 (0)1264 332424
E-mail: salesorder.tandf@thomsonpublishingservices.co.uk

Composition by Wearset Ltd, Boldon, Tyne & Wear, UK

Printed and bound in Malta by Gutenberg Press

Contents

Section III: Psychiatric disturbances in Parkinson's disease

Section IV: Special topics in Parkinson's disease

Foreword

Parkinson's disease (PD) is a progressive neurodegenerative disorder with a plethora of clinical manifestations including motor system dysfunction, autonomic abnormalities, cognitive decline, and a variety of neuropsychiatric manifestations. The behavioral and neuropsychiatric aspects of PD represent an important clinical challenge in optimizing the quality of life of patients and their caregivers. This dimension of the illness frequently accounts for a substantial portion of the distress associated with the disease, the burden experienced by caregivers, and the requirement for institutionalization or nursing home placement. The pharmacologic issues regarding appropriate management of the neuropsychiatric aspects are particularly complex since some of the medications used to treat PD aggravate neuropsychiatric symptoms, and agents used to control behavioral disturbances in PD may increase parkinsonism.

It is to this complex set of problems that *Psychiatric Issues in Parkinson's Disease* edited by Matthew Menza and Laura Marsh is devoted. The volume begins with updates on the basic neurology of PD, the treatment of the movement disorder of PD, challenges in the management of advanced PD, and optimal control of non-motor somatic symptoms of PD. Next, the array of signs and symptoms associated with cognitive impairment in PD are considered. Cognitive impairment not reaching criteria for dementia is explicated, followed by a discussion of the dementia that commonly occurs in PD and a consideration of the relationship of dementia of PD to dementia with Lewy bodies (DLB). In recent years the many clinical and pathological similarities between the dementia of PD and the syndrome of DLB have become apparent with only the initial symptom differing in the two disorders. The evolving understanding of the relationship between the dementia of PD and DLB is considered in detail.

Mood disorders including anxiety and depression in PD are described along with the current strategies for optional management. Treatment of psychosis is one of the most challenging aspects involved in caring for a patient with PD. Conventional neuroleptic agents commonly exaggerate parkinsonism and may produce such profound motor disabilities as to hasten death. Atypical antipsychotic medication must be used with caution in the elderly, since there is an increased risk of both cerebrovascular disease and death associated with these medications. On the other hand, few non-antipsychotic medications have a meaningful effect in reducing psychotic symptoms and, left untreated, psychosis in PD can create a behavioral state unacceptable to patient, caregiver, and care environment. Substantial clinical experience and wisdom is required to resolve this clinical conundrum individually for each patient manifesting psychotic symptoms. Guidelines for responding to the complicated challenges surrounding the management of psychosis in PD are provided.

Sleep abnormalities are increasingly recognized in PD, particularly rapid eye movement (REM) sleep behavior disorder. This sleep disturbance representing the acting out of dreams has been associated uniquely with disorders produced by abnormalities of alpha-synuclein protein metabolism. REM sleep behavior disorder has been observed in PD, DLB and the multiple system atrophies. It is rarely seen in other neurodegenerative disorders, even those manifesting aspects of parkinsonism. The neurobiology and management of REM sleep behavior disorder and other sleep abnormalities encountered in patients with PD are described. Behavior disturbances such as agitation, obsessive-compulsive disorder, and pathological gambling are discussed in the chapter pertaining to behavioral disturbances in PD.

Wider issues bearing on the management of PD are considered in the final set of chapters, addressing disability, coping with therapy, personality issues, rehabilitation, long term care and nursing homes, advocacy groups, and caregiver issues. These chapters define the complex ecology of care that is required for optimal quality of life of a patient with PD.

Together the chapters of *Psychiatric Issues in Parkinson's Disease* provide a comprehensive overview of our evolving understanding of the neurobiology, clinical manifestations, and treatment (both pharmacologic and non-pharmacologic) of psychiatric manifestations of PD. Each of the chapters is contributed by an experienced individual qualified to provide in-depth understanding, describe the application of guidelines, and bring critical expertise to bear. The chapters provide both a scientific perspective and important practical clinical guidance. This volume represents an important milestone in advancing understandings of the neurobiology of behavioral changes in PD and is a clinical companion that can help practitioners provide improved care to victims of this disease and their caregivers.

Jeffrey L. Cummings, MD.
Los Angeles, California
2005.

Preface

Parkinson's disease (PD) is now the second most common neurodegenerative disease in the elderly. About one million Americans have the illness and it is projected that this number will increase considerably as our population ages. Once rarely discussed in public, the many courageous and well-known individuals who have talked about their own struggles with PD have increased awareness of this disorder. This heightened profile has led to a decrease in stigma and increased support for research on mechanisms and treatment of the disease. With this new emphasis on research comes a greater sense of hope for a cure as well as for better ways to manage PD.

The impact of PD on individuals is as wide-ranging as the clinical manifestations of the disease itself. While it affects nearly all aspects of life for most people, those without PD often fail to appreciate that the disease can make even the most mundane daily activity a challenge. In addition, most discussion of PD focuses on its motor features, such as tremor, slowness, and imbalance. Yet the so-called "non-motor" aspects of the illness, such as depression, anxiety, memory difficulties, sleep disturbances, etc., are often prominent and can cause as much or more difficulty for individuals struggling with the disease.

While we anticipate that a cure for PD will come eventually, we remain faced with the question of what to do now that will ease the burden of the illness. Often, clinicians and patients approach us with the question, "What do I do about . . .?" These questions cover nearly every aspect of PD, from diagnosis and medication to coping and the value of advocacy. In order to understand, treat, or cope with PD, it is important to understand the various manifestations of the illness, particularly the clinical presentations and management of psychiatric disturbances. Accordingly, we hope that clinicians, patients and their families will be helped by the practical approach to understanding and treating PD that you will find in this book.

It is for these reasons that we have gathered together a group of experts on PD to address reducing the burden of the illness. We have found, in our many years of treating individuals with PD, that the impact of the non-motor aspects and how they relate to the motor aspects is often underappreciated, by both the family and the physician. One goal of this book is to provide our readers with a better understanding of the neuropsychiatric and quality-of-life struggles that affect individuals living with PD. Furthermore, we aim to provide guidance to clinicians from multiple disciplines about managing these problems. While this book is intended for a clinically trained audience, we expect that many patients, families, and other caregivers will benefit from the information provided and use this book as a resource for subsequent discussions with their treating clinicians.

Because many of the motor and psychiatric issues are interrelated, their optimal management requires coordination between those who provide neurological care, psychiatric care, family support, and other services. The book begins, therefore, with chapters that discuss the neurology of PD and the latest treatments for its primary motor features. Subsequent chapters in Section I of the book discuss the motor complications of antiparkinsonian medications and the other non-motor physical symptoms that are common in PD patients, such as constipation, dry skin, and blurred vision. These chapters are intended to serve as a primer on the treatment of the typical motor and associated symptoms of PD from the neurologist's perspective. Such an understanding should enhance co-management of PD by those whose primary focus is on the psychiatric aspects of PD.

Sections II and III of the book are devoted to information and guidance on the neuropsychiatric disturbances that can occur in PD. Awareness of these phenomena should facilitate their early identification and suitable interventions. Section II provides discussions and advice on cognitive impairment and dementia that should help in understanding the common presentations and various manifestations of cognitive difficulties. These chapters will also offer practical advice on management. In Section III, you will find chapters on depression and on anxiety, common problems experienced by those with PD. These problems greatly affect quality of life and attention to them can lessen the burdens of the illness. Our belief, and experience, is that addressing these problems successfully improves all aspects of an individual's and their family's life. There are also chapters devoted to psychosis and to other behavioral disturbances including disinhibition. Problems such as hallucinations, delusions, and gambling often seem completely out of character for the individual with PD, but they are in large part related to the medications used to treat PD. We spend considerable time explaining these problems and offering advice on treatment.

The chapters in Section IV focus on a variety of matters that are less likely to be discussed in medical textbooks of this sort. However, we included these topics because they are integral to patient care and are of great relevance to the long-term management of PD by clinicians, patients and their families. To that end, we provide perspectives and advice on learning to cope with the illness, disability, and the value of rehabilitation. We also discuss the role of nursing homes in the later stages of the illness and pay special attention to the issues faced by caregivers. Lastly, we discuss the value of advocacy. Advocacy groups offer the comfort and collective optimism of a shared purpose and provide opportunities for individuals to become better informed about PD and involved in changing the future for individuals with PD.

Our expectation for this book is that it will help you to better understand and manage the various faces of PD. If you are a clinician, we hope that it will also help you to provide advice and comprehensive guidance to patients and their families, as well as to members of other clinical disciplines involved in the care of these patients. If PD affects you or a loved one, we also hope that this book will, in some way, help to ease your burden.

Matthew Menza
Laura Marsh

Contributors

Dag Aarsland, *Centre for Neuro and Geriatric Psychiatric Research, Stavanger University Hospital, Stavanger, Norway*

Susan Spear Bassett, *Associate Professor of Psychiatry, Department of Psychiatry, Johns Hopkins Hospital, Baltimore, MD, USA*

Kevin M Biglan, *Assistant Professor, University of Rochester Neurology Associates, Rochester, NY, USA*

David J Burn, *Consultant Neurologist & Reader in Movement Disorder Neurology, Newcastle General Hospital, Newcastle upon Tyne, UK*

Laura Jane Cohen, *Director of Outreach, Parkinson's Action Network, Washington DC, USA*

Amy L Comstock, *Executive Director, Parkinson's Action Network, Washington DC, USA*

Roseanne DeFronzo Dobkin, *Professor, Department of Psychiatry, Robert Wood Johnson Medical School, Piscataway, NJ, USA*

S Rebecca Dunlop, *Reasearch Nurse, Johns Hopkins National Parkinson Foundation Center for Excellence, Baltimore, MD, USA*

Leslie D Frazier, *Associate Professor, Department of Psychology, Florida International University, Miami, FL, USA*

Melissa Gerstenhaber, *Research Nurse Coordinator, Department of Psychiatry and Behavioral Sciences, Johns Hopkins University School of Medicine, Baltimore, MD, USA*

Paul E Holtzheimer III, *Assistant Professor, Department of Psychiatry and Behavioral Sciences, Emory University School of Medicine, Atlanta, GA, USA*

Lee Hyer, *Professor of Psychiatry, University Behavioral Healthcare Center, University of Medicine and Dentistry of New Jersey, Piscataway, NJ, USA*

Daniel I Kaufer, *Department of Neurology, University of North Carolina School of Medicine, Chapel Hill, NC, USA*

Benjamin J Kirby, *Communications Director, Parkinson's Action Network, Washington DC, USA*

Geoffrey W Lane, *Research Fellow, Geropsychology, University of Rochester Medical Center, Rochester, NY, USA*

Gerald Leventhal, *Professor, Department of Psychiatry, UMDMJ – New Jersey Medical School, Newark, NJ, USA*

Humberto Marin, *Department of Psychiatry, Robert Wood Johnson Medical School, Piscataway, NJ, USA*

Margery H Mark, *Associate Professor of Neurology and Psychiatry, Department of Neurology, New Brunswick, NJ, USA*

Laura Marsh, *Associate Professor, Department of Psychiatry and Neurology, Johns Hopkins University School of Medicine, Baltimore, MD, USA*

William M McDonald, *Associate Professor, Department of Psychiatry and Behavioral Sciences, Emroy University School of Medicine, Atlanta, GA, USA*

Matthew Menza, *Professor and Vice Chair, Department of Psychiatry and Neurology, Robert Wood Johnson Medical School, Piscataway, NJ, USA*

Nasir S Mirza, *Foundation Programme 1 doctor, Guy's and St Thomas' NHS Trust, London, UK*

E D Playford, *Senior Lecturer/Honorary Consultant Neurologist, Institute of Neurology, National Hospital for Neurology and Neurosurgery, London, UK*

Irene Hegeman Richard, *Associate Professor, Department of Neurology and Psychiatry, University of Rochester School of Medicine and Dentistry, New York, NY, USA*

Alexander I Tröster, *Associate Professor, Department of Neurology, University of North Carolina, Chapel Hill, NC, USA*

Daniel Weintraub, *Assistant Professor, Departments of Psychiatry and Neurology, University of Pennsylvania School of Medicine, Philadelphia, PA, USA*

chapter 1

Pathogenesis, diagnosis, and treatment

Margery H Mark

In the last decade, enormous strides have been made in understanding and treating Parkinson's disease (PD). Most importantly, with the significant involvement of cognition, behavior, and mood, PD is now recognized as more than just a motor disorder and the nigrostriatal dopamine system is just one of many pathways involved. Progress in understanding the disease process itself has been made possible by the identification of genes causing PD (such as mutations in α-synuclein and parkin) and the implications for α-synuclein aggregation and impairment of the ubiquitin/proteasome pathway in cell death. Ultimately, knowing why the cells degenerate will allow targeted drug therapy and interrupt the process.

The neurologic syndrome of PD is characterized by bradykinesia, rigidity, tremor, and, in later stages, postural instability. PD must be differentiated from the "Parkinson-plus" syndromes of dementia with Lewy bodies, multiple system atrophy, progressive supranuclear palsy, and corticobasal degeneration.

For the cardinal neurologic features of PD, levodopa remains the most efficacious treatment, but recent trends have turned to initial therapy with direct-acting dopamine agonists in younger patients, although new problems with these drugs have become recognized in the last few years. Peripheral inhibition of catechol-O-methyltransferase (COMT inhibitors) allowing prolongation of levodopa action is another therapeutic alternative added in the last decade. An older drug, amantadine, has found new life in reducing dyskinesias, possibly through its mechanism as an *N*-methyl-D-aspartate (NMDA)-receptor antagonist. Despite the popularity of treatment algorithms, there is no single, correct answer for treating PD; medication regimens need to be individualized for all PD patients, focusing on the motor as well as cognitive function and dysfunction of the patient.

Introduction

Parkinson's disease (PD) is a chronic, progressive neurodegenerative disorder, classically affecting the nigrostriatal dopaminergic system; its primary pathology is loss of dopamine-producing cells in the pars compacta of the substantia nigra. Prevalence rates vary, but it is estimated that about one million Americans have PD, with an annual incidence of just over 13/100 000 person-years (age-adjusted) in the US. Epidemiologic studies of age-adjusted incidence reveal an incidence rate of 9.7/100 000 in Sweden, and just over 11/100 000 in both Taiwan and Japan.[1] Age-adjusted prevalence rates (per 100 000 population) range from 104.7 (Japan), 114.6 (US), 168.8 (Taiwan), to 258.8 (Sicily). The average age of onset is about 60 years, with a slight male predominance, although between 5% and 10% of patients may begin before age 40, defined as young-onset PD. The majority of patients in the US with PD are over age 65, making it the second most common neurodegenerative disease (after Alzheimer's disease) of the elderly, resulting in a significant impact on the financial resources of a progressively aging population.[2]

Etiology and pathogenesis

Evidence for both genetic and environmental factors in the pathogenesis of PD accumulates daily; most likely, age-dependent genetic factors with cumulative environmental influences are responsible for the majority of cases. Oxidative stress, mitochondrial dysfunction, and apoptosis have been implicated in cell death via both exogenous (e.g., toxic) and endogenous (e.g., genetic) mechanisms.[3]

In the last decade, multiple genes for PD have been identified (Table 1.1). The first, and possibly the most significant, was a mutation in the α-synuclein gene, termed the *PARK1* gene, found in a large Italian family with autosomal dominant PD, called the Contursi kindred.[4–6] Since its initial identification in 1997, there have been two further point mutations as well as

Table 1.1 Genetics of PD

Locus	Designation	Transmission	Gene/linkage
4q21-23	PARK1	AD	α-synuclein
6q25-27	PARK2	AR	parkin
4q21	PARK4(1)*	AD	α-synuclein
4p14	PARK5	AD	UCHL1
1p36	PARK6	AR	PINK1
1p36	PARK7	AR	DJ-1
12p11.2-q13.1	PARK8	AD	LRRK2
2p13	PARK3	AD	linkage
1p36	PARK9	AR	linkage
1p32	PARK10	Suscept	linkage (late-onset)
2q36-37	PARK11	Suscept	linkage
2q22-23	none	Suscept	NR4A2
5q23.1-23.3	none	Suscept	synphilin-1
17q21	none	Suscept	tau
Mitochondrial mutations			complex 1

* PARK4 was the designation for linkage originally thought to be on 4p, but recently found to be a triplication of the α-synuclein gene.
AD: autosomal dominant; AR: autosomal recessive; Suscept: susceptibility gene.

both gene triplication and duplication.[7] A central role for α-synuclein in all patients with PD is suggested by its biochemistry. Alpha-synuclein aggregates, or more specifically, oligomeric aggregates called protofibrils, have been demonstrated to cause cell membrane (including mitochondrial membrane) disruption and cell death. It is a major component of Lewy bodies, the pathognomonic feature of PD (see Pathology). In addition, aggregation of α-synuclein is enhanced in an oxidative milieu (both in the presence of toxins and in endogenous systems), and overexpression of α-synuclein yields a clinical picture of parkinsonism in transgenic animal models.[8]

More commonly occurring mutations exist in autosomal recessive genes with early-onset PD, those for parkin (*PARK2*),[9] DJ-1 (*PARK7*),[10] and PINK1 (*PARK6*).[11,12] Parkin is an enzyme in the ubiquitin/proteasome system, DJ-1 has a putative role in a cell's oxidative stress response, and PINK1 is a mitochondrial protein kinase; in recessive disorders, loss of function results in loss of protective mechanisms provided by these enzymes.

The newest mutation to be reported is in the gene for the enzyme LRRK2 (leucine-rich repeat kinase 2).[13] Labeled *PARK8* is located on chromosome

12p, LRRK2 encodes for a newly described protein, dardarin. It appears to function as a tyrosine kinase, and the reported mutations may have an activating effect on the kinase activity of LRRK2,[14] thus expanding the pathogenetic possibilities to include phosphorylation of key proteins involved in PD. Age of onset in individuals with this mutation is variable (35–78 years),[15] but the clinical phenotype is fairly characteristic for typical PD. The neuropathology, however, is quite variable,[16] with α-synuclein-positive Lewy bodies in the brainstem, widespread Lewy bodies throughout the cortex, tau-positive pathology as in other Parkinson-plus syndromes, or just nigral degeneration without any distinctive histopathology. This autosomal dominant mutation accounts for about 5–6% of familial and 1–2% of apparently sporadic cases, making it the most common known genetic cause of PD.[17]

Despite genetic heterogeneity, biochemical properties of the mutant genes suggest a common pathogenetic mechanism in PD. A likely scenario is that cell death results from common mechanisms (with or without mutations) involving protein folding and/or degradation through the ubiquitin/proteasome pathway as well as oxidative stress. Future drug therapy may be directed at these targets to slow down or even prevent cell death in both inherited and sporadic forms of PD.

Diagnosis

Typical PD may begin with subtle, unilateral symptoms and signs such as unilateral hand tremor, decreased arm swing, micrographia, and loss of facial expression (hypomimia). Depression, anxiety, and sleep abnormalities may also be early complaints. The diagnostic criteria of PD (defined for research protocols to minimize inclusion of patients with atypical parkinsonisms) include the cardinal triad of rest tremor, akinesia or bradykinesia (lack of movement or slow movement), and rigidity; two of the three are required for diagnosis.[18] Later in disease, loss of postural reflexes may occur. PD typically begins unilaterally and usually remains asymmetric throughout the course of disease, often with the initially affected side showing greater severity of signs and symptoms. Course of disease is variable among patients, but is usually slowly progressive. While life-span is generally reduced, younger-onset patients may live for decades after the onset of symptoms with appropriate treatment.

Cardinal signs[19]

The tremor of PD is most often seen at rest, in which the body part is not voluntarily activated and is completely supported against gravity. It is classically a 4–6 Hz rest tremor, but a postural and/or a simple kinetic tremor may also be seen. Tremor at rest is seen most easily when the patient rests his hand in his lap, or dangles it freely while walking; it usually abates when the patient performs a purposeful movement. Rarely, some PD patients have a greater postural/kinetic tremor (and even rarer, only a posture/kinetic tremor). Tremor most often occurs in the hands, but may also affect the feet and lips and jaw, but not the head and neck or voice, as seen in essential tremor. Some patients may complain of the sensation of an internal tremor, even if it is not visible. Tremor occurs in over 75% of PD patients, and tremor-predominant PD at onset often predicts a more benign course.[20] Absence of tremor does not rule out PD, but it is a red flag to consider an atypical parkinsonism (see Differential Diagnosis, below).

The akinesia/bradykinesia is manifested by general slowing of movements, decreases in fine motor control and rapid alternating movements (e.g., buttoning clothes, cutting meat) and hypomimia, or the mask-like facies, which is exemplified by decreased blink rates. The more problematic symptoms involve limitations in initiating movements (start hesitation). This causes difficulties getting out of a chair or getting started walking. As a result of the akinesia/bradykinesia, the gait is characterized by dragging a leg or short, shuffling steps. Pivoting while turning becomes difficult and patients may need to take small, marching steps to complete a turn (turning *en bloc*).

Rigidity, or "lead-pipe" rigidity, is a uniform increase in tone of a limb that is the same throughout the range of motion around a joint (e.g., wrist, elbow, shoulder, knee). It should be differentiated from upper motor neuron spasticity in which there is a catch and release of tone. The term "cogwheeling" does not refer to a type of rigidity, but rather indicates tremor superimposed on tone and should be avoided.

Postural instability gradually becomes a considerable problem in PD. Initially it may be manifest as minor retropulsion in which the patient may stumble backwards or take multiple steps backward on the "pull test" (a clinical test of postural stability in which the examiner evaluates the patient's righting reflexes by pulling backwards sharply on the standing patient's shoulders). Eventually, the patient will lose the righting reflex and be unable to prevent falling (usually backwards). In the latest stages, patients are unable to stand or walk without assistance and are unable to find their vertical position in space.

Features consistent with PD[19]

Disorders of mood (depression, anxiety) and cognition, as well as psychosis (primarily visual hallucinations) are common in PD and the focus of this volume; they will be discussed at length in subsequent chapters.

Some patients with typical PD may have, either in the treated or untreated state, a secondary dystonia that is manifested generally by painful cramping of muscles. Curling of toes, especially upon arising in the morning (when the patient is at his lowest dopamine level) is typical, but cramping of calves, thighs, and the neck are also common. Nonmotor features that can also occur in PD include disorders of autonomic function, manifested by orthostatic hypotension (usually asymptomatic in typical PD), sweating abnormalities, bladder dysfunction such as urgency and frequency, impotence, and gastrointestinal complaints, such as abdominal bloating and constipation. These are discussed further in Chapter 4.

Differential diagnosis

The diagnosis of PD is almost exclusively clinical, based on history and neurological examination. Approximately 15–25% of patients with a parkinsonism will have an atypical parkinsonian syndrome.[21] Appropriate inquiry should be made as to the medications that the patient is taking or has taken, as drug-induced parkinsonism is largely reversible; it is usually secondary to neuroleptic medications, but any medication that blocks D_2 dopamine receptors (including phenothiazine antiemetics and metoclopramide) may be a culprit. Vascular parkinsonism may be non-progressive or progress in a step-wise fashion; vascular risk factors will be present and prevention of further cardio- and cerebrovascular events may prevent further insult. Most of the remainder of the patients with atypical parkinsonian syndromes will have a primary neurodegenerative disorder. There are, however, currently no reliable, commercially available tests that can diagnose PD or differentiate it from the atypical neurodegenerative parkinsonisms, or Parkinson-plus syndromes. Red flags that suggest an alternate diagnosis include early postural instability, absence of rest tremor, early dementia, rapid progression of symptoms, early or severe dysautonomia, and involvement of other neurologic systems (for example, corticospinal tract involvement, peripheral neuropathy, supranuclear gaze abnormalities, or cerebellar features). The primary neurodegenerative parkinsonisms include dementia with Lewy bodies (DLB), multiple system atrophy (MSA), progressive supranuclear palsy (PSP), and corticobasal degeneration (CBD).[22] Tables 1.2–1.5 list the major clinical features of each of these four disorders. Although tremor may occur in all four disorders (most prevalent in DLB, next in MSA, less common in PSP, and rare in CBD), it is less common than in PD.[22] Except for DLB, the parkinsonism is generally unresponsive to treatment with levodopa.[23]

Table 1.2 Dementia with Lewy bodies (DLB)

Significant cognitive dysfunction
With: Parkinsonism
      Visual hallucinations
      Fluctuations (defined as marked variation in a patient's cognitive or functional abilities, or periods of confusion or decreased responsiveness alternating with lucidity and attentiveness)

Note: Parkinsonism preceding dementia by an interval of 1 year or more is termed PD-dementia (PD-D), while dementia that precedes or accompanies the onset of parkinsonism is labeled DLB.

Table 1.3 Multiple system atrophy (MSA)

Parkinsonism
With: Poor response to levodopa
      Autonomic features
      Speech or bulbar dysfunction
      Absence of dementia
      Absence of levodopa-induced confusion
      Falls

Three clinical subtypes of MSA are:
Shy-Drager syndrome: primary dysautonomia with parkinsonism
Striatonigral degeneration: akinetic-rigid syndrome with no improvement on levodopa but with dyskinesias (grimacing)
Olivopontocerebellar atrophy: cerebellar features with parkinsonism

Table 1.4 Progressive supranuclear palsy (PSP)

Parkinsonism that usually presents with falling
With: Supranuclear ophthalmoplegia
      Dystonic rigidity of neck (hyperextension)
      Pseudobulbar palsy
      Dysarthria progressing to anarthria
      Dysphagia
      Axial > appendicular rigidity
      Mental disturbance; but dementia may be mild

Table 1.5 Corticobasal degeneration (CBD)

Parkinsonism
With: Asymmetric features
      Dystonia
      Apraxia
      Alien limb phenomenon
      Cortical sensory loss
      Dysarthria
      Dysphagia
      Oculomotor abnormalities
      Dementia

Pathology

It is been estimated that by the time of onset of motor symptoms in PD, at least 50% of substantia nigra pars compacta neurons are lost. There is also cell loss in the locus coeruleus, dorsal raphe nuclei, nucleus basalis of Meynert, and dorsal motor nucleus of the vagus. The pathognomonic feature of PD (as well as DLB) is the Lewy body, a characteristic cytoplasmic inclusion body (Figure 1.1a). In DLB and PD with dementia (PD-D), Lewy bodies can be found diffusely throughout the brain, including the cortex.[24] (Similarities and differences between DLB and PD-D are discussed further in Chapter 7.)

Immunocytochemical studies originally were not particularly helpful in characterizing Lewy bodies. They contained ubiquitinated protein and,

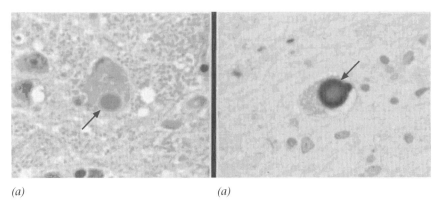

(a)   *(a)*

Figure 1.1 *Photomicrographs of Lewy bodies in the substantia nigra of a patient with Parkinson's disease. (a) H&E stain. The Lewy body is seen as a typical, intracytoplasmic inclusion with a pale pink halo and a dense eosinophilic core. (b) α-synuclein immunostain. The Lewy body stains intensely with antibodies for α-synuclein; the pale halo seen on routine stains is most prominently seen with α-synuclein immunocytochemistry. (Photomicrographs courtesy of Dennis W Dickson, MD.)*

unlike the neurofibrillary tangles of Alzheimer's disease, PSP, and CBD, they are tau-negative. But in the last few years, following the identification of the first gene for PD as a mutation in α-synuclein, antibodies to this protein demonstrated highly sensitive staining of Lewy bodies (Figure 1.1b).[25] It is also nearly specific, as only the glial cytoplasmic inclusions seen in MSA are also synuclein-positive. We now identify PD, DLB, and MSA as synucleinopathies and distinguish them from the parkinsonism tauopathies, PSP and CBD.[22]

Treatment of PD

Treatment of early PD

(Chapter 2 discusses initial management of PD in further detail.)

When a patient first presents with motor symptoms of PD, there are several treatment options. If the patient is extremely mildly affected (e.g., has a subtle, non-bothersome rest tremor and little else symptomatically), one may choose to delay therapy until such time as a proven neuroprotective agent is available. A medication for mild symptoms may be in order, such as selegiline, a centrally acting monoamine oxidase type B (MAO-B) inhibitor. Anticholinergic drugs are only effective for tremor and come with a host of side effects; therefore, these agents should be prescribed with care and reserved for younger patients who have a pronounced and bothersome rest tremor. Certainly, if depression or anxiety are prominent complaints early on, they should be treated symptomatically.

Once a patient develops functionally disabling motor symptoms, however, therapy should begin with either a dopamine agonist or levodopa.[26] Polytherapy is not needed in early PD, and indeed starting more than one medication simultaneously may be confusing if side effects ensue. The decision regarding which drug to start is largely a matter of choice. As a rule, many experts will use dopamine agonists as initial monotherapy in mild, younger-onset patients, whereas older patients or those with baseline cognitive difficulties should be started on a levodopa preparation from the beginning. Nevertheless, using agonists as first-line treatment continues to generate controversy and many experts recommend more critical examination of this approach.[27]

Dopamine agonists[28]

Dopamine agonists have less antiparkinson effect than levodopa, but also have a longer duration of action and are less likely to cause dyskinesias. Two ergot-derivative dopamine agonists, bromocriptine and pergolide, and two non-ergot drugs, pramipexole and ropinrole, are currently marketed in the US. Bromocriptine is seldom used for treatment of PD anymore since it is the least potent of the agonists. The two non-ergot agonists are approved for treatment of both early (as monotherapy) and advanced disease (with levodopa).[29] Long-term studies with pramipexole[30] and ropinirole[31] have shown ongoing improvement in motor symptoms, although in all studies, levodopa remained more effective at all time points. Over time, virtually all patients on agonists require the addition of levodopa.

Side effects of dopamine agonists include nausea, somnolence and postural hypotension, confusion and toxic psychosis, and potentiation of dyskinesias in patients on levodopa. Sudden sleep attacks are an infrequent but potential adverse effect of all dopaminergic drugs, most commonly seen with dopamine agonists;[32] all patients on dopaminergic therapy who drive should be made aware of sedation and sleep attacks as side effects of their treatment. A recently reported, uncommon but increasingly recognized and potentially serious side-effect of dopamine agonist therapy is pathologic gambling;[33] although this also appears to occur with other dopaminergic drugs, reduction of the agonist is usually effective in eliminating the problem. Of increasing concern are recent reports of several cases of heart valvular disease, some requiring surgery, in patients on high doses of pergolide,[34] suggesting that all patients on pergolide should undergo baseline echocardiographic evaluation with yearly follow-up or discontinuation of the drug in patients with evidence of valve abnormalities.

Levodopa[28]

The most effective drug to treat PD is levodopa, the immediate precursor of dopamine, which crosses the blood–brain barrier. Levodopa must be used in combination with carbidopa, a peripheral decarboxylase inhibitor. Levodopa is effective for most patients during at least the first 5 years of treatment.[35] Later, as the disease progresses, the duration of benefit from each dose may shorten (the "wearing off" effect), and still later some patients develop sudden, unpredictable fluctuations between mobility and immobility (the "on-off" effect). After about 5–8 years of levodopa therapy, patients may have either dose-related clinical fluctuations, dose-related dyskinesias (chorea, dystonia) or inadequate response (see Table 1.6). Carbidopa/levodopa is available in an immediate-release (IR) and controlled-release (CR) form; either one may be used initially, and they may be used together for a quick "kick-in" (IR) and for more sustained serum levels (CR).

Table 1.6 Definitions

On: improvement in parkinsonian signs and symptoms when the medication is working optimally

Off: the state of re-emergence of parkinsonian signs and symptoms when the medication's effect has waned

Motor (response) fluctuations: the complications of the treatment of PD affecting ability to move

Treatment of PD: Definitions

Wearing off: a loss of benefit from a dose of levodopa, typically at the end of a few hours

On-off phenomenon: unpredictable, usually abrupt oscillations in motor state

Dyskinesias: abnormal involuntary movements, usually associated with high levodopa levels (high dopa dyskinesias, or HDD), but frequently occurring when plasma levodopa levels are dropping (low dopa dyskinesias, or LDD)

Side effects of levodopa include anorexia, nausea and vomiting, and orthostatic hypotension, vivid dreams, hallucinations, delusions, confusion, and sleep disturbance.

Levodopa has been implicated as a source of oxidative stress, but there is no clear evidence that levodopa causes neurotoxicity in humans.[36] A recent National Institutes of Health (NIH)-sponsored, double-blind study of levodopa vs placebo in early, mild PD patients demonstrated clear superiority of levodopa in a dose-dependent manner over placebo, including after 2 weeks of washout, indicating no clinical acceleration of disease.[37]

Treatment of advanced PD

(Management of advanced stage PD is discussed further in Chapter 3.)

Early on, patients respond to dopaminergic replacement therapy with a smooth, stable improvement in symptoms and signs. With time, however, the therapeutic window narrows. Those on dopamine agonists as monotherapy will require addition of a levodopa preparation; those already on levodopa may develop response fluctuations, beginning with simple wearing-off. Strategies for compensating for these problems center around the concept of continuous dopaminergic stimulation.[38] To accomplish this, the levodopa dose may be increased or the dosage interval may be narrowed to compensate for the shorter duration of response. CR may be added to IR preparations, or vice versa. As peripheral methylation of levodopa decreases the available drug for transport from the gut to the blood, inhibition of intestinal catechol-O-methyltransferase (COMT) with entacapone or tolcapone allows for more sustained levodopa levels, decreasing off time.[28] If patients are not yet on an agonist, the addition of one of these drugs may also result in improved on time. An old drug, apomorphine, a non-specific dopamine agonist, can be used parenterally, and has recently been approved and marketed in a subcutaneous injectable form for "rescue therapy" for off periods in advanced PD.[39]

If dyskinesias develop, levodopa may be reduced while adjunctive drugs may be adjusted up or down as needed for reduction in fluctuations. Another older drug, amantadine, originally developed as an antiviral agent, has been used to treat mild symptoms of PD. More recently, it has also been found to be effective in reducing dyskinesias,[40] probably via its putative mechanism as an antagonist of striatal interneuronal N-methyl-D-aspartate (NMDA) receptors.

For appropriate candidates (relatively young and healthy, cognitively intact, on optimal medication treatment, with significant fluctuations and dyskinesias), bilateral deep brain stimulation (DBS) of the subthalamic nucleus appears to be at least as effective as thalamic stimulation in controlling parkinsonian tremor, and has been shown to be more than twice as effective as pallidotomy in treating all the symptoms of PD (Figure 1.2).[41] Bilateral stimulation improves tremor, rigidity, and bradykinesia and allows sustainable postoperative reduction in levodopa dosage.[42] Despite a more complex process for programming the electrical stimulator, DBS of the subthalamic nucleus has proven long-term efficacy and has supplanted all other surgical procedures. In general, it is the current surgical treatment of choice for PD.[43]

Unfortunately, not all motor complications of PD respond to dopaminergic therapy; these include freezing of gait, falling and balance problems, and speech abnormalities. Non-motor complications, including the

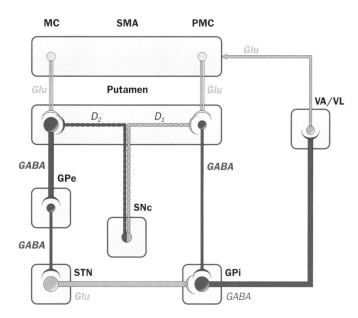

Figure 1.2 *A simplified schematic of the basal ganglia circuitry. Lighter blue efferents indicate excitatory pathways; darker blue lines indicate inhibitory pathways. In this schema, the subthalamic nucleus (STN) and globus pallidus interna (GPi) are disinhibited, resulting in overactivity of both the STN and GPi. The rationale for lesioning these nuclei to treat PD arises from this proposed circuit. SNc: substantia nigra pars compacta; GPe: globus pallidus externa; VA/VL: ventroanterior and ventrolateral nuclei of the thalamus; MC: motor cortex; SMA: supplementary motor area; PMC: premotor cortex; Glu: glutamate; GABA: gamma-aminobutyric acid. (By Margery H Mark, after Alexander & Crutcher.[44])*

psychiatric disorders as well as autonomic dysfunction (orthostatic hypotension, bladder frequency and urgency, impotence, and constipation) should all be addressed and treated symptomatically.

Despite the popularity of treatment algorithms, there is no single, correct answer for treating PD; one of multiple treatment choices may be the right one for an individual, and indeed medication regimens need to be individualized for all PD patients. The most important principle in medication adjustment is to "start low and go slow." The chief complaint (e.g., too much off time, disabling dyskinesias, or hallucinations) should be addressed first, and one new medication should be added or adjusted at a time, focusing on the drug interval as well as the dose. Finally, one should be alert for "red flags," such as advanced age, vivid dreams, hallucinations, and confusion. When these problems occur or threaten, drugs with an unfavorable risk:benefit ratio should be reduced or eliminated first: anticholinergics, MAO-B inhibitors, amantadine followed by dopamine agonists, leaving levodopa as monotherapy if necessary.

Conclusions

PD is a chronic, progressive neurodegenerative disease. The main pathology targets the nigrostriatal dopamine system, with motor signs and symptoms of rest tremor, akinesia, rigidity, and postural instability the clinical hallmarks. More recent evidence shows that PD is a much more diffuse condition, with involvement of cognitive processes the rule rather than the exception. Current treatment of the motor disorder is aimed at replacing the dopamine deficiency with levodopa, the immediate precursor of dopamine that crosses the blood–brain barrier, and other strategies such as direct-acting dopamine agonists, central MAO-B inhibitors, peripheral COMT inhibitors, and NMDA-receptor antagonists. Appropriate candidates may benefit from DBS of the subthalamic nucleus. Finally, the cause of PD remains to be elucidated, but clues from the first cloned genes in familial PD cases suggest that cell death results from common mechanisms involving the ubiquitin/proteasome pathway and oxidative stress. Future drug therapy may be directed at these targets to slow down or even prevent cell death in both inherited and sporadic forms of PD.

References

1. Korell M, Tanner CM, Epidemiology of Parkinson's disease: An overview. In: Ebadi MPR (ed.) *Parkinson's Disease*. CRC Press: Boca Raton, 2005; 39–50.
2. Lang AE, Lozano AM, Parkinson's disease. First of two parts. *New Engl J Med* 1998; **339**:1044–1053.
3. Huang Z, de la Fuente-Fernandez R, Stoessl AJ, Etiology of Parkinson's disease. *Can J Neurol Sci* 2003; **30**:S10–S18.
4. Golbe LI, Di Iorio G, Bonavita V, Miller DC, Duvoisin RC, A large kindred with autosomal dominant Parkinson's disease. *Ann Neurol* 1990; **27**:276–282.
5. Polymeropoulos MH, Higgins JJ, Golbe LI et al, A gene for Parkinson's disease maps to 4q21-q23. *Science* 1996; **274**:1197–1199.
6. Polymeropoulos MH, Lavedan C, Leroy E et al, Mutation in alpha synuclein identified in families with Parkinson's disease. *Science* 1997; **276**:2045–2047.
7. Golbe LI, Mouradian MM, Alpha-synuclein in Parkinson's disease: Light from two new angles. *Ann Neurol* 2004; **55**:153–156.
8. Mouradian MM, Recent advances in the genetics and pathogenesis of Parkinson disease. *Neurology* 2002; **58**:179–185.
9. Lücking CB, Durr A, Bonifati V et al, Association between early-onset Parkinson's disease and mutations in the parkin gene. French Parkinson's Disease Genetics Study Group. *New Engl J Med* 2000; **342**:1560–1567.
10. Bonifati V, Rizzu P, Squtieri F et al, DJ-1 (PARK7), a novel gene for autosomal recessive, early onset parkinsonism. *Neurol Sci* 2003; **24**:159–160.
11. Valente EM, Abou-Sleiman PM, Caputo V et al, Hereditary early-onset Parkinson's disease caused by mutations in PINK1. *Science* 2004; **304**:1158–1160.
12. Hatano Y, Li Y, Sato K, Asakawa S et al, Novel PINK1 mutations in early-onset parkinsonism. *Ann Neurol* 2004; **56**:424–427.
13. Paisan-Ruiz C, Saenz A, de Munain AL et al, Familial Parkinson's disease: clinical and genetic analysis of four Basque families. *Ann Neurol* 2005; **57**(3):365–372.
14. Kachergus J, Mata IF, Hulihan M et al, Identification of a novel LRRK2 mutation linked to autosomal dominant parkinsonism: evidence of a common founder across European populations. *Am J Hum Genet* 2005; **76**(4):672–680.
15. Di Fonzo A, Rohe CF, Ferreira J et al, A frequent LRRK2 gene mutation associated with autosomal dominant Parkinson's disease [see comment]. *Lancet* 2005; **365**(9457):412–415.
16. Zimprich A, Biskup S, Leitner P et al, Mutations in LRRK2 cause autosomal-dominant parkinsonism with pleomorphic pathology [see comment]. *Neuron* 2004; **44**(4):601–607.
17. Brice A, How much does dardarin contribute to Parkinson's disease? *Lancet* 2005; **365**:363–364.
18. Ward CD, Gibb WR, Research diagnostic criteria for Parkinson's disease. *Adv Neurol* 1990; **53**:245–249.
19. Paulson HL, Stern MB, Clinical manifestations of Parkinson's disease. In: Watts RL, Koller WC (eds) *Movement Disorders. Neurologic Principles and Practice*, 2nd edn. McGraw-Hill: New York, 2004; 233–245.
20. Frucht SJ, Clinical assessments. In: Pahwa R, Lyons KE, Koller WC (eds) *Therapy of Parkinson's Disease*, 3rd edn. Marcel Dekker Inc: New York, 2004; 37–52.
21. Hughes AJ, Daniel SE, Kilford L et al, Accuracy of clinical diagnosis of idiopathic Parkinson's disease: a clinico-pathological study of 100 cases. *J Neurol Neurosurg Psychiatry* 1992; **55**:181–184.
22. Mark MH, Lumping and splitting the Parkinson plus syndromes. *Neurol Clin* 2001; **3**:607–627.

23. Louis ED, Klatka LA, Liu Y et al, Comparison of extrapyramidal features in 31 pathologically confirmed cases of diffuse Lewy body disease and 34 pathologically confirmed cases of Parkinson's disease. *Neurology* 1997; **48**:376–380.

24. Lowe J, Lennox G, Leigh PN, Disorders of movement and system degeneration. In: Graham DJ, Lantos P (eds) *Greenfield's Neuropathology*. Arnold: London, 1997; 285–290.

25. Spillantini MG, Schmidt ML, Lee VM, Troganowski JQ, Jakes R, Goedert M, Alpha-synuclein in Lewy bodies. *Nature* 1997; **388**:839–840.

26. Miyasaki JM, Martin W, Suchowersky O et al, Practice parameter: Initiation of treatment for Parkinson's disease: An evidence-based review: Report of the Quality Standards Subcommittee of the American Academy of Neurology. *Neurology* 2002; **58**:11–17.

27. Wooten GF, Agonists vs levodopa in PD: the thrilla of whitha. *Neurology* 2003; **60**:360–362.

28. Poewe W, Granat R, Geser F, Pharmacologic treatment of Parkinson's disease. In: Watts RL, Koller WC (eds) *Movement Disorders. Neurologic Principles and Practice*, 2nd edn. McGraw-Hill: New York, 2004; 247–271.

29. Lambert D, Waters CH, Comparative tolerability of the newer generation antiparkinsonian agents. *Drugs Aging* 2000; **16**:55–65.

30. Parkinson Study Group, Pramipexole vs levodopa as initial treatment for Parkinson disease: A randomized controlled trial. *JAMA* 2000; **284**:1931–1938.

31. Rascol O, Brooks DJ, Korczyn AD, De Deyn PP, Clarke CE, Lang AE, A five-year study of the incidence of dyskinesia in patients with early Parkinson's disease who were treated with ropinirole or levodopa. 056 Study Group. *New Engl J Med* 2000; **342**:1484–1491.

32. Paus S, Brecht HM, Koster J, Seeger G, Klockgether T, Wullner U, Sleep attacks, daytime sleepiness, and dopamine agonists in Parkinson's disease. *Mov Disord* 2003; **18**:659–667.

33. Driver-Dunckley E, Samanta J, Stacy M, Pathological gambling associated with dopamine agonist therapy in Parkinson's disease. *Neurology* 2003; **61**:422–423.

34. Van Camp G, Flamez A, Cosyns B, Goldstein J, Perdaens C, Schoors D, Heart valvular disease in patients with Parkinson's disease treated with high-dose pergolide. *Neurology* 2003; **61**:859–861.

35. Koller WC, Hutton JT, Tolosa E, Capildeo R, the Carbidopa/Levodopa Study Group, Immediate-release and controlled-release carbidopa/levodopa in PD. A 5-year randomized multicenter study. *Neurology* 1999; **53**:1012–1019.

36. Agid Y, Chase T, Marsden D, Adverse reactions to levodopa: drug toxicity or progression of disease? *Lancet* 1998; **351**:851–852.

37. Parkinson Study Group, Does levodopa slow or hasten the rate of progression of Parkinson disease? The results of the ELLDOPA trial. *Neurology* 2003; **60**:A80–A81.

38. Sage JI, Mark MH, The rationale for continuous dopaminergic stimulation in patients with advanced Parkinson's disease. *Neurology* 1992; **42**(Suppl 1):23–28.

39. Dewey RB, Jr, Hutton JT, LeWitt PA, Factor SA, A randomized, double-blind, placebo-controlled trial of subcutaneously injected apomorphine for parkinsonian off-state events. *Arch Neurol* 2001; **58**:1385–1392.

40. Verhagen Metman L, Del Dotto P, van den Munckhof P, Fang J, Mouradian MM, Chase TN, Amantadine as treatment for dyskinesias and motor fluctuations in Parkinson's disease. *Neurology* 1998; **50**:1323–1326.

41. Esselink RA, de Bie RM, de Haan RJ et al, Unilateral pallidotomy versus bilateral subthalamic nucleus stimulation in PD: a randomized trial. *Neurology* 2004; **62**:201–207.

42. Kleiner-Fisman G, Fisman DN, Sime E, Saint-Cyr JA, Lozano AM, Lang AE, Long-

term follow up of bilateral deep brain stimulation of the subthalamic nucleus in patients with advanced Parkinson disease. *J Neurosurg* 2003; **99**:489–495.

43. Rodriguez-Oroz MC, Zamarbid EI, Guridi J, Palmero MR, Obeso JA, Efficacy of deep brain stimulation of the subthalamic nucleus in Parkinson's disease 4 years after surgery: double blind and open label evaluation. *J Neurol Neurosurg Psychiatry* 2004; **75**:1382–1385.

44. Alexander GE, Crutcher MD, Functional architecture of basal ganglia circuits: neural substrates of parallel processing. *Trends Neurosci* 1990; **13**:266–271.

An update on the medical management

David J Burn

Introduction

This chapter focuses upon the management, and particularly the drug treatment of early PD. For the purposes of clarity, early PD is defined here as the diagnostic and maintenance disease phases, according to classification of MacMahon and Thomas (Figure 2.1).[1] The management of the complex disease phase, and the motor fluctuations, postural instability, etc. associated with this stage is discussed in Chapter 3.

The anti-parkinsonian drugs considered in detail are symptomatic therapies, since no agent has yet been shown beyond reasonable doubt to have disease-modifying or "neuroprotective" properties. Non-medical

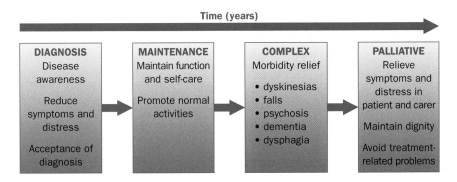

Time (years)

DIAGNOSIS	MAINTENANCE	COMPLEX	PALLIATIVE
Disease awareness	Maintain function and self-care	Morbidity relief	Relieve symptoms and distress in patient and carer
Reduce symptoms and distress	Promote normal activities	• dyskinesias • falls • psychosis • dementia • dysphagia	Maintain dignity
Acceptance of diagnosis			Avoid treatment-related problems

Figure 2.1 *Pathway of disease progression in PD (modified from reference 1).*

interventions are discussed, as is the means of assessing the patient's response to treatment in the early stages. Finally, a number of new symptomatic and potentially neuroprotective drugs at different stages of development are reviewed.

Setting the scene: Drug treatment of early PD

In 1967, Cotzias and co-workers described the efficacy and tolerability of levodopa in PD patients, when the drug was started in low doses and gradually increased thereafter.[2] Unfortunately, despite dramatic initial benefits, workers quickly came to realize the limitations of levodopa treatment, and to recognize a phenomenon termed the "long-term levodopa syndrome." This "syndrome," in brief, comprises a premature wearing-off of the anti-parkinsonian effects of levodopa, and response fluctuations. The latter can include dramatic swings between gross hyperkinetic involuntary movements (dyskinesias) and a "frozen," immobile state (akinesia). These problems emerge at a rate of approximately 10% per year, so that by 10 years into the illness virtually all PD patients can expect to experience such unpredictable responses.[3] Notably, however, younger PD patients tend to develop levodopa-induced dyskinesias and fluctuations earlier after diagnosis than older patients.[4] Not surprisingly, therefore, research into the medical management of early PD has focused upon the use of alternative agents to levodopa in order to delay this long-term levodopa syndrome, whilst still providing adequate symptomatic benefit. It might be argued that such alternatives are of particular importance in the younger patient, in whom life expectancy is correspondingly greater.

There is no universally applicable, evidence-based algorithm for the management of early PD; treatment should be tailored to the individual patient's requirements and their progress monitored regularly to assess response and possible side-effects. Since comparable motor deficits have differential effects on actual functioning, patient input is exceedingly important. A number of other factors, including age, severity, type of disease (tremor-dominant versus bradykinesia-dominant), occupational status, and psychiatric and medical co-morbidities must also be taken into account when deciding about initiating medical therapy. The evidence-based report of the Quality Standards Subcommittee of the American Academy of Neurology provides a useful framework of three broad guidelines to consider when prescribing early drug treatment (Table 2.1).[5]

Table 2.1 Evidence-based review of initiation of treatment for PD[5]

1. Initiate Selegiline:
   • has very mild symptomatic benefit
   • has no evidence for neuroprotective benefit

2. For PD patients requiring initiation of symptomatic therapy:
   • either levodopa or a dopamine agonist can be used
   • levodopa provides superior motor benefit but is associated with a higher risk of dyskinesias

3. There is no evidence that initiating treatment with sustained-release levodopa provides an advantage over immediate-release levodopa

Psychiatric issues relevant to early PD management

Up to 30% of patients have psychological symptoms or psychiatric disturbances such as depression or anxiety during the 4–8 year prodromal period before the onset of overt motor signs and diagnosis[6] that affect early PD management, including treatment compliance. Some patients will defer initiating symptomatic therapy even when motor symptoms interfere with working or the ability to tend to daily functions. This may be because of concerns about long-term levodopa effects. Others may view the need to start symptomatic therapy as a "concession" to the disease, a belief that warrants exploration if the patient has disability resulting from the lack of treatment. Patients with mood disturbances may cope sub-optimally with the diagnosis and decline or delay antiparkinsonian therapy because of nihilistic or hopeless feelings. In such cases, primary treatment of the affective disturbance will usually improve overall function, including motor symptoms.[7] Both depressive and anxiety disturbances influence a patient's perspective and predilection for somatic complaints. Any mismatch between impairments on the physical exam and reported disability should raise concerns about a comorbid affective disturbance.

Anti-parkinsonian drugs

Immediate-release levodopa

Despite ongoing debate regarding early or late levodopa therapy, there is no doubt that levodopa remains the most effective oral symptomatic treatment for PD.[8] Levodopa is administered with a peripheral dopa-decarboxylase inhibitor (DDI). The available formulations are carbidopa plus levodopa or co-careldopa (Sinemet) and benserazide plus levodopa or co-beneldopa (Madopar). The most common formulation includes 25 mg carbidopa and 100 mg levodopa (Sinemet 25/100). Carbidopa/levodopa 10/100 and 25/250 formulations are also available. The DDI prevents the formation of dopamine peripherally, thereby allowing a lower dose of levodopa to be administered and reducing the risk of associated nausea or vomiting. Levodopa crosses the blood–brain barrier, where it is converted by endogenous aromatic amino acid decarboxylase to dopamine, and then stored in surviving nigrostriatal neuronal terminals.

While there is some variation in clinical practice, immediate-release levodopa is usually commenced in a dose of 50–100 mg per day, increasing every 3–4 days until a dose of 50–100 mg three times daily is reached. The patient should be instructed in the early stage of their illness to take the drug with food to minimize nausea. If there is little or no response to 50 mg three times daily, the unit dose may be doubled to 100 mg. Should no significant motor response occur despite increasing the daily levodopa dose to 600 mg or more, the diagnosis of PD should be questioned, as an alternative diagnosis such as multiple system atrophy, progressive supranuclear palsy or vascular parkinsonism may be more likely.

Side-effects

Levodopa, commenced in the above way, is usually well tolerated. Nausea, vomiting, and orthostatic hypotension are the most commonly encountered side-effects. They may be minimized by increasing the levodopa dose more gradually, or co-prescribing domperidone 10 mg or 20 mg three times daily. Domperidone is available in Canada, Mexico, and Europe, but not in the US. Later in the course of the illness, levodopa is associated with mental changes, including vivid dreams, nightmares, psychosis, behavioral changes, and even a toxic confusional state (delirium), as discussed in Chapters 10 and 12. In early PD, onset of such symptoms spontaneously, or in response to antiparkinsonian medications, would strongly suggest an alternative diagnosis such as dementia with Lewy bodies.

Drug interactions

Clinically relevant interactions with levodopa include hypertensive crises with monoamine oxidase type A inhibitors (MAOI-A). It is therefore advised that levodopa be avoided for at least 2 weeks after stopping a MAOI-A. MAOI agents currently available in the US include phenelzine sulfate (Nardil), tranylcypromine sulfate (Parnate), isocarboxazid (Marplan), and selegiline (specific for the monoamine oxidase-B enzyme), all of which irreversibly bind to monoamine oxidase (MAO). Reversible MAO inhibitors are available in Europe (e.g., brofaromine, cimoxatone, clorgyline, lazabemide, moclobemide). Substances such as St. John's wort that may have MAOI-like activity may be used for self-treatment of depression and should be discontinued. Levodopa can also enhance the hypotensive effects of antihypertensive agents and antagonize the action of anti-psychotics. The absorption of levodopa may be reduced by concomitant administration of oral iron preparations, and an interval of two or more hours in-between dosing is therefore advised.

Controlled-release levodopa preparations

Both Sinemet and Madopar are available as controlled release (CR) preparations. The nomenclature for Sinemet CR is particularly confusing. In the United Kingdom, the drug is marketed as Sinemet CR (carbidopa/levodopa 50/200) and also as Half Sinemet CR (carbidopa/levodopa 25/100). Trying to prescribe Half Sinemet CR unambiguously can be difficult: if the instruction is misinterpreted and a tablet of Sinemet CR is halved, the slow-release mechanism is disrupted. In the US, Sinemet CR is available as carbidopa/levodopa 50/200, carbidopa/levodopa 25/100, and carbidopa/levodopa 50/250.

The levodopa in CR preparations has approximately 60–70% bioavailability, which is less than the 90–100% obtained from immediate release formulations. In contrast with immediate-release levodopa, the bioavailability of CR preparations is increased in the presence of food. No benefit for CR over immediate-release levodopa has been demonstrated in terms of dyskinesias and response fluctuation frequency at 5 years.[9,10] CR preparations, by virtue of their prolonged response duration (2–4 hours for CR versus 1–3 hours for immediate release), may be of help, however, in simplifying drug regimens, in relieving nocturnal akinesia, and in prescribing with immediate-release levodopa during the day to relieve end-of-dose deterioration.

Two commonly encountered problems with CR preparations are, first, changing the patient from all immediate-release to all CR levodopa. This is often poorly tolerated as the CR levodopa has a longer latency than immediate-release levodopa to turn the patient "on" (typically 60–90 versus

30–50 minutes), and the patient's perception is that the quality of the "on" period is poorer. Second, CR preparations should not be prescribed more than four times a day, as levodopa concentrations may build up unpredictably, causing increased dyskinesias and confusion.

Dopamine agonists (oral)

In 1973, bromocriptine was found to cause prolonged dopamine receptor stimulation, and the following year beneficial effects of bromocriptine in PD were reported.[11] Theoretically, dopamine agonists, which stimulate dopamine receptors both pre- and post-synaptically, are an attractive therapeutic option in PD, since they may "by-pass" the degenerating nigrostriatal dopaminergic neurons.[12] Unfortunately, experience to date has generally revealed dopamine agonists to be less potent than levodopa and also to be less well tolerated. The dopamine agonists differ in their affinity for a number of receptors, including the dopamine receptor family (see Table 2.2). It is not yet known whether these differences are clinically significant.

All dopamine agonists can significantly improve motor function in early PD, although as the disease progresses only a small minority of patients will derive sufficient benefit from the agonist alone to avoid the introduction of levodopa. There have been very few comparative studies performed between the dopamine agonists, so it is not possible to state which drug should be recommended. Pergolide and ropinirole appear to have some advantages over bromocriptine (although they are also more expensive). In practice, it is often worth changing from one agonist to another if side-effects are a problem, since there is variability in a given patient's tolerance to the different drugs.

Table 2.2 Dopamine agonists: dopamine receptor profiles

Agonist	*Ergot derivative*	D_1	D_2	D_3
Bromocriptine	Yes	–	+ +	+ +
Pergolide	Yes	+ +	+ + +	+ + +
Ropinirole	No	0	+ + +	+ + + +
Cabergoline	Yes	+ +	+ + + +	?
Pramipexole	No	–	+ + +	+ + + +

+: minimal agonist effect; + + + +: maximal agonist effect; –: antagonist activity; 0: no affinity for receptor.

Side-effects

The principal side-effects of the dopamine agonists are nausea and vomiting, postural hypotension, hallucinations and confusion, and exacerbation of dyskinesias. There is also a low but definite risk of fibrotic reactions (restrictive cardiac valvulopathy and pleuropulmonary fibrosis) occurring in patients taking dopamine agonists. Recent data suggest that clinically important restrictive cardiac valvulopathy can occur in up to 20% of patients prescribed pergolide, with significant correlation between cumulative agonist dose and tenting area of the mitral valve. Although ergot derivatives (see Table 2.2) have been mainly associated with fibrotic problems, possibly via 5-HT_{2B} mediated modification of fibroblast mitogenesis, it is by no means certain that the non-ergot agonists are free from this side-effect. Monitoring for fibrotic reactions varies enormously, with no international standard regimen available. Given the generally low frequency of the problem, it is our current practice to screen all patients commencing any agonist with a chest X-ray, urea and electrolytes and ESR, and to ask about potentially relevant clinical symptoms at follow-up visits. Others, however, recommend more intensive screening and monitoring. Large, prospective pharmacovigilance studies are required to clarify this issue.[13] Additionally, there is also an increased risk of toxicity when erythromycin is co-prescribed with an agonist.

The dopamine agonists have been implicated in causing "sleep attacks," with sudden onset of drowsiness, leading to driving accidents in some cases.[14] The term "sleep attack" is almost certainly a misnomer, however, as patients do have warning of impending sleepiness, though may subsequently be amnesic for up to several minutes whilst in this state. It is sensible to advise all patients commencing an agonist that excessive drowsiness may occur, particularly during up-titration of the dose. This may be compounded by the use of other sedative drugs and alcohol.

Occasionally, dopamine agonists may be associated with hypersexuality, pathological gambling and repetitive, purposeless motor acts (punding). Younger, male patients seem to be particularly at risk of these phenomena.

Selegiline

Selegiline is a selective, irreversible inhibitor of monoamine oxidase (MAO) type B. Inhibition of this enzyme slows the breakdown of dopamine in the striatum. A dose of 5–10 mg of selegiline per day is normally prescribed. Higher doses are associated with only minimal additional inhibition of MAO type B.

Following the publication of the UK Parkinson's Disease Research Group study in 1995, where an excess mortality in the group of patients taking selegiline was demonstrated, prescriptions for the drug in the UK (but not in the USA) dropped by nearly 50%.[15] This study drew much criticism from some quarters, both in its design and also in the data analysis. The reason for the possible excess mortality is uncertain, but it has been suggested that the drug should be avoided in patients with known falls, confusion and postural hypotension. The use of selegiline in younger patients with early PD, with or without a dopamine agonist, as a means of deferring levodopa treatment still has its advocates.

Side-effects

The mild amfetamine-like effects of metabolites of selegiline account for some of the side-effects, which include hallucinations and confusion, particularly in moderate to advanced disease. Withdrawal of selegiline in such patients may also be associated with a significant deterioration in motor function.

Interactions

It is frequently recommended that selegiline as a co-prescription with selective serotonin re-uptake inhibitors (SSRIs) is best avoided. A hypertensive reaction that may include neuropsychiatric features has been reported in a small minority of cases. A serotonin syndrome is also possible with the combination. However, in clinical practice, these interactions are rare and the combination of selegiline at no more than the usual dose of 10 mg daily with SSRIs is well-tolerated.[16]

Amantadine

Amantadine was introduced as an anti-parkinsonian treatment in the late 1960s. It has a number of putative mechanisms of action, including the facilitation of pre-synaptic dopamine release, blocking dopamine re-uptake, an anticholinergic effect, and also as an N-methyl-D-aspartate (NMDA) receptor antagonist. Initially employed in the early stages of treatment, where its effects are mild and relatively short-lived, interest has recently focused upon the use of amantadine as an anti-dyskinetic agent in advanced disease.[17] The dose range for amantadine is 100–300 mg, although the lower end of the range is more commonly used, due to increased side-effects at higher dosages.

Side-effects

These include confusion and hallucinations, peripheral edema and livedo reticularis. There may be significant worsening of parkinsonism when amantadine is withdrawn.

Anticholinergic drugs

The availability of anticholinergic drugs such as benzhexol and orphenadrine predated the introduction of levodopa. The prescription of these drugs has fallen markedly, however, because of troublesome side-effects, including cognitive impairment and frank confusional states. In selected younger patients the tremorlytic effect of these agents may still be helpful, but close monitoring is advised. Cognitive deficits have been documented on formal neuropsychological testing even in younger PD patients receiving anticholinergics. A recent pathological study has suggested that chronic use of this class of drug may be associated with increased cerebral amyloid plaque formation, further questioning the place for anticholinergics in the management of early PD.[18]

Catechol-*O*-methyl transferase (COMT) inhibitors

The introduction of COMT inhibitors to the market has been nothing if eventful. After a long gestation as a class of drugs, second-generation inhibitors were developed in the 1980s. Unlike the first-generation COMT inhibitors used in Europe (gallates and tropolone), these agents were shown to be potent, reversible and highly specific inhibitors of COMT. The first commercial COMT inhibitor available, tolcapone, lasted only a few months before the European Union suspended the drug in November 1998 because of reports of fatal hepatotoxicity. Tolcapone can still be prescribed in the USA, under careful supervision. A second COMT inhibitor, entacapone, was released shortly after tolcapone, and is the only drug of this class currently available in Europe.

COMT is a ubiquitous enzyme, found in gut, liver, kidney, and brain, amongst other sites. In theory, COMT inhibition may occur both centrally (where the degradation of dopamine to homovanillic acid is inhibited) and peripherally (where conversion of levodopa to the inert 3-*O*-methyldopa is inhibited) to benefit the patient with PD. In practice, both tolcapone and entacapone act primarily as peripheral COMT inhibitors.[19] When entacapone is prescribed, a 200 mg dose is used with each dose of levodopa administered, up to a frequency of ten doses per day. Recently, entacapone has been combined with levodopa and carbidopa (Stalevo) in a number of fixed-dose preparations, thereby reducing the total daily number of tablets necessary. Tolcapone is prescribed as either 100 mg or 200 mg three times per day. Because of increased dyskinesias, an overall reduction of 10–30% in the daily dose of levodopa needs to be anticipated. While entacapone may be employed with any other anti-parkinsonian drug (although caution may be needed with apomorphine), the optimal use of entacapone in early PD is uncertain. Interest has arisen, however, from the ability of COMT inhibition to smooth out plasma (and presumably brain) levodopa fluctuations. Since the latter is thought to be fundamental in the genesis of dyskinesias, it has been suggested that the early use of COMT inhibition with levodopa could delay the onset of motor complications.

Side-effects
Other than hepatotoxicity and exacerbation of dyskinesias, COMT inhibitors may also cause diarrhea (particularly with tolcapone; the mechanism for this is unknown), abdominal pain, and a dryness of the mouth. If tolcapone is prescribed, liver function tests need to be monitored regularly. Harmless urine discoloration caused by metabolites of COMT inhibitors is reported in approximately 8% of patients.

Interactions
Non-selective MAO inhibitors, or a daily dose of selegiline in excess of 10 mg should be avoided when using entacapone. The British National Formulary also advises caution in the co-prescription of venlafaxine with entacapone, as there is a theoretical risk of increased adrenergic side-effects. Patients taking iron preparations should be advised to separate this medication and entacapone by at least 2 hours.

Non-medical treatments

The modern management of PD centers on pharmacological therapy, although it has been suggested that physiotherapy can improve the disabilities associated with the condition, as an adjunct to drug treatment. The purpose of physiotherapy is to maximize functional ability and minimize secondary complications through movement rehabilitation within a context of education and support for the whole person. Physiotherapy for PD covers a number of different treatment techniques, all centered on active exercises and re-education of mobility.

Studies and questionnaires from specialist societies indicate that only a third or fewer of people with PD actually see a physiotherapist, at least in the UK. Reasons for this may include perception of lack of benefit and limited access due to high demands on physiotherapy services. Regarding the former, there is insufficient evidence at the present time to support or refute the efficacy of physiotherapy in PD.[20] Until such evidence is forthcoming, it is considered desirable that patients with PD are seen at an early stage in their disease course by a physiotherapist with experience of the condition, so that appropriate education and exercises may be initiated.

Most people with PD have speech difficulties, typically worsening as the disease progresses. Of these, 90% have involvement of laryngeal function and 45% have additional articulatory dysfunction. Early assessment by a speech and language therapist (SALT) is to be encouraged, but probably only 20% of patients are actually referred. Although there is currently a lack of evidence to support or refute the efficacy of one form of SALT over another, or indeed the efficacy of SALT in PD, a number of techniques, such as Lee-Silverman Voice Therapy, which emphasizes increased vocal effort, have shown promise in clinical trials.

Assessing the patient's response to treatment

Whilst the diagnosis of PD may be beyond reasonable doubt, not all patients necessarily require immediate treatment. After diagnosis, an explanation of the condition, education, and support are essential. If available, a PD nurse specialist is invaluable at this early stage. Depending upon the country in question, patients who drive may need to be advised to inform their insurance company and also the driving licensing authorities.

The patient's response to treatment may be assessed at three levels: impairment, disability, and handicap (reflected by health-related quality of life). Table 2.3 gives some examples of instruments that may be used, as they relate to PD. A systematic evaluation of rating scales for impairment and disability in PD found that, in contrast to their widespread clinical use, the majority of rating scales had either not been subjected to extensive clinometric evaluation or had demonstrated clinometric shortcomings.[21] Nevertheless, instruments such as the Unified Parkinson's Disease Rating Scale (UPDRS) have been validated and shown to have good inter-rater reliability.

Table 2.3 Assessment instruments for PD

Measures	*Examples*	*Comments*
Impairment	• UPDRS[a] part III (motor) • Short Parkinson's evaluation scale • Webster rating scale	Validated, with good inter-rater reliability
Disability	• UPDRS part II	Includes ADLs[b] but also some impairments
	• Northwestern University Disability Scale	Moderate to good reliability and validity for PD
	• Ten-meter walking time • Nine-hole peg test	
Quality of life	• EuroQol-5D & SF-36 • PDQ-39 or PDQ-8	Generic scales Disease-specific, validated scale for PD

[a] Unified Parkinson's Disease Rating Scale.
[b] Activities of daily living.

Recently, there has been a rapid growth in the use of health-related quality of life measures, both generic and specific, in clinical trials and research studies addressing the impact of PD. In part, this derives from deficiencies in rating scales for impairment and disability that do not reflect the significant effects upon quality of life that, for instance, depression may have. Health-related quality of life instruments can also be useful in determining health policy, due to the association between perceived state of health and demand for resources, prediction of risks and mortality. Additionally, assessing the patient's response to treatment may require the use of additional instruments in specific non-motor domains, such as sleep, depression, and cognitive function. The use of these scales will be discussed elsewhere.

In clinical practice, it is neither practical nor desirable to perform a battery of scales that are time-consuming and which may not actually reflect the change in status compared with a previous visit. The emphasis should be on functional change: "What *can* you do now that you couldn't before?" or, conversely, "What *can't* you do now or do you require assistance in carrying out?" The decision to start or change treatment should be made after full and frank discussion with the patient and their family. Consistency of who sees the patient at each visit is desirable but not always possible. Realistic goals need to be set out; for example, severe tremor may be very difficult to treat medically and escalating levodopa dosage to high levels may not be justified in this situation, bearing in mind the limited therapeutic gain versus potential long term problems associated with an increased cumulative dose. Concomitant depression and sleep disturbance should always be considered, since both are common in PD, can be severe, and may "mask" responses to change in motor status.

Pipeline drug therapies for early Parkinson's disease

A number of drugs at various stages of development are under consideration for the symptomatic management of early PD. Rotigotine is a dopamine agonist delivered through a silicone-based transdermal patch that is replaced every 24 hours. Recent trials have shown that this agent can be safely administered once daily and improves parkinsonian signs in patients with early PD. Rasagiline mesylate is an irreversible monoamine oxidase type B inhibitor. It improves the symptoms of early PD while both preclinical and clinical studies indicate that it may also modify the progression of PD. Istradefylline (KW-6002) is a selective adenosine A_{2A} antagonist that may increase "on" time in patients without troublesome dyskinesias. The drug may also prove to be useful as an adjunct to levodopa in the treatment of early PD.

In addition to symptomatic therapies, there is an urgent need to identify therapies that slow down the progression of PD. The use of such agents early in the disease course is clearly logical, to preserve as large a remaining neuronal pool as possible. There have, however, been very few clinical trials aimed at demonstrating neuroprotection. Reasons for this include the size and complexity of the design required demonstrating such an effect over and above possible symptomatic benefits. Table 2.4 shows a number of drugs considered to have potential as neuroprotective agents. This list, whilst not exhaustive, is derived from a recent systematic review of the topic.[22]

Conclusion

The treatment of early PD represents a significant challenge. When to introduce treatment and which drug to use should be tailored to the individual. Although the assessment of drug effects and disease progression may be helped by scales that record impairment, disability, and health-related quality of life, simple questions targeting day-to-day functioning can be

Table 2.4 Potential neuroprotective drugs for PD

Drug	Primary mechanism
Caffeine	Adenosine antagonist
Coenzyme Q10	Anti-oxidant/mitochondrial stabilizer
Creatine	Mitochondrial stabilizer
Estrogen (17β estradiol)	Undetermined/multiple
GM-1 ganglioside	Trophic factor
GPI 1485	Trophic factor
Minocycline	Anti-inflammatory/anti-apoptotic
Nicotine	Unknown (?anti-oxidant, ?anti-excitotoxic)
Rasagiline/selegiline	Anti-oxidant/anti-apoptotic
Ropinirole/pramipexole	Anti-oxidant/mitochondrial membrane

extremely helpful in informing treatment decisions. Early referral for physiotherapy and speech and language therapy assessments is to be encouraged, although more evidence is required to confirm or refute the benefits that may accrue from these interventions in PD.

Whilst the therapeutic armory continues to expand, direct comparison between drugs within a particular class is generally lacking (dopamine agonists, for example), and it is uncertain when one class of drug should be introduced compared with another (dopamine agonists versus COMT inhibitors, for example). Finally, the challenge of developing effective neuroprotective therapy for PD remains an exciting, and increasingly visible, goal.

References

1. MacMahon DG, Thomas S, Practical approach to quality of life in Parkinson's disease. *J Neurol* 1998; **245**:S19–S22.
2. Cotzias GC, Van Woert MH, Schiffer LM, Aromatic amino acids and modification of parkinsonism. *New Engl J Med* 1967; **276**:374–379.
3. Marsden CD, Parkes JD, "On-off" effects in patients with Parkinson's disease on chronic levodopa therapy. *Lancet* 1976; **1**:292–296.
4. Quinn NP, Critchley P, Marsden CD, Young onset Parkinson's disease. *Mov Disord* 1987; **1**:209–219.
5. Miyasaki JM, Martin W, Suchowersky O, Weiner WJ, Lang AE, Practice parameter: initiation of treatment for Parkinson's disease: an evidence-based review. *Neurology* 2002; **58**:11–17.
6. Gonera EG, van't Hof M, Berger HJ et al, Symptoms and duration of the prodromal phase in Parkinson's disease. *Mov Disord* 1997; **12**:871–876.
7. Starkstein SE, Preziosi TJ, Bolduc PL, Robinson RG, Depression in Parkinson's disease. *J Nerv Ment Dis* 1990; **178**:27–31.

8. Weiner WJ, The initial treatment of Parkinson's disease should begin with levodopa. *Mov Disord* 1999; **14:**716–724.

9. Block G, Liss C, Reines S et al, Comparison of immediate-release and controlled-release carbidopa/levodopa in Parkinson's disease. *Eur Neurol* 1997; **37:**23–27.

10. Dupont E, Andersen A, Boas J et al, Sustained-release Madopar HBS compared with standard Madopar in the long-term treatment of *de novo* parkinsonian patients. *Acta Neurol Scand* 1996; **93:**14–20.

11. Calne DB, Teychenne PF, Claveria LE, Eastmen R, Greenacre JK, Petrie A, Bromocriptine in parkinsonism. *Br Med J* 1974; **4:**442–444.

12. Montastruc JL, Rascol O, Senard JM, Treatment of Parkinson's disease should begin with a dopamine agonist. *Mov Disord* 1999; **14:**725–730.

13. Rascol O, Pathak A, Bagheri H, Montastruc JL, New concerns about old drugs: valvular heart disease on ergot derivative dopamine agonists as an exemplary situation of pharmacovigilance. *Mov Disord* 2004; **6:**611–613.

14. Frucht S, Rogers JD, Greene PE, Gordon MF, Fahn S, Falling asleep at the wheel: motor vehicle mishaps in persons taking pramipexole and ropinirole. *Neurology* 1999; **52:**1908–1910.

15. Lees AJ, on behalf of the Parkinson's Disease Study Group of the UK, Comparison of therapeutic effects and mortality data of levodopa and levodopa combined with selegiline in patients with early, mild Parkinson's disease. *Br Med J* 1995; **311:**1602–1607.

16. Richard IH, Kurlan R, Tanner C et al, Serotonin syndrome and the combined use of deprenyl and an antidepressant in Parkinson's disease. *Neurology* 1997; **48:**1070–1077.

17. Blanchet PJ, Verhagen-Metman L, Chase TN, Renaissance of amantadine in the treatment of Parkinson's disease. *Adv Neurol* 2003; **91:**251–257.

18. Perry EK, Kilford L, Lees AJ, Burn DJ, Perry RH, Increased Alzheimer pathology in Parkinson's disease related to antimuscarinic drugs. *Ann Neurol* 2003; **54:**235–238.

19. Martínez-Martín P, O'Brien CF, Extending levodopa action: COMT inhibition. *Neurology* 1998; **50**(Suppl 6):S27–S32.

20. Deane KHO, Jones D, Playford ED, Ben-Shlomo Y, Clarke CE, Physiotherapy versus placebo or no intervention in Parkinson's disease. *Cochrane Review*. Issue 1. John Wiley & Sons, Ltd, Chichester, UK, 2004.

21. Ramaker C, Marinus J, Stiggelbout AM, van Hilten BJ, Systematic evaluation of rating scales for impairment and disability in Parkinson's disease. *Mov Disord* 2002; **17:**867–876.

22. Ravina BM, Fagan SC, Hart RG et al, Neuroprotective agents for clinical trials in Parkinson's disease: a systematic assessment. *Neurology* 2003; **60:**1234–1240.

chapter 3

Management of advanced-stage disease

Irene Hegeman Richard

Introduction

Advancing Parkinson's disease (PD) is associated with a variety of motor and non-motor symptoms that are quite unique to this illness and pose difficult clinical challenges. Most patients with advanced PD would benefit from having a neurologist specializing in movement disorders as part of their care team. The majority of patients eventually develop motor complications related to disease progression and dopaminergic pharmacotherapy (Table 3.1). Motor complications include dyskinesias, wearing-off of medication effect prior to the next scheduled dose and unpredictable shifts in mobility referred to as the "on-off" phenomenon. Some patients also develop fluctuations in emotional states (e.g. mood, anxiety) and other non-motor domains (e.g. pain, autonomic function). In addition to these fluctuating symptoms generally thought to be secondary to dopaminergic dysfunction, patients develop impairments that appear to be less related to dopamine neurotransmission, namely dysarthria, dysphagia, and impairments in gait and balance (Table 3.2). This chapter provides an overview of the phenomenology and treatment approaches to motor and emotional fluctuations, dysarthria, dysphagia and gait and balance problems.

Motor complications

Motor complications of therapy in PD include motor fluctuations ("wearing off" and "on-off") and dyskinesias. After being treated with levodopa for a

Table 3.1 Dopamine-related motor symptoms of advanced PD

Symptom	Description	Therapeutic options
Wearing off/ end of dose deterioration	• Re-emergence of PD symptoms prior to next scheduled levodopa dose • Associated with declining plasma levodopa levels • Typically involves motor symptoms (bradykinesia, tremor) • May also include changes in mood, level of anxiety • May include pain and autonomic symptoms	• Consider more frequent dosing of levodopa (e.g change from TID to QID) • Consider adding a COMT inhibitor (entacapone) to enhance action of levodopa • Consider adding an agent with a different mechanism of action (e.g. dopamine agonist, MAOB inhibitor, amantadine)
Peak dose dyskinesias	• Excessive, involuntary movements • Associated with peak levodopa levels • May be focal (e.g. one foot) or diffuse (involving face, head, trunk, extremities) • May also involve respiratory muscles • Usually choreic and painless	• May not need to do anything since they are often mild and not disturbing to patients • Consider reducing amount of levodopa per dose and decreasing interval between doses (e.g. change from two tablets TID to one and a half tablets QID) • Consider reducing the amount of levodopa relative to agonist • Consider adding amantadine
Early morning akinesia	• Immobility upon awakening • May be associated with painful dystonia (often involving the foot)	• Consider adding controlled-release levodopa preparation at bedtime (may help with symptoms during the night but unlikely to last until morning) • Set alarm and take levodopa $\frac{1}{2}$–1 hour prior to getting out of bed

Table 3.1 continued

Symptom	Description	Therapeutic options
"Off" periods	• Immobility that is often accompanied by non-motor symptoms (e.g. anxiety, pain) • Related to low levodopa levels but may not have obvious relationship with timing of doses • Effect of levodopa dose may be delayed (delayed on) or absent (dose failure)	• Consider apomorphine injection as "rescue" therapy

period of several years, many patients no longer have a smooth, stable, effective response.[1] Younger patients are more likely than older patients to develop motor fluctuations and dyskinesias.[2] There is uncertainty as to whether these complications relate solely to the duration and dosage of levodopa or whether they relate, at least in part, to the increasing severity of disease. It is likely that a combination of the disease itself and the medication is responsible.[3]

When initially treated with levodopa, patients do not notice any fluctuations in their motor response (Figure 3.1a). After several years of treatment, patients begin to notice a gradual "wearing off" of the beneficial effect of their doses and some shortening of their duration of action. As time progresses, patients may develop "on-off" fluctuations. These are rather abrupt changes in motor function, seemingly unrelated to the timing of medication. Patients can quickly change from the "on" (mobile) state to the "off" (immobile, or nearly so) state. The "off" state can be accompanied by other non-motor symptoms as well. Autonomic changes may include flushing or sweating, some patients experience abdominal bloating and a number experience pain. The "on" state is often associated with dyskinesias, leaving the patient with little or no periods of "normal" mobility (Figure 3.1b).

Dyskinesias are involuntary movements that come in a variety of forms.[4–6] The most commonly encountered are peak-dose dyskinesias, generally thought to reflect excessive dopaminergic tone. Peak-dose dyskinesias are usually choreic and painless. In fact, except in extremely severe cases where function is limited or in people who are very self-conscious, patients themselves tend not to be bothered by the dyskinesias. It is usually those around them who are concerned. As time progresses, the therapeutic window narrows such that the dosage of levodopa needed to improve motor function equals that required to induce dyskinesias. Diphasic dyskinesias occur at the beginning and/or end of dose. These are often the most severe dyskinesias seen in PD patients, mainly affecting subjects with early-onset disease.[7] They are often stereotypic or ballistic, and are difficult to manage. Dystonia, a sustained increase in tone that results in a fixed posture, can be a manifestation of the disease itself but is typically seen as medication is wearing-off.[8] It often occurs first thing in the morning.[9] Dystonia frequently affects the foot and can be quite painful.

Emotional fluctuations

Up to two-thirds of PD patients with motor fluctuations can experience marked fluctuations in mood.[10,11] Many patients also develop fluctuations in levels of anxiety. It is not clear why virtually all patients develop motor fluctuations while only some develop emotional fluctuations. The relationship between mood and anxiety fluctuations and between emotional fluctuations and more pervasive depressive or anxiety disorders remains to be determined. Mood changes can be so profound that patients transition from depressed and suicidal to euphoric and hypomanic within minutes, with these emotional fluctuations often being more disabling and distressing to patients than the motor changes. Mood fluctuations can occur several times a day. The most typically reported pattern is for patients to be depressed and anxious while "off " (parkinsonian, immobile) and normal or euphoric while "on".[10,11] Other investigators have, however, reported that mood is worse during periods of either immobility ("off") or excessive mobility ("on with dyskinesias")[12] and in some cases, there may be little temporal correlation between mood and motor states.[13] Although mood fluctuations have been noted mostly in patients who experience motor fluctuations, there is evidence that mood fluctuations may predate motor fluctuations in some patients.[11]

Research involving the phenomenology and underlying mechanisms of emotional fluctuations in PD has been limited. The presumption that emotional fluctuations are associated with motor fluctuations[10,11,14–16] has led to the hypotheses that mood and anxiety fluctuations are either: (1) a psychological reaction to motor dysfunction, or (2) an independent result of changing brain dopamine levels. Research involving levodopa infusions

Table 3.2 Physical symptoms of advanced PD unrelated to dopamine

Symptom	Description	Therapeutic options
Freezing	• Sudden, transient inability to walk or great difficulty with walking • Often occurs when going through doorways or trying to walk through a crowd • May occur in "on" or "off" states	• Try to optimize "on" time • Consider visual cues/sensory tricks (e.g. stepping over light from laser pointed at floor)
Speech difficulties	• Hypophonia • Dysarthria	• Speech therapy
Swallowing difficulties	• Problems with various phases of swallowing • Choking, risk of aspiration	• Consider referral to speech/swallowing therapist • Radiological swallowing study (pharyngogram) • May need to change head position during swallowing • Alter food consistency • May need feeding tube
Postural instability	• Tendency to retropulse (fall backwards)	• Consider physical therapy referral • May benefit from gait training, assistive device or assistance from others when ambulating

demonstrated, however, that changes in emotional states may precede changes in motor state by several minutes.[17] This finding as well as diary evidence of temporal dissociation between mood, anxiety, and motor states in some patients[13] makes a purely reactive hypothesis less tenable.

The optimal treatment of emotional fluctuations is unclear but attempts to reduce motor fluctuations (as discussed later in the chapter) may be particularly beneficial in patients for whom emotional and motor states are temporally correlated. It would also be wise to evaluate patients with emotional fluctuations for an underlying mood or anxiety disorder and consider the use of antidepressant or anxiolytics medications.

Disorders of speech and swallowing

Dysarthria is a common manifestation of PD that worsens with disease progress.[18] Patients with PD are often said to manifest a "hypophonic dysarthria," the characteristics of which include monotony of pitch (dysprosody) and volume (hypophonia), imprecise articulation, variations in speed resulting in both inappropriate silences and rushes of speech (sometimes referred to as "festination" of speech). Patients with PD frequently demonstrate pallilalia (the tendency to repeat the final syllable or sound of a word). Orolingual dyskinesias can also affect speech. Communication is further impaired in PD by the tendency of patients to use fewer facial expressions and hand gestures that often accompany and clarify the meaning of speech.[19] Speech therapists can provide evaluation and training techniques for patients to practice at home.

Dysphagia is another symptom that worsens with disease progression. Although the majority of patients have evidence of abnormal swallowing on formal testing, many are unaware of the problem[20] which can lead to aspiration. Dysphagia in PD is characterized by abnormalities in various phases of swallowing, including abnormal bolus formation, transfer and esophageal dysmotility.[21] Sialorrhea (drooling) in PD appears to be due to reduced swallowing and forward head posture, rather than increased saliva production.[22,23] There is some evidence to suggest that levodopa increases swallowing speed[24] but in general, attempts to adjust medications prove ineffective. Speech/swallowing therapists can provide careful assessments and diagnosis of swallowing problems. They provide advice on swallowing techniques and exercises and may offer dietary alternatives and advice on food consistency.[19,25] Some patients require surgical placement of a feeding tube.

Disorders of gait and balance

Postural instability is often considered a cardinal feature of PD but generally does not occur until later in the illness.[26] It is thought to result from widespread neuronal loss. Patients have a tendency to fall backward (retropulse). Postural instability contributes to gait impairment, which is a frequent cause of disability in advanced PD.[27] Other features of gait disturbances in PD include reduced velocity, reduced stride and step length, increased trunk flexion and decreased arm swing.[28] Patients use extra steps and turn "en bloc," rather than pivoting on one foot. Difficulty monitoring the timing of stride is associated with falls but it does not appear to correlate well with tremor, rigidity, or bradykinesia.[29]

Freezing is the occurrence of a sudden inability to move. Many patients develop freezing only when "off" or "wearing off," and they can be helped by increasing "on" time. Other patients develop freezing that is independent of "on-off" status and is not predictably influenced by any modification in drug treatment.[4] Although a small number of patients develop freezing early, it is usually a later manifestation. Examples of freezing include "start hesitation" (inability to initiate gait, "like a car being stuck in neutral") and getting "stuck" through doorways. Sometimes motor/sensory tricks or cues are helpful.[4,30] Techniques may include imagining high stepping marching, walking over a strip on the floor or using a laser pointed at the ground. Though mechanical walkers may stabilize patients and increase confidence, a study by Cubo et al[31] suggests that PD patients may walk more slowly with them and that standard walkers (without wheels) may aggravate freezing.

Pharmacotherapy in advanced PD

Levodopa is known to be the single most effective treatment to improve motor symptoms in PD.[32,33] Concerns regarding its use have arisen, however. One concern is that, by increasing dopamine metabolism and oxidative stress, levodopa may actually be toxic to nigral neurons and that it may hasten disease progression. The other concern is that, whether or not it is actually toxic to neurons, it may play a role in the evolution of motor fluctuations and dyskinesias. The hypothesis that levodopa is toxic to neurons is based primarily on preclinical studies.[34–36] Data from healthy animals and humans does not convincingly demonstrate levodopa toxicity and there is no evidence of levodopa-induced neurotoxicity in patients with PD.[34] Despite the lack of evidence for a toxic effect in patients with PD, it appears as though levodopa may contribute to long-term complications like motor fluctuations and dyskinesias. Levodopa's involvement in the emergence of long-term motor complications appears to be related to a combination of presynaptic and postsynaptic changes in the striatum. Both duration of treatment and disease progression and severity may be important determinants.[37–39] Approaches to treatment in early PD, including "levodopa-sparing" strategies with the use of dopamine agonists as monotherapy early on, have been proposed as a method to prevent motor fluctuations.[40] At this point, however, the influence that early treatment approaches have on

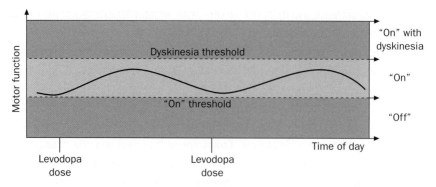

Figure 3.1a *Early PD: relatively stable motor function in response to levodopa. In early PD, motor function remains fairly stable and patients experience optimal motor function without "off" periods or dyskinesias.*

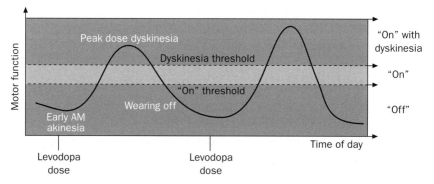

Figure 3.1b *Advanced PD: fluctuating motor function in response to levodopa. With advancing disease, patients experience less "on" time (optimal mobility) and more time "off" (poor mobility) or "on" with dyskinesias (excessive mobility).*

longer-term functioning is not clear and all patients ultimately require levodopa treatment.

Once patients have developed motor complications, the general approach to treatment has been to alter levodopa administration so as to minimize the peaks and troughs in plasma (and presumably brain) levodopa levels, thereby providing more continuous dopaminergic stimulation to the striatum.[41–43] Support for this approach comes from research studies in which continuous levodopa administration (intraduodenal or intravenous) has been shown to minimize or even eliminate motor fluctuations.[38,44] Unfortunately, there is no way to provide continuous levodopa administration currently outside of the research setting. Controlled release formulations of carbidopa/levodopa have not had a great impact on reducing motor fluctuations, attributable in part to issues with unpredictable gastrointestinal absorption.[45,46] An important fact to remember about controlled release formulations of carbidopa/levodopa (particularly when switching from one formulation to the other) is that the bioavailability of controlled release tablets is less than that of immediate release tablets. A controlled release carbidopa/levodopa tablet (one of the 50/200 strength or two of the 25/100 strength) is comparable in potency to about $1\frac{1}{2}$ (not two) of the 25/100 strength immediate-release tablets. One approach is to lower the dosage and increase the frequency of carbidopa/levodopa dosing. Some patients with advanced disease take tablets of carbidopa/levodopa every hour while others may liquefy and sip it to hasten absorption throughout the day (ten tablets of 10/100 strength mixed with one liter of water with 2000 mg of ascorbic acid).

Adding a catechol-*O*-methyltranferase (COMT) inhibitor to carbidopa/levodopa is another means by which the effect of levodopa can be enhanced. Levodopa is converted to dopamine by aromatic acid decarboxylase (inhibited by carbidopa) and levodopa is also peripherally metabolized to 3-*O*-methyldopa (3-OMD) by COMT. In addition to reducing the systemic elimination of levodopa and enhancing its response, COMT inhibitors reduce variations in plasma levodopa levels.[42,43] Although tolcapone is rarely used now due to reports of liver toxicity,[47,48] entacapone is a frequently prescribed and generally well-tolerated COMT inhibitor that has been demonstrated to reduce motor fluctuations in clinical trials.[49,50] Entacapone is usually given at a dose of 200 mg with each individual levodopa intake. Diarrhea and harmless urine discoloration are the most common non-dopaminergic side-effects[43,51] and the most common dopaminergic side-effects are dyskinesia and nausea. Many clinicians decrease the daily dosage of levodopa by 10–30% (either by decreasing dosages or increasing dosing intervals) when starting entacapone in order to minimize anticipated increases in dyskinesia.[43,52] Lower entacapone dosages can also be used.

Another approach to maximizing motor function includes the use of additional anti-parkinsonian agents in combination with carbidopa/levodopa. Of course, polypharmacy is not without risks and clinicians are often limited by the development of side-effects such as confusion, hallucinations, or orthostatic hypotension. Agents frequently added to the levodopa regimen include dopamine agonists, MAO-B inhibitors (e.g. selegiline, rasagiline) and amantadine. There is some preliminary evidence to suggest that higher dosages of amantadine may have particular efficacy in reducing dyskinesias, perhaps related to NMDA receptor antagonist properties.[53] The FDA recently approved the non-ergot dopamine receptor agonist apomorphine for use as an intermittent subcutaneous injection for the acute treatment of "off" episodes. This medication has been used in Europe for many years. It is usually quite effective in treating "off" symptoms within 10–15 minutes, the effect lasting 1–2 hours and the drug can be self-administered periodically as needed throughout the day. Because of its strong emetic effects domperidone 20 mg TID (available in Canada) or trimethobenzamide (Tigan) 300 mg TID should be started 3 days prior to the initiation of apomorphine[54-58] and continued throughout the duration of apomorphine treatment.

Deep brain stimulation surgery

Surgical treatments of Parkinson's disease now mainly involve deep brain stimulation (DBS) of the globus pallidus interna (GPi) or subthalamic nucleus (STN). DBS of either area can improve motor function (primarily by decreasing "off" time) and reduce dyskinesias, but the advantages of one of the two anatomical sites over the other have not yet been established.[59,60] Although the precise mechanism of DBS is not known, high-frequency stimulation of a brain target simulates effects of a functional lesion. In this way, circuitry can be manipulated bilaterally with a lower risk of permanent adverse events. Furthermore, adjustment of stimulator settings can be made at any time to maximize benefit and minimize side-effects. Candidates for DBS are patients with advanced PD who cannot be managed effectively with medications. One of the major risks of surgery is intracerebral hemorrhage but it should also be noted that reports of depressed[61,62] and abnormally elevated mood[63,64] have been reported in association with DBS. Due to the risk of worsening cognitive function, it is generally recommended that patients with cognitive impairment do not undergo the procedure. DBS is a welcome option but it remains a costly procedure and requires that a center have surgical, neurological, and neurophysiological expertise.

Conclusion

Advanced PD is associated with a variety of symptoms that present difficult clinical challenges. The majority of patients ultimately develop motor complications including dyskinesias and motor fluctuations. These symptoms are thought to be related to a combination of disease progression and dopamin-ergic therapy. In addition, many patients develop fluctuations in emotional and other non-motor functions such as pain. Patients also develop symptoms thought to be less closely related to dopaminergic dysfunction including impairments in speech, swallowing, balance, and gait. Approaches to the treatment of motor complications currently involve attempts to provide more continuous dopaminergic stimulation that include adjustments in carbidopa/levodopa dosing and addition of other medications including the COMT inhibitor entacapone, dopamine agonists, MAO-B inhibitors, and amantadine (which may be helpful in reducing dyskinesias). The FDA has approved apomorphine as a PRN (pro re nata) subcutaneous injection to alleviate "off" periods. Current surgical approaches include DBS of the GPi and STN, which are reserved for patients whose symptoms cannot be effectively treated with medications. In particular, DBS can reduce dyskinesias and "off" time. The treatment of non-motor fluctuations remains unclear and the management of dysphagia, dysarthria, postural instability, and gait problems has been largely non-pharmacologic, involving various forms of therapy, patient training. and lifestyle modifications. Research currently underway includes alternative approaches to the treatment of advanced PD including transplantation (fetal midbrain neurons, stem cells) and gene therapy using viral vectors to deliver proteins to the basal ganglia in order to enhance dopamine availability or restore function of damaged neurons.

References

1. Poewe W, L-dopa in PD: Mechanisms of action on and pathophysiology of levodopa failure. In: Jankovic J, Tolosa E (eds) *Parkinson's Disease and Movement Disorders*, 2nd edn. Williams and Wilkins; Baltimore, 1993.
2. Kostic V, Przedborski S, Flaster E, Sternick N, Early development of levodopa-induced dyskinesias and response fluctuations in young-onset Parkinson's disease. *Neurology* 1991; **41**:202–205.
3. Fahn S, Parkinson disease, the effect of levodopa, and the ELLDOPA trial. *Arch Neurol* 1999; **56**:529–535.
4. Quinn NP, Classification of fluctuations in patients with Parkinson's disease. *Neurology* 1998; **51**:S25–S29.
5. Nutt JG, Levodopa-induced dyskinesia: review, observations, and speculations. *Neurology* 1990; **40**:340–345.
6. Marsden CD, Parkes JD, Quinn N, Fluctuations of disability in Parkinson's disease: Clinical aspects. In: Marsden CD, Fahn S (eds) *Movement Disorders*. Butterworth; London, 1981; 96–122.
7. Quinn NP, Critchley P, Marsden CD, Young onset Parkinson's disease. *Mov Disord* 1987; **2**:73–91.

8. Poewe WH, Lees AJ, Stern GM, Dystonia in Parkinson's disease: clinical and pharmacological features. *Ann Neurol* 1988; **23**:73–78.

9. Melamed E, Early-morning dystonia: a late side effect of long term levodopa therapy in Parkinson's disease. *Arch Neurol* 1979; **36**:308–310.

10. Hardie RJ, Lees AJ, Stern GM, On-off fluctuations in Parkinson's disease. A clinical and neuropharmacological study. *Brain* 1984; **107**:487–506.

11. Nissenbaum H, Quinn NP, Brown RG et al, Mood swings associated with the "on-off" phenomenon in Parkinson's disease. *Psychol Med* 1987; **17**:899–904.

12. Menza MA, Sage J, Marshall E et al, Mood changes and "on-off" phenomena in Parkinson's disease. *Mov Disord* 1990; **5**:148–151.

13. Richard IH, Justus AW, Kurlan R, The relationship between mood and motor fluctuations in Parkinson's disease. *J Neuropsychiatry Clin Neurosci* 2001; **3**:35–41.

14. Friedenberg DL, Cummings JL, Parkinson's disease, depression and the on-off phenomenon. *Psychosomatics* 1989; **30**:94–99.

15. Lees AJ, The on-off phenomenon. *J Neurol Neurosurg Psychiatry* 1989; Suppl:29–37.

16. Cantello R, Gilli M, Riccio A et al, Mood changes associated with "end-of-dose deterioration" in Parkinson's disease. *J Neurol Neurosurg Psychiatry* 1986; **49**:1182–1190.

17. Maricle RA, Nutt JG, Valentine RJ et al, Dose–response relationship of levodopa with mood and anxiety in fluctuating Parkinson's disease: A double-blind, placebo controlled study. *Neurology* 1995; **45**:1757–1760.

18. Streifler M, Hofman S, Disorders of verbal expression in parkinsonism. *Adv Neurol* 1984; **40**:385–393.

19. Deane KHO, Whurr R, Playford ED, Ben-Shlomo Y, Clarke CE, Speech and language therapy versus placebo or no intervention for dysarthria in Parkinson's disease. *The Cochrane Database of Scientific Reviews* 2004; 2.

20. Robbins JA, Logermann JA, Kirshner HS, Swallowing and speech production in Parkinson's disease. *Ann Neurol* 1986; **19**:283–287.

21. Bushmann M, Dobmeyer SM, Leeker L, Perlmutter JS, Swallowing abnormalities and their response to treatment in Parkinson's disease. *Neurology* 1989; **39**:1309–1314.

22. Johnston BT, Li Q, Castell JA, Castell DO, Swallowing and esophageal function in Parkinson's disease. *Am J Gastroenterol* 1995; **90**:1741–1746.

23. Begheri H, Damase-Michel C, Lapeyre-Mestre M et al, A study of salivary secretion in Parkinson's disease. *Clin Neuropharmacol* 1999; **22**:213–215.

24. Clarke CE, Gullaksen E, Macdonald S, Lowe R, Referral criteria for speech and language therapy assessment of dysphagia caused by idiopathic Parkinson's disease. *Acta Neurol Scand* 1998; **97**:27–35.

25. Deane KHO, Whurr R, Playford ED, Ben-Shlomo Y, Clarke CE, Speech and language therapy for dysarthria in Parkinson's disease: a comparison of techniques. *The Cochrane Database of Scientific Reviews* 2004; 2.

26. Paulson HL, Stern MB, Clinical manifestations of Parkinson's disease. In: Watts RL, Koller WC (eds) *Neurological Principles and Practice.* McGraw-Hill; New York, 1997; 183–199.

27. Schrag A, Ben-Shlomo Y, Guinn N, How common are complications of Parkinson's disease? *J Neurol* 2002; **249**:419–423.

28. Krystkowiak P, Blatt JL, Bourriez JL et al, Effects of subthalamic nucleus stimulation and levodopa treatment on gait abnormalities in Parkinson disease. *Arch Neurol* 2003; **60**:80–84.

29. Schaafsma JD, Giladi N, Balash Y, Bartels AL, Gurevich T, Hausdorff JM, Gait dynamics in Parkinson's disease: relationship to Parkinsonian features, falls and response to levodopa. *J Neurol Sci* 2003; **212**:47–53.

30. Rubinstein TC, Giladi N, Hausdorff JM, The power of cueing to circumvent

dopamine deficits: a review of physical therapy treatment of gait disturbances in Parkinson's disease. *Mov Disord* 2002; **17**:1148–1160.

31. Cubo E, Moore CG, Leurgans S, Goetz CG, Wheeled and standard walkers in Parkinson's disease patients with gait freezing. *Parkinsonism and Related Disorders* 2003; **10**:9–14.

32. Koller WC, Hubble JP, Levodopa therapy in Parkinson's disease. *Neurology* 1990; **40**:40–47.

33. Poewe WH, Wenning GK, The natural history of Parkinson's disease. *Neurology* 1996; **47**:146–152.

34. Weiner WJ, The initial treatment of Parkinson's disease should begin with levodopa. *Mov Disord* 1999; **14**:716–724.

35. Fahn S, Levodopa-induced neurotoxicity: does it represent a problem for the treatment of Parkinson's disease? *CNS Drugs* 1997; **8**:376–393.

36. Mena MA, Casarejos MJC, Paino CL, deYebenes JG, Glia conditioned medium protects fetal rat midbrain neurones in culture from L-DOPA toxicity. *Neuroreport* 1996; **7**:441–445.

37. Shulman L, Levodopa toxicity in Parkinson's disease: Reality or myth?: Reality–practice patterns should change. *Arch Neurol* 2000; **57**:407–408.

38. Mouradian MM, Heusen IJE, Baronto F et al, Modifications of central dopaminergic mechanisms by continuous levodopa therapy for advanced Parkinson's disease. *Ann Neurol* 1990; **27**:18–23.

39. Chase TN, Engber TM, Mouradian NM, Palliative and prophylactic benefits of continuously administered dopaminomimetics in Parkinson's disease. *Neurology* 1994; **44**:515–518.

40. Montastruc JL, Rascol O, Senard J-M, Treatment of PD should begin with a dopamine agonist. *Mov Disord* 1999; **14**:725–730.

41. Stocchi F, Olanow CW, Continuous dopaminergic stimulation in early and advanced Parkinson's disease. *Neurology* 2004; **62**(Suppl):S56–S63.

42. Nutt JG, Woodward WR, Beckner RM et al, Effect of peripheral catechol-O-methyl transferase inhibition on the pharmacokinetics and pharmacodynamics of levodopa in parkinsonian patients. *Neurology* 1994; **44**:913–919.

43. Brooks DJ, Safety and tolerability of COMT inhibitors. Neurology 2004; **62**(Suppl):S39–S46.

44. Syed N, Murphy J, Zimmerman TJ, Mark MH, Sage LI, Ten years' experience with enteral levodopa infusions for motor fluctuations in Parkinson's disease. *Mov Disord* 1998; **13**:336–338.

45. Hutton JT, Morris JL, Bush DF, Smith ME, Liss CL, Reines S, Multicenter controlled study of Sinemet CR vs. Sinemet (25/100) in advanced Parkinson's disease. *Neurology* 1989; **39**(Suppl):67–72.

46. Shults C, Treatments of Parkinson's disease: Circa 2003. *Arch Neurol* 2003; **60**:1680–1684.

47. Assal F, Spahr L, Hadengue A, Rubbia-Brandt L, Burkhard PR, Rubbici-Brandt L, Tolcapone and fulminant hepatitis. *Lancet* 1998; **352**:958.

48. Benabou R, Waters C, Hepatotoxic profile of catechol-*O*-methyltransferase inhibitors in Parkinson's disease. *Expert Opinion on Drug Safety* 2003; **2**:263–267.

49. Parkinson Study Group, Entacapone improves motor fluctuations in levodopa-treated Parkinson patients. *Ann Neurol* 1997; **42**:747–755.

50. Rinne UK, Larsen JP, Siden A, Worm-Petersen J, NOMECOMT Study Group, Entacapone enhances the response to levodopa in parkinsonian patients with motor fluctuations. *Neurology* 1998; **51**:1309–1314.

51. Poewe W, The role of COMT inhibition in the treatment of Parkinson's disease. *Neurology* 2004; **62**(Suppl):S31–S38.

52. Brooks DJ, Sagar H, the UK-Irish Entacapone Study Group, Entacapone is beneficial in both fluctuating and non-fluctuating patients with Parkinson's disease. A randomized, placebo-controlled, double-blind six-month study. *J Neurol Neurosurg Psychiatry* 2003; **74**:1064–1072.

53. Metman LV, DelDotto P, van den Munckhof P, Fang J, Mouradian MD, Chase TN, Amantadine as treatment for dyskinesias and motor fluctuations in Parkinson's disease. *Neurology* 1998; **50**:1323–1326.

54. Verhagen Metman L, Locatelli ER, Bravi D, Apomorphine responses in Parkinson's disease and the pathogenesis of motor complications. *Neurology* 1997; **48**:369–372.

55. Dewey RBJ, Hutton JT, LeWitt PA, Factor SA, A randomized, double-blind, placebo-controlled trial of subcutaneously injected apomorphine for parkinsonian on-state events. *Arch Neurol* 2001; **58**:1385–1392.

56. Factor SA, Literature review: Intermittent subcutaneous apomorphine therapy in Parkinson's disease. *Neurology* 2004; **62**(Suppl):S12–S17.

57. Swope DM, Rapid treatment of "wearing off" in Parkinson's disease. *Neurology* 2004; **62**(Suppl):S27–S31.

58. Stacy M, Apomorphine: North American clinical experience. *Neurology* 2004; **62**(Suppl):S18–S21.

59. The Deep-Brain Stimulation for Parkinson's Disease Study Group, Deep-brain stimulation of the subthalamic nucleus or the pars interna of the globus pallidus in Parkinson's disease. *New Engl J Med* 2001; **345**:956–963.

60. Olanow CW, Present and future directions in the management of motor complications in patients with advanced PD. *Neurology* 2003; **61**(Suppl):S24–S33.

61. Kumar RLA, Sime E, Halket E, Lang AE, Comparative effects of unilateral and bilateral subthalamic nucleus deep brain stimulation. *Neurology* 1999; **53**:561–566.

62. Bagheri H, Damase-Michel C, Lapeyre-Mestre M et al, A study of salivary secretion in Parkinson's disease. *Clin Neuropharmacol* 1999; **22**:213–215.

63. Ghika J, Vingerhoets F, Albanese A, Villmeure JG, Bipolar swings in mood in a patient with bilateral subthalamic deep brain stimulation (DBS) free of antiparkinsonian medication. *Parkinsonism and Related Disorders* 1999; **5**(Suppl 1):104.

64. Krack P, Kuman R, Ardouin C et al, Mirthful laughter induced by subthalamic nucleus stimulation. *Mov Disord* 2002; **16**:867–875.

chapter 4

Non-motor somatic symptoms

Nasir Mirza and Kevin M Biglan

Introduction

While Parkinson's disease (PD) is defined by its motor symptoms (i.e. tremor, bradykinesia, and rigidity) and most therapeutic interventions target motor impairment, non-motor symptoms are common and a source of major disability.[1,2] In addition to the psychiatric, behavioral, and sleep manifestations discussed elsewhere in this text, somatic complaints including dysautonomia and sensory phenomena represent significant challenges in the management of Parkinson's disease. Table 4.1 presents an overview of these somatic complaints. This chapter reviews the frequency, manifestations and treatment of autonomic dysfunction and sensory disorders in patients with PD.

Autonomic nervous system dysfunction

Autonomic nervous system dysfunction affects 70–80% of PD patients, and causes significant morbidity and discomfort.[3,4] Symptoms attributable to the autonomic nervous system were recognized by James Parkinson in his original 1817 monograph on "The Shaking Palsy" where he reported on severe constipation and urinary incontinence as prominent features of the illness.[5] In addition to gastrointestinal disorders and urinary symptoms, dysautonomia in PD can produce sexual dysfunction, defects in thermoregulation, and often most problematic, defects in cardiovascular regulation.

Table 4.1 Overview of somatic symptoms in Parkinson's disease

Autonomic dysfunction	Gastrointestinal dysfunction	Dysphagia
		GI dysmotility
	Urinary dysfunction	Nocturia
		Frequency/urgency
		Incontinence
	Sexual dysfunction	Impotence
		Diminished libido
	Impaired thermoregulation	Hyperhidrosis
		Heat/cold intolerance
	Orthostatic hypotension	
Sensory phenomenon	Pain	Musculoskeletal
		Dystonic
		Primary – "off" Pain
	Akathisia	
	Restless legs syndrome	

Gastrointestinal dysfunction

Gastrointestinal dysfunction may be the most common non-motor feature of PD with the entire GI axis being affected.[6]

Dysphagia

Swallowing difficulties are a common but generally late complication of PD.[7] While clinical symptoms occur in 50% of PD patients, nearly 90% of patients will have evidence of dysphagia using videofluoroscopy.[8,9] Dysphagia may result in weight loss, malnutrition, inability to take medications, and aspiration pneumonia. In addition, this problem has clinical relevance as a recent study suggests that the median survival time after the onset of symptomatic dysphagia in PD patients is only 24 months.[7]

As with most motor disturbances in PD, the history should be aimed at determining whether swallowing function varies in response to on–off phenomena. Certainly dysphagia is usually worse during "off" time and significant improvement of swallowing is usually seen after levodopa or apomorphine administration.[10,11] Therefore, maximizing therapy to minimize off time is often the first and most important strategy in managing "off" dysphagia. When this is not feasible patients should be instructed to eat only during "on" time.

All PD patients who experience clinically significant swallowing dysfunction should be evaluated by a speech and swallowing therapist. Soft diets and thickened liquids help many patients. Behavioral treatments, such as neck flexion during swallowing and not mixing solid and liquid foods, may also be useful. In rare instances, when adequate nutrition cannot be maintained despite optimal medical and behavioral management, percutaneous endoscopic gastrostomy (PEG) may be required.

Constipation

Constipation is ubiquitous in PD and a major source of patient dissatisfaction.[12] Unlike many somatic symptoms in PD, constipation can occur at any stage of illness and may even predate the development of more classic motor symptoms.[13] While generally considered only a nuisance, serious and life-threatening complications can arise from untreated constipation, including megacolon, bowel rupture, and acute abdomen.

Constipation results from both the gastrointestinal hypomotility and paradoxical contraction of sphincter muscles during defecation (anismus).[14] Gastrointestinal hypomotility is characterized by infrequent defecation and anismus by excessive straining, pain, and a sense of incomplete evacuation.

The history should differentiate abnormalities of colonic transit from those of defecation as treatment approaches may vary. A review of medications that may potentiate constipation (e.g. anticholinergics) is mandatory. In patients with an acute or subacute history of constipation, a full investigation of the colon by either colonoscopy or barium enema is necessary in order to exclude organic obstruction by neoplasms or inflammatory disease. If outlet obstruction is suspected, further investigations may be performed, including defecography, anorectal manometry, electromyography, or balloon expulsion tests.

Reducing or eliminating medications, specifically anticholinergics, that may exacerbate constipation is an important first step in management. Dietary modification including increasing fluid and dietary fiber intake through dietary changes or supplementation (psyllium or methylcellulose) should be considered in all patients. Lack of physical activity is a frequent contributor to constipation in PD and patients should be encouraged to implement a program of regular physical activity with walking or swimming being excellent and safe choices for PD patients. If necessary a stool softener, such as docusate, can be used on a daily basis. If further treatment is required, an osmotic laxative can be used. A polyethylene glycol electrolyte-balanced solution used on a regular basis is effective in patients with PD.[15] Irritant laxatives or enemas should be used sparingly and only when other measures have failed. Pyridostigmine bromide[16] and colchicine[17] have been noted anecdotally to be of benefit in some patients. In rare cases where megacolon or volvulus has developed, surgical referral is necessary.

If constipation is caused by anismus, the preferred therapy is botulinum toxin injection into the striated pelvic floor musculature.[18,19] Although this may occasionally be followed by fecal incontinence, this side-effect is short-lived and less frequent than after alternative therapies such as sphinctero-tomies. Table 4.2 outlines additional potential uses of botulinum toxin injections in PD management.

Urinary symptoms

Bladder dysfunction is common and under-recognized in PD.[3] Nocturia is the earliest urinary problem in patients with PD, followed by symptoms of urgency and frequency and difficulty voiding. The severity of urinary symptoms is related to the severity of PD.[20]

The most common neurogenic cause of bladder symptoms in PD is detrusor hyperreflexia,[21] followed by impaired pelvic floor muscle relaxation or sphincter bradykinesia.[22] This can result in voiding dysfunction due to bladder outflow obstruction.[23] The effect of levodopa on bladder function is unclear, though bradykinesia or imbalance may impair an individual's ability to get to a toilet in a timely fashion, resulting in incontinence.

The evaluation aims to exclude other causes of urinary dysfunction, such as diabetes, prostatic hypertrophy, or gynecologic surgeries. Most patients should undergo a thorough urological evaluation. For nocturnal frequency fluid intake should be limited after the evening meal. In cases where this is not effective, peripherally acting anticholinergics, such as oxybutynin,

---

Table 4.2 Select uses of botulinum toxin in PD management

Constipation/anismus
Neurogenic bladder/urinary retention
Musculoskeletal pain due to muscle spasm/rigidity
Dystonia and dystonic pain
Excessive salivation/drooling

propantheline, or tolterodine, can be used to treat symptoms of frequency and urgency. Hyoscyamine can be tried as a second-line agent. Anticholinergic agents should be used cautiously as they can precipitate worsening cognition, hallucinations, and may even worsen voiding problems or produce urinary retention in patients who have detrusor hypoactivity or outlet obstruction. Antidepressants, such as imipramine, nortryptiline, and doxepin, may help incontinence and may be considered in patients with sleep or behavioral indications for these drugs.[24] Botulinum toxin injections (usually targeting the detrusor muscle) may also be effective for urinary difficulties associated with PD, particularly in patients who can not tolerate or fail oral alternatives.[25] Finally, any abrupt change in urinary function should raise the possibility of a urinary tract infection.

Sexual problems

A total of 60–80% of male PD patients[26] and 40–80% of female PD patients[27] display moderate to severe sexual problems and reduced sexual activity. Women with sexual dysfunction most commonly report difficulties with arousal (87.5%), while men report erectile dysfunction (68.4%).[28] Comorbid illnesses, concomitant medications, and severity of PD all contribute to sexual dysfunction.

Psychiatric disorders are common causes of sexual dysfunction in Parkinson's patients. Depression and anxiety should be screened for and treated appropriately. Many drugs can cause erectile dysfunction and impaired libido, and a thorough medication history is essential. Drugs that can induce impotence include α- and β-adrenergic blockers, guanethidine, thiazide diuretics, anxiolytics, digoxin, cimetidine, and some antidepressants. Selective serotonin re-uptake inhibitors are commonly used in PD and associated with a variety of sexual side-effects including loss of libido, anorgasmia, and impotency.[29] Medical evaluation of the impotent patient should also be performed. Vascular disease, diabetes, thyroid disease and other endocrinological causes should be ruled out.

In patients where medical or psychiatric causes are treated, several therapeutic options for sexual dysfunction exist. Previously untreated or undertreated PD patients may find that dopaminergic therapy helps sexual functioning, through enhanced libido.[30] Sildenafil and related compounds, intracavernous injections, or transurethral suppositories of alprostadil, and penile implants are widely used and effective for impotency.[31] The dopamine agonists, apomorphine[32] and pergolide,[33] are also effective for treating impotency, and may have some additional utility in PD patients with sexual dysfunction.[34]

As discussed elsewhere, some patients on high doses of antiparkinsonian therapy become hypersexual, even in the face of an inability to perform, and dose reductions or psychiatric treatment may be beneficial.

Thermoregulation

Thermoregulatory disturbances, hyperhidrosis, hypothermia, and feeling abnormally hot or cold are well-recognized features of PD.[35] Sweating disturbances are usually associated with other symptoms of autonomic dysfunction and tend to occur in more advanced disease. Sweating dysfunction may present as whole body or drenching sweats, asymmetrical sweating, or localized sweating predominantly involving the head, neck, and trunk. Hyperhidrosis may impair social functioning, cause sleep disruption, and cause significant burden due to the need to change and wash clothing frequently.

Sweating episodes occur most commonly as a wearing "off" phenomenon, but may also accompany peak-dose dyskinesias.[36] Management can be aided by avoiding hot and humid environments and strenuous physical activity, wearing well-ventilated clothes, and keeping well hydrated. The management of off-period sweating may respond favorably to strategies aimed at reducing or minimizing "off" time. In addition to attempts to minimize dopaminergic therapy, β-adrenergic blockers may be effective against on-period sweating.

Orthostatic hypotension

Orthostatic hypotension (OH) is defined as a fall in blood pressure of at least 20 mmHg systolic or 10 mmHg diastolic during standing or head-up tilt-table testing.[37] However, symptoms of OH are not always directly proportional to blood pressure readings, and OH by blood pressure may be asymptomatic. The estimated prevalence of OH varies, ranging from 20% to greater than 60%.[3]

OH presents clinically as light-headedness or frank syncope occurring shortly upon changing from a supine or sitting position to standing and usually resolves upon resumption of a recumbent position. Importantly OH may present with atypical symptoms including weakness, "coat hanger" distribution ache across the shoulders, chest discomfort, lower back ache, calf claudication, light-headedness, diaphoresis, pallor, graying out of vision, weakness, and mental clouding.[38] OH is often worse first thing in the morning, and may be exacerbated by heat, food, alcohol, vasoactive medications, exercise, and valsalva manuevers.

OH in PD patients is often due to impaired vasoconstriction because of decreased sympathetic outflow. Complicating matters is that many medications used in PD (levodopa, dopamine agonists, atypical antipsychotics, monoamine oxidase inhibitors, and catechol-O-methyl transferase inhibitors) can precipitate or exacerbate OH.[3]

Patients should be treated for OH only if symptomatic and symptoms impair activities of daily living or quality of life. The goal of treatment is to improve the patient's functional capacity and symptoms, rather than to achieve any particular target blood pressure. A complete medication history should be obtained from the patient to identify and eliminate agents that can cause OH, specifically antihypertensive agents or diuretics. Levodopa and dopamine agonists may exacerbate OH, therefore, gradual dosage increases when initiating therapy or dose reductions in established patients can sometimes be useful.

Behavioral and non-pharmacological approaches are the mainstays of therapy. Avoiding triggers such as sudden head-up postural changes, early morning physical activity, hot environments, and alcohol. Lying flat at night exacerbates the loss of intravascular volume, therefore, elevating the head of the bed by 30–40° is useful for morning orthostatic hypotension and avoiding complications of supine hypertension.[38] Postprandial hypotension may be improved by having several small meals instead of a few heavy meals, and drinking water before meals.[39] Increased salt and water intake is a general recommendation to patients with OH. In patients with autonomic failure, drinking about 500 ml water leads to a significant increase in blood pressure, and might work best when ingested in the early morning at least 30 minutes before getting out of bed and before meals. On the other hand, fluid intake should be avoided before sleep, as it can worsen supine hypertension causing nocturnal diuresis and subsequent worsening of OH. Waist-high stockings or abdominal binders are often recommended. Leg-crossing, squatting, thigh contractions and toe extension are useful maneuvers to avoid OH.[40]

If conservative measures are insufficient to alleviate the symptoms of OH, pharmacologic intervention with medications should be considered. In general, fludrocortisone is the first-line treatment. Side-effects include hypokalemia and excessive water retention and edema. Direct- or indirect-acting sympathomimetics represent a second group of drugs to combat OH.

Several studies have confirmed the ability of midodrine to improve OH in autonomic failure.[41,42] It may be used alone or in conjunction with fludrocortisone. The main side-effects include pruritus and urinary retention in men. Domperidone, a peripheral dopamine receptor antagonist, may be useful in levodopa or dopamine agonist induced OH.[43] Similarly additional carbidopa with each dose of levodopa may be useful.

Desmopressin may be useful in patients with early morning drops in blood pressure due to nocturnal polyuria. Erythropoietin has been used to treat OH on the basis of its capacity to increase red blood cell mass and blood viscosity.[44] Octreotide, a somatostatin analog, is reported to prevent postprandial OH in patients with autonomic neuropathy but its use is limited by expense and need for parenteral administration.[45] Selective serotonin-reuptake inhibitors have also been used to treat OH in patients with PD.[46]

Sensory phenomena and pain

Surveys of PD patients suggest a prevalence of pain in PD of around 38–50%.[47–49] PD-related pain may be categorized as musculoskeletal pain, neuritic or radicular pain, dystonia-associated pain, primary or central pain, and akathitic discomfort.[50] Most pain in PD appears to be related to musculoskeletal causes or dystonia, though pain can be a common manifestation of the "off" phenomenon.

Pains of musculoskeletal origin often presage the appearance of the cardinal features of the disease, e.g. a stiff or frozen shoulder may be the first symptom of PD.[51] This type of pain is described as aching, cramping, arthralgic, and myalgic in character. Associated findings may include skeletal deformity, limited joint mobility, and even contractures.[50] Musculoskeletal pains are best treated by maximizing motor function and reducing "off" time. Physical therapy and an exercise program are critical. Directed botulinum toxin injections (see Table 4.2) in select painful muscles associated with severe rigidity and stiffness may be useful.[52]

Pain caused by dystonia can be diagnosed in cases in which there is visible twisting, cramping, or posturing of the painful extremity or body part. Dystonia frequently occurs as an early morning manifestation of dopaminergic deficiency, as a wearing-off phenomenon later in the day, as a diphasic dyskinesia (beginning and end of dose phenomenon), or as a peak-dose dyskinesia associated with levodopa treatment. In general "off" dystonia is treated by attempts to minimize "off" time through the use of dopamine agonists, COMT-inhibitors, and MAO-B inhibitors. Second-line agents for treating dystonia in PD include anticholinergics, baclofen and lithium.[50] Injections of botulinum toxin (see Table 4.2) may produce dramatic relief of pain in cases of focal dystonia refractory to pharmacotherapy.[53] Pallidotomy and bilateral subthalamic nucleus stimulation have also been reported to relieve painful dystonia in PD.[54,55]

Central or primary pain in PD is presumed to be a direct consequence of the disease itself, and not a secondary phenomenon of the motor manifestations. It is often linked to "off" periods or inadequate dopaminergic dosages. Primary pain is usually a non-specific, poorly localized, cramp-like, and aching sensation, and seems to be worse on the side of the body more affected by motor symptoms but can occur in any body region.[56] Patients may also describe paresthesias, burning dysesthesias, coldness, and numbness. Central pain in PD often responds to optimization of anti-parkinsonian medication. Conventional analgesics, opiates, tricyclic agents, lithium, gabapentin, methylphenidate, and atypical neuroleptics may be helpful in cases where dopaminergic agents are ineffective. Deep brain stimulation to the pallidum or the subthalamic nucleus has been advocated for treating central pain syndromes in PD, though this has not been systematically evaluated.[57]

Akathisia is a subjective sense of inner restlessness, resulting in an inability to remain still, and manifests as a constant need to move or change positions.[58] Akathisia is usually related to periods of dopaminergic deficiency, and is often relieved by dopaminergic treatment. Restlessness is also a core element of the restless legs syndrome, in which patients experience an intense and irresistible urge to move the legs accompanied by sensory complaints.[59] Characteristically, the symptoms are worse at rest, in the evening or at night, and may be relieved dramatically by levodopa or dopamine agonists. Resistant cases may respond to opiates or gabapentin at bedtime.[60,61]

Overlap with psychiatric symptoms

A high comorbidity of psychiatric and non-motor somatic features in PD patients could be predicted from the high prevalence rates of these disorders in PD. In fact, a number of studies have reported a significant association between psychiatric disease and autonomic dysfunction in PD.[4,62] In addition, certain somatic symptoms may be a manifestation of psychiatric disease, for example, while diaphoresis may be a symptom of anxiety, and diminished libido, impotence and constipation may be features of depression, they can also be manifestations of autonomic dysfunction. The clinician, therefore, must remain watchful of dysautonomia as a possible alternative explanation of various psychiatric complaints and vice versa.

Also, clinically significant interactions between psychiatric and sensory symptoms of PD likely exist. Persistent pain of any cause can precipitate depression. Depression is more severe in patients with PD who experience pain than in those who do not.[62] Conversely, depression may heighten the severity of a pain syndrome. Pain is more common in depressed PD patients than in non-depressed PD patients. It is important, therefore, that any assessment of pain in a PD patient take into account the potential contributing role of depression, and vice versa.

References

1. Karlsen KH, Larsen JP, Tandberg E, Maeland JG, Influence of clinical and demographic variables on quality of life in patients with Parkinson's disease. *J Neurol Neurosurg Psychiat* 1999; **66**:431–435.
2. Shulman LM, Taback RL, Rabinstein AA, Weiner WJ, Non-recognition of depression and other non-motor symptoms in Parkinson's disease. *Parkinsonism and Related Disorders* 2002; **8**(3):193–197.
3. Zesiewicz TA, Baker MJ, Wahba M, Hauser RA, Autonomic nervous system dysfunction in Parkinson's disease. *Curr Treat Options Neurol* 2003; **5**(2):149–160.
4. Hobson P, Islam W, Roberts S, Adhiyman V, Meara J, The risk of bladder and autonomic dysfunction in a community cohort of Parkinson's disease patients and normal controls. *Parkinsonism & Related Disorders* 2003; **10**(2):67–71.
5. Parkinson J, *An Essay on the Shaking Palsy.* Whittingham & Rowland for Sherwood, Neely & Jones: London, 1817.
6. Byrne KG, Pfeiffer R, Quigley EM, Gastrointestinal dysfunction in Parkinson's disease. A report of clinical experience at a single center. *J Clin Gastroenterol* 1994; **19**(1):11–16.
7. Muller J, Wenning GK, Verny M et al, Progression of dysarthria and dysphagia in postmortem-confirmed parkinsonian disorders. *Arch Neurol* 2001; **58**(2): 259–264.
8. Edwards LL, Quigley EM, Pfeiffer RF, Gastrointestinal dysfunction in Parkinson's disease: frequency and pathophysiology. *Neurology* 1992; **42**(4):726–732.
9. Stroudley J, Walsh M, Radiological assessment of dysphagia in Parkinson's disease. *Br J Radiol* 1991; **64**(766):890–893.
10. Bushmann M, Dobmeyer SM, Leeker L, Perlmutter JS, Swallowing abnormalities and their response to treatment in Parkinson's disease. *Neurology* 1989; **39**(10): 1309–1314.
11. Tison F, Wiart L, Guatterie M et al, Effects of central dopaminergic stimulation by apomorphine on swallowing disorders in Parkinson's disease. *Mov Disord* 1996; **11**(6):729–732.
12. Jost WH, Eckardt VF, Constipation in idiopathic Parkinson's disease. *Scand J Gastroenterol* 2003; **38**(7):681–686.

13. Abbott RD, Petrovitch H, White LR et al, Frequency of bowel movements and the future risk of Parkinson's disease. *Neurology* 2001; **57**(3):456–462.
14. Pfeiffer RF, Gastrointestinal dysfunction in Parkinson's disease. *Lancet Neurology* 2003; **2**(2):107–116.
15. Eichhorn TE, Oertel WH, Macrogol 3350/electrolyte improves constipation in Parkinson's disease and multiple system atrophy. *Mov Disord* 2001; **16**(6):1176–1177.
16. Sadjadpour K, Pyridostigmine bromide and constipation in Parkinson's disease. *JAMA* 1983; **249**(9):1148.
17. Sandyk R, Gillman MA, Colchicine ameliorates constipation in Parkinson's disease. *J R Social Med* 1984; **77**(12):1066.
18. Jost WH, Schrank B, Herold A, Leiss O, Functional outlet obstruction: anismus, spastic pelvic floor syndrome, and dyscoordination of the voluntary sphincter muscles. Definition, diagnosis, and treatment from the neurologic point of view. *Scand J Gastroenterol* 1999; **34**(5):449–453.
19. Albanese A, Maria G, Bentivoglio AR, Brisinda G, Cassetta E, Tonali P, Severe constipation in Parkinson's disease relieved by botulinum toxin. *Mov Disord* 1997; **12**(5):764–766.
20. Araki I, Kuno S, Assessment of voiding dysfunction in Parkinson's disease by the international prostate symptom score. *J Neurol Neurosurg Psychiat* 2000; **68**(4): 429–433.
21. Fowler CJ, Urinary disorders in Parkinson's disease and multiple system atrophy. *Funct Neurol* 2001; **16**(3):277–282.
22. Pavlakis AJ, Siroky MB, Goldstein I, Krane RJ, Neurourologic findings in Parkinson's disease. *J Urology* 1983; **129**(1):80–83.
23. Singer C, Weiner WJ, Sanchez-Ramos JR, Autonomic dysfunction in men with Parkinson's disease. *Eur Neurol* 1992; **32**(3):134–140.
24. Andersson KE, Drug therapy for urinary incontinence. *Baillères Best Pract Res Clin Obstet Gynaecol* 2000; **14**(2):291–313.
25. Leippold T, Reitz A, Schurch B, Botulinum toxin as a new therapy option for voiding disorders: Current state of the art. *Eur Urol* 2003; **44**(2):165–174.
26. Nappi RE, Detaddei S, Veneroni F et al, Sexual disorders in Parkinson's disease. *Funct Neurol* 2001; **16**(3):283–288.
27. Welsh M, Hung L, Waters CH, Sexuality in women with Parkinson's disease. *Mov Disord* 1997; **12**(6):923–927.
28. Bronner G, Royter V, Korczyn AD, Giladi N, Sexual dysfunction in Parkinson's disease. *J Sex Marital Ther* 2004; **30**(2):95–105.
29. Kennedy SH, Eisfeld BS, Dickens SE, Bacchiochi JR, Bagby RM, Antidepressant-induced sexual dysfunction during treatment with moclobemide, paroxetine, sertraline, and venlafaxine. *J Clin Psychiatry* 2000; **61**(4):276–281.
30. Brown E, Brown GM, Kofman O, Quarrington B, Sexual function and affect in parkinsonian men treated with L-dopa. *Am J Psychiatry* 1978; **135**(12):1552–1555.
31. Montorsi F, Salonia A, Deho F et al, Pharmacological management of erectile dysfunction. *BJU Int* 2003; **91**(5):446–454.
32. Dula E, Bukofzer S, Perdok R, George M, Double-blind, crossover comparison of 3 mg apomorphine SL with placebo and with 4 mg apomorphine SL in male erectile dysfunction. *Eur Urol* 2001; **39**:558–564.
33. Pohanka M, Kanovsky P, Bares M, Pulkrabek J, Rektor I, Pergolide mesylate can improve sexual dysfunction in patients with Parkinson's disease: the results of an open, prospective, 6-month follow-up. *Eur J Neurol* 2004; **11**(7):483–488.
34. O'Sullivan JD, Apomorphine as an alternative to sildenafil in Parkinson's disease. *J Neurol Neurosurg Psychiat* 2002; **72**(5):681.

35. Swinn L, Schrag A, Viswanathan R, Bloem BR, Lees A, Quinn N, Sweating dysfunction in Parkinson's disease. *Mov Disord* 2003; **18**(12):1459–1463.

36. Sage JI, Mark MH, Drenching sweats as an off phenomenon in Parkinson's disease: treatment and relation to plasma levodopa profile. *Ann Neurol* 1995; **37**(1):120–122.

37. The Consensus Committee of the American Autonomic Society and the American Academy of Neurology, Consensus statement on the definition of orthostatic hypotension, pure autonomic failure, and multiple system atrophy. *Neurology* 1996; **46**(5):1470.

38. Oldenburg O, Kribben A, Baumgart D, Philipp T, Erbel R, Cohen MV, Treatment of orthostatic hypotension. *Curr Opin Pharmacol* 2002; **2**(6):740–747.

39. Shannon JR, Diedrich A, Biaggioni I et al, Water drinking as a treatment for orthostatic syndromes. *Am J Med* 2002; **112**(5):355–360.

40. Bouvette CM, McPhee BR, Opfer-Gehrking TL, Low PA, Role of physical counter-maneuvers in the management of orthostatic hypotension: efficacy and biofeedback augmentation. *Mayo Clin Proc* 1996; **71**(9):847–853.

41. Low PA, Gilden JL, Freeman R, Sheng KN, McElligott MA, Efficacy of midodrine vs placebo in neurogenic orthostatic hypotension. A randomized, double-blind multicenter study. Midodrine Study Group. *JAMA* 1997; **277**(13):1046–1051.

42. Wright RA, Kaufmann HC, Perera R et al, A double-blind, dose-response study of midodrine in neurogenic orthostatic hypotension. *Neurology* 1998; **51**(1):-120–124.

43. Lang AE, Kujawa K, Goetz CG, Acute orthostatic hypotension when starting dopamine agonist therapy in Parkinson disease: The role of domperidone therapy. *Arch Neurol* 2001; **58**(5):835.

44. Perera R, Isola L, Kaufmann H, Effect of recombinant erythropoietin on anemia and orthostatic hypotension in primary autonomic failure. *Clin Auton Res* 1995; **5**(4):211–213.

45. Hoeldtke RD, Boden G, O'Dorisio TM, Treatment of postprandial hypotension with a somatostatin analogue (SMS 201-995). *Am J Med* 1986; **81**(6B):398–402.

46. Montastruc JL, Pelat M, Verwaerde P et al, Fluoxetine in orthostatic hypotension of Parkinson's disease: a clinical and experimental pilot study. *Fundam Clin Pharmacol* 1998; **12**(4):398–402.

47. Goetz CG, Tanner CM, Lew M, Wilson RS, Garron DC, Pain in Parkinson's disease. *Mov Disord* 1986; **1**(1):45–49.

48. Koller WC, Sensory symptoms in Parkinson's disease. *Neurology* 1984; **34**(7):957–959.

49. Snider SR, Fahn S, Isgreen WP, Cote LJ, Primary sensory symptoms in parkinsonism. *Neurology* 1976; **26**(5):423–429.

50. Ford B, Pain in Parkinson's disease. *Clin Neurosci* 1998; **5**(2):63–72.

51. Cleeves L, Findley L, Frozen shoulder and other shoulder disturbances in Parkinson's disease. *J Neurol Neurosurg Psychiat* 1989; **52**(6):813–814.

52. Grazko MA, Polo KB, Jabbari B, Botulinum toxin A for spasticity, muscle spasms, and rigidity. *Neurology* 1995; **45**(4):712–717.

53. Pacchetti C, Albani G, Martignoni E, Godi L, Alfonsi E, Nappi G, "Off" painful dystonia in Parkinson's disease treated with botulinum toxin. *Mov Disord* 1995; **10**(3):333–336.

54. Laitinen LV, Bergenheim AT, Hariz MI, Leksell's posteroventral pallidotomy in the treatment of Parkinson's disease. *J Neurosurg* 1992; **76**(1):53–61.

55. Limousin P, Krack P, Pollak P et al, Electrical stimulation of the subthalamic nucleus in advanced Parkinson's disease. *New Engl J Med* 1998; **339**(16):1105–1111.

56. Quinn NP, Koller WC, Lang AE, Marsden CD, Painful Parkinson's disease. *Lancet* 1986; 1(8494):1366–1369.
57. Sage JI, Pain in Parkinson's disease. *Curr Treat Option Neurol* 2004; 6(3):191–200.
58. Sachdev P, Loneragran C, The present status of akathisia. *J Nervous Mental Dis* 1991; 179(7):381–389.
59. Walters AS, Toward a better definition of the restless legs syndrome. The International Restless Legs Syndrome Study Group. *Mov Disord* 1995; 10(5):634–642.
60. Hening WA, Walters A, Kavey N, Gidro-Frank S, Cote L, Fahn S, Dyskinesias while awake and periodic movements in sleep in restless legs syndrome: treatment with opioids. *Neurology* 1986; 36(10):1363–1366.
61. Adler CH, Treatment of restless legs syndrome with gabapentin. *Clin Neuropharmacol* 1997; 20(2):148–151.
62. Berrios GE, Campbell C, Politynska BE, Autonomic failure, depression, and anxiety in Parkinson's disease. *Br J Psychiatry* 1995; 166(6):789–792.

chapter 5

Cognitive impairment

Susan Spear Bassett

Introduction

While it is a minority of patients that will develop a frank dementia, most patients with Parkinson's disease (PD) will experience changes in intellectual function, often early in the course of their illness. These changes, or cognitive impairments, manifest themselves primarily as difficulties in executive function and their effect on daily life can be profound. Such impairments significantly interfere with occupational and social functioning, often leading to loss of employment and family conflict. This picture is complicated by the fact that some medications can exacerbate existing cognitive difficulties or precipitate their development.

This paper provides a description of the impairments, the underlying pathology, clinical evaluation, and current treatments for cognitive impairments in this population. While psychiatrists are not often initially focused on cognitive aspects of the illness, treatment of the psychiatric complications requires an understanding of the role cognitive status plays in the patient's presentation. In addition, where it might be expected that successful treatment of depression would restore cognitive function; this is often not the case in Parkinson's disease. However, since for most PD patients the cognitive deficits are restricted to executive functions, individual strategies can be developed to circumvent many of the life problems that result from these impairments.

Selective cognitive impairments

Although Parkinson's original essay "The Shaking Palsy" reported that the intellect remained intact,[1] in fact, Parkinson's disease (PD) is associated with some degree of cognitive impairment in the majority of those affected with this disorder.[2-4] Typically, the impairment is evident early in the course of the illness and is more selective and less severe than that found in PD patients who develop overt dementia.[5,6]

Parkinson's patients, even those with mild disease, exhibit patterns of cognitive deficits that include decrements in planning, sequencing, concept formation, and working memory,[7-18] all tasks associated with frontal lobe dysfunction. Whether cognitive deficits are restricted solely to those associated with frontal lobe dysfunction, however, is not clear. Reports from studies that have examined performance on memory tests, including both immediate and delayed recall of material differ.[2,11,18] Sullivan (1989) suggested that memory deficits were directly related to overall disease severity, with mildly impaired patients showing no decrements in memory performance, while Goldman found increasing memory deficits with increasing disease severity, including deficits among those very mildly affected. A recent study by Locascio and colleagues[19] found decrements in verbal memory for all patients, however decrements in visual memory appear to occur later and vary with age of disease onset. Reports of cognitive slowing are also inconsistent,[20,21] as are reports of decrements in verbal fluency and confrontational naming.[2,22] It is unclear whether these impairments correlate with age of disease onset or the eventual development of dementia.[19,23] In global terms many of these deficits reflect an inability to spontaneously self-generate efficient task-specific strategies.[14,24]

Pathophysiology of cognitive impairments in PD

While basal ganglia pathology and degeneration of dopaminergic neurons in the substantia nigra is central to the pathogenesis of PD, theories suggest that the diverse disturbances present in this disease likely involve disruption in functionally segregated neuronal circuits involving different components of the basal ganglia, thalamus, and cerebral cortex.[25,26] This model of basal ganglia function involves five segregated circuits – motor, oculomotor, orbitofrontal, dorsolateral prefrontal, and anterior cingulate loops – of which three, the orbitofrontal, dorsolateral prefrontal, and anterior cingulate, appear integral to cognitive function.

Recent functional brain imaging studies have examined responses to cognitive tasks in an effort to understand the effects of basal ganglia pathology on cognition. PET and fMRI studies have shown that specific cognitive tasks produce different metabolic or activation patterns, distinguishing these circuits. PET studies have demonstrated independent metabolic patterns associated with specific cognitive functions.[27,28] For example, a gambling task requiring judgment and set-shifting, found decreased metabolism in the orbitofrontal circuit whereas the connections between the dorsolateral prefrontal cortex and thalamus via left caudate were unchanged.[27] fMRI studies have also shown the dissociation of frontal and medial dopomergeric projections in mild PD cases using an implicit rule-learning paradigm, with decreased activation in the inferior frontal region, while activation in the medial frontal cortex and cingulate, areas related to memory function, did not differ.[29] Further support for the differential dysfunction of these circuits was evident in another fMRI study where a reduction in activation in specific striatal and frontal lobe areas was apparent during a working memory task, but only among those PD patients with cognitive impairment.[30] This differential involvement of the cortical loops may reflect the progressive nature of the disease and prove useful for targeting therapies.

While dysfunction in the cortico circuits may underlie cognitive deficits apparent on executive and other frontal tasks, the dopaminergic system is likely not the only neurotransmitter disruption in this disease. Among newly diagnosed and previously unmedicated PD patients, for example, dopaminergic and anticholinergic medications improve motor control, dopaminergic treatment improves performance on a working memory and cognitive sequencing task, while anticholinergic agents adversely affect immediate recall.[5] Other cognitive processes were not affected, however, suggesting that some cognitive functions (e.g., short-term memory) are served both by dopamine and cholinergic subcortical-frontal systems, and others are independent of nigrostriatal pathology and may be related to primary cortical dysfunction. While the primary degeneration seen in PD may contribute to the development of dementia, it is likely that Alzheimer-type pathology and/or cortical limbic Lewy body degeneration are significant factors.[31] Support for the involvement of Alzheimer-type pathology includes reports of decreased hippocampal volumes in PD[32] related to memory performance rather than frontal tasks[33] and a decrease in posterior cingulate gyrus metabolites.[34]

Changes in cognition in response to PD treatments

Surgical interventions

Pallidotomy, an ablation procedure performed for patients with severe motor symptoms that have not responded to standard treatment, in general appears to have little long-term effect on cognition. Studies have reported initial changes in working memory, visuospatial learning and visuo-construction. At 3-month to 1-year follow-up, most studies report most cognitive functions return to baseline,[35–37] although there are reports of sustained impairment in verbal learning for those with a left-sided procedure.[37] Longer-term follow-up, up to 4 years, finds that for most patients cognitive functions have returned to pre-surgery levels.[38,39]

Deep brain stimulation, another procedure for treatment refractory PD patients, is successful in reducing the range of motor symptoms that afflict patients. It does not appear to produce global cognitive decline, however, there is general agreement that specific language dysfunction, namely verbal fluency, commonly occurs.[40–43] In addition, there have been reports of impairments of attention, verbal memory and executive function[41,42,44] and conversely reports of improvement in memory and executive function.[42,45] Imaging studies of patients following DBS have noted a correspondence between improvements in learning performance and increases in brain networks thought to be involved in these functions.[46] A recent 3-year follow-up of 70 patients, employing an extensive neuropsychological battery, found that for all cognitive areas tested, the majority of patients showed no change from baseline. For each test there were selected individuals that improved and declined. Only verbal fluency showed a significant number of patients declining from baseline, with no improvement over the 3-year period.[40]

Medications for motor impairments

L-dopa is the standard treatment for motor complications of PD and there is evidence that such treatment also affects cognition, improving a number of aspects of executive function and verbal fluency as well as sentence comprehension and short-term memory,[47–51] while possibly impairing inhibitory control.[52] However it is likely that the impact of L-dopa therapy on cognition may relate either to (1) individual drug responsiveness with de nova patients showing an improvement in cognition, those who stabilize on therapy showing no change and those whose status fluctuates actually continuing to show cognitive impairment[50] or (2) to the differential dopamine depletion on individual cortico-striatal circuits.[52] Recently, clinicians have been prescribing dopamine agonists initially for patients instead of L-dopa because of the reported lower incidence of dyskinesias in patients whose initial therapy is a dopamine agonist.[53] However, a recent comparison of L-dopa and the dopamine agonist pramipexole, showed that the agonist impaired executive functions, verbal fluency and memory performance.[54]

Clinical presentation

The most common complaints from PD patients include a decline or change in the ability to organize and complete activities both at home and at work. This appears related to a decrease in not only organizational skills but also in attention and concentration, with increased distractibility. Reports to physicians include responses such as this recent communication from a 55-year-old female patient:

> "When I woke up at 7:45 this morning my priority was to finish making a card for a sick friend and then work on finishing my Christmas 2003 cards ... but FIRST I needed to get my shower and get dressed. Before I got out of bed though I wanted to go through a pile of catalogs and yesterday's mail. At 9:30 I was interrupted by a phone call for information that made me come downstairs. And I never went back up to get ready for the day."

The selective cognitive impairments that affect most patients have the greatest impact on social and occupational functioning. Patient interviews indicate that these difficulties are significant and quality-of-life studies find a direct association between poorer cognitive function and compromised life quality.[55-58] Indirect evidence for the link between cognition and social function comes from several treatment outcome studies following levodopa, pallidotomy, and implants, where improvements in cognition and social functioning are reported.[59-62] The impact of cognitive dysfunction on occupational functioning obviously varies with the demands of specific jobs, but can be significant. Patients often complain of being unable to organize and plan their workday. This includes difficulty structuring tasks into consistent components, sequencing these tasks, maintaining sustained focus, and completing tasks on time. Difficulties even extend to maintaining order in their workspace.

Assessment, management and treatment of cognitive impairments in PD

Management and treatment of cognitive dysfunction in PD requires a multi-faceted approach. Patient and family education are crucial. Patients often are not told that cognitive impairment can be a part of their disease. Patients are generally relieved to learn that they are "not losing my mind" and that problems with their thinking are not unexpected. For family members as well, understanding that the cognitive capacity of their relative is compromised helps them understand behaviors and develop plans to accommodate these dysfunctions. Each patient requires individual strategies to compensate for these impairments and one important strategy is to utilize external cues which are effective for improving organizing and planning. In addition, regularizing sleep and exercise can maximize functioning.

Assessment of cognitive impairments

A thorough and targeted neuropsychological evaluation is required to quantitatively document and track the selective cognitive impairments that affect most patients. Such a targeted evaluation is outlined by Zgaljardic and colleagues and includes tests which are related to the integrity of each of the three cortico-striatal loops important for cognition.[7] While this would provide detailed information, for most patients ordering an extensive neuropsychological evaluation is not feasible. Instead, information regarding cognitive dysfunction is most often gathered through interviews with the patient and family members as well as the use of brief assessment measures. Most PD patients are well aware of the cognitive difficulties they are experiencing and usually report these in terms of their impact on occupational and social functioning. A brief cognitive assessment tool, developed specifically for PD from the Mini-Mental State Examination, may be useful to document and track cognitive problems.[63] The IQCODE provides a means for rating changes in cognition by family members and can also be used to track changes over time.[64,65]

Cholinesterase inhibitors

Pharmacologic treatment of cognitive impairments in PD has been focused primarily on the use of cholinesterase inhibitors in patients with dementia. A retrospective study of 160 consecutive patients treated for dementia with cholinesterase inhibitors, found that those with a diagnosis of PD dementia showed improvement in global cognitive function and global clinical assessment.[66] Two double-blind trials of donepezil have now been completed and both show improvement in cognition. The first included 16 PD patients on 5–10 mg/day for 10 weeks and found significant improvement in global cognition, with the effect being larger than that seen in AD.[67] The second, an 18 week study of donepezil (2.5–10 mg/day) including 16 PD patients with dementia or serious cognitive impairment found improvements in memory, processing speed, and attention. While not all patients were able to tolerate the medication, all adverse side-effects were rapidly reversible.[68]

Rivastigmine (Exelon), a drug that inhibits both acetylcholinesterase and butyrylcholinesterase, shown to be effective in delaying cognitive decline in AD patients, appears promising for use in PD.[69] An open-label study of 12 patients showed improvement in cognition as well as neuropsychiatric complications.[70] A case series of patients with cognitive and behavioral problems showed improvement both in cognition and functional abilities as well as resolution of visual hallucinations.[71] A second open-label study of rivastigmine in 28 PD patients with mild to moderate dementia (13–25 MMSE) treated for 26 weeks found significant improvements in attention, concentration, memory, and word-finding, with no worsening of motor symptoms.[72]

There have also been recent studies of cholinesterase inhibitors that include nicotonic activity as well as nicotine itself. This is of interest because stimulation of nicotinic receptors may assist with dopamine release. A recent study of 16 patients with galantamine, a cholinesterase inhibitor with additional nicotinic activity, found two-thirds of the patients showed an improvement in global cognitive function.[73] However, a study utilizing transdermal nicotine treatment did not find any effect on cognition.[74]

Other medications

There are other medications that have potential use in PD. These include the drug modafinil, a novel wake-promoting agent, currently used for narcolepsy, which has been shown to significantly improve performance on tests of memory, planning, and stop-inhibition.[75] A second medication, atomoxetine, a norepinephrine (noradrenaline) reuptake inhibitor, currently used for attention deficit hyperactivity disorder, may be particularly useful for improving attention and concentration, as it increases extracellular levels of both norepinephrine and dopamine.[76,77] It does, however, occasionally cause urinary retention in some elderly patients, so caution is advised.

Finally, memantine, an NMDA receptor blocker that neutralizes the effects of glutamate and has been used to treat dyskinesia in PD patients[78,79] has recently been shown to improve cognition in patients with both AD and vascular dementia.[80,81]

Cognitive rehabilitation

While there have been several studies of comprehensive, multidisciplinary rehabilitation programs for individuals with PD, none included any cognitive assessments nor interventions aimed at cognitive rehabilitation.[82,83] We have to examine studies in Alzheimer's disease to explore the potential of cognitive therapy and its potential for PD. A recent study of mildly impaired AD patients on stable doses of cholinesterase inhibitors evaluated three techniques which have been shown to enhance learning in these patients; spaced retrieval, dual cognitive support, and procedural memory training. The 12-week study compared the cognitive rehabilitation program with a program of mental stimulation and found gains in orientation, associate learning, processing speed, and functional tasks that were evident at the conclusion of the program and at 3-month follow-up.[84] While this type of program would need to be evaluated and tailored for PD patients with selective cognitive deficits, the program as outlined may be useful for PD patients, particularly because the use of explicit cues has been shown to improve performance on tests of learning in PD.[85]

In summary, Parkinson's disease (PD), a neurodegenerative disorder characterized by motor impairments including bradykinesia, cogwheel rigidity, and resting tremor, produces cognitive impairment as well. Almost all patients suffer selective cognitive impairments, including difficulties with attention, concentration, problem solving, set shifting, and memory, which are thought to reflect dysfunction of cortical circuits subserving frontal brain regions. These impairments are most often reported by patients in terms of the disabilities they cause, such as difficulties in paying attention at work, problems handling more than one project at a time, inability to sequence, plan and organize tasks at work and home, and problems completing tasks which have been started and in fact starting several at the same time without finishing any. At the present time, treatment of cognitive dysfunction relies primarily on patient and family education, behavioral interventions and the use of cholinesterase inhibitors.

References

1. Parkinson J, *An Essay on the Shaking Palsy*. Sherwood, Neely, and Jones: London, 1817.
2. Goldman WP, Baty JD, Buckles VD, Sahrmann S, Morris JC, Cognitive and motor functioning in Parkinson disease: subjects with and without questionable dementia. *Arch Neurol* 1998; 55(5):674–680.
3. Lees AJ, Smith E, Cognitive deficits in the early stages of Parkinson's disease. *Brain* 1983; 106(Pt 2):257–270.
4. Cooper JA, Sagar HJ, Jordan N, Harvey NS, Sullivan EV, Cognitive impairment in early, untreated Parkinson's disease and its relationship to motor disability. *Brain* 1991; 114(Pt 5):2095–2122.
5. Cooper JA, Sagar HJ, Doherty SM, Jordan N, Tidswell P, Sullivan EV, Different effects of dopaminergic and anticholinergic therapies on cognitive and motor function in Parkinson's disease. A follow-up study of untreated patients. *Brain* 1992; 115(Pt 6):1701–1725.
6. Levin BE, Katzen HL, Early cognitive changes and nondementing behavioral abnormalities in Parkinson's disease. *Adv Neurol* 1995; 65:85–95.
7. Zgaljardic DJ, Borod JC, Foldi NS, Mattis P, A review of the cognitive and behavioral sequelae of Parkinson's disease: relationship to frontostriatal circuitry. *Cogn Behav Neurol* 2003; 16(4):193–210.
8. Higginson CI, King DS, Levine D, Wheelock VL, Khamphay NO, Sigvardt KA, The relationship between executive function and verbal memory in Parkinson's disease. *Brain Cogn* 2003; 52(3):343–352.
9. Green J, McDonald WM, Vitek JL et al, Cognitive impairments in advanced PD without dementia. *Neurology* 2002; 59(9):1320–1324.
10. Owen AM, Iddon JL, Hodges JR, Summers BA, Robbins TW, Spatial and non-spatial working memory at different stages of Parkinson's disease. *Neuropsychologia* 1997; 35(4):519–532.
11. Farina E, Cappa SF, Polimeni M et al, Frontal dysfunction in early Parkinson's disease. *Acta Neurol Scand* 1994; 90(1):34–38.
12. Ogden JA, Growdon JH, Corkin S, Deficits on visuospatial tests involving forward planning in high-functioning Parkinsonians. *Neuropsychiat Neuropsychol Behav Neurol* 1990; 3:125–139.
13. Morris RG, Downes JJ, Sahakian BJ, Evenden JL, Heald A, Robbins TW, Planning and spatial working memory in Parkinson's disease. *J Neurol Neurosurg Psychiatry* 1988; 51:757–766.
14. Taylor AE, Saint-Cyr JA, Lang AE, Frontal lobe dysfunction in Parkinson's disease. The cortical focus of neostriatal outflow. *Brain* 1986; 109(Pt 5):845–883.
15. Cools AR, van den Bercken JH, Horstink MW, van Spaendonck KP, Berger HJ, Cognitive and motor shifting aptitude disorder in Parkinson's disease. *J Neurol Neurosurg Psychiatry* 1984; 47(5):443–453.
16. Flowers KA, Robertson C, The effect of Parkinson's disease on the ability to maintain a mental set. *J Neurol Neurosurg Psychiatry* 1985; 48(6):517–529.
17. Gotham AM, Brown RG, Marsden CD, "Frontal" cognitive function in patients with Parkinson's disease "on" and "off" levodopa. *Brain* 1988; 111(Pt 2):299–321.
18. Sullivan EV, Sagar HJ, Gabrieli JD, Corkin S, Growdon JH, Different cognitive profiles on standard behavioral tests in Parkinson's disease and Alzheimer's disease. *J Clin Exp Neuropsychol* 1989; 11(6):799–820.
19. Locascio JJ, Corkin S, Growdon JH, Relation between clinical characteristics of Parkinson's disease and cognitive decline. *J Clin Exp Neuropsychol* 2003; 25(1): 94–109.

20. Smith MC, Goldman WP, Janer KW, Baty JD, Morris JC, Cognitive speed in non-demented Parkinson's disease. *J Int Neuropsychol Soc* 1998; **4**:584–592.

21. Berry EL, Nicolson RI, Foster JK, Behrmann M, Sagar HJ, Slowing of reaction time in Parkinson's disease: the involvement of the frontal lobes. *Neuropsychologia* 1999; **37**:787–795.

22. Azuma T, Cruz RF, Bayles KA, Tomoeda CK, Montgomery EB Jr, A longitudinal study of neuropsychological change in individuals with Parkinson's disease. *Int J Geriatr Psychiatry* 2003; **18**(11):1043–1049.

23. Janvin C, Aarsland D, Larsen JP, Hugdahl K, Neuropsychological profile of patients with Parkinson's disease without dementia. *Dement Geriatr Cogn Disord* 2003; **15**(3):126–131.

24. Kulisevsky J, Avila A, Barbanoj M, Antonijoan R, Berthier ML, Gironell A, Acute effects of levodopa on neuropsychological performance in stable and fluctuating Parkinson's disease patients at different levodopa plasma levels. *Brain* 1996; **119**(Pt 6):2121–2132.

25. Alexander GE, DeLong MR, Strick PL, Parallel organization of functionally segregated circuits linking basal ganglia and cortex. *Annu Rev Neurosci* 1986; **9**:357–381.

26. Wichmann T, DeLong MR, Functional and pathophysiological models of the basal ganglia. *Curr Opin Neurobiol* 1996; **6**(6):751–758.

27. Thiel A, Hilker R, Kessler J, Habedank B, Herholz K, Heiss WD, Activation of basal ganglia loops in idiopathic Parkinson's disease: a PET study. *J Neural Transm* 2003; **110**(11):1289–1301.

28. Lozza C, Baron JC, Eidelberg D, Mentis MJ, Carbon M, Marie RM, Executive processes in Parkinson's disease: FDG-PET and network analysis. *Hum Brain Mapp* 2004; **22**(3):236–245.

29. Werheid K, Zysset S, Muller A, Reuter M, von Cramon DY, Rule learning in a serial reaction time task: an fMRI study on patients with early Parkinson's disease. *Brain Res Cogn Brain Res* 2003; **16**(2):273–284.

30. Lewis SJ, Dove A, Robbins TW, Barker RA, Owen AM, Cognitive impairments in early Parkinson's disease are accompanied by reductions in activity in fronto-striatal neural circuitry. *J Neurosci* 2003; **23**(15):6351–6356.

31. Emre M, What causes mental dysfunction in Parkinson's disease? *Mov Disord* 2003; **18**(Suppl 6):S63–S71.

32. Camicioli R, Moore MM, Kinney A, Corbridge E, Glassberg K, Kaye JA, Parkinson's disease is associated with hippocampal atrophy. *Mov Disord* 2003; **18**(7): 784–790.

33. Riekkinen P Jr, Kejonen K, Laakso MP, Soininen H, Partanen K, Riekkinen M, Hippocampal atrophy is related to impaired memory, but not frontal functions in non-demented Parkinson's disease patients. *Neuroreport* 1998; **9**(7):1507–1511.

34. Camicioli RM, Korzan JR, Foster SL et al, Posterior cingulate metabolic changes occur in Parkinson's disease patients without dementia. *Neurosci Lett* 2004; **354**(3):177–180.

35. Vingerhoets G, van der LC, Lannoo E et al, Cognitive outcome after unilateral pallidal stimulation in Parkinson's disease. *J Neurol Neurosurg Psychiatry* 1999; **66**(3):297–304.

36. Perrine K, Dogali M, Fazzini E et al, Cognitive functioning after pallidotomy for refractory Parkinson's disease. *J Neurol Neurosurg Psychiatry* 1998; **65**(2):150–154.

37. Trepanier LL, Saint-Cyr JA, Lozano AM, Lang AE, Neuropsychological consequences of posteroventral pallidotomy for the treatment of Parkinson's disease. *Neurology* 1998; **51**(1):207–215.

38. Alegret M, Valldeoriola F, Tolosa E et al, Cognitive effects of unilateral pos-

teroventral pallidotomy: a 4-year follow-up study. *Mov Disord* 2003; **18**(3): 323–328.

39. Valldeoriola F, Martinez-Rodriguez J, Tolosa E et al, Four year follow-up study after unilateral pallidotomy in advanced Parkinson's disease. *J Neurol* 2002; **249**(12):1671–1677.

40. Funkiewiez A, Ardouin C, Caputo E et al, Long term effects of bilateral subthalamic nucleus stimulation on cognitive function, mood, and behaviour in Parkinson's disease. *J Neurol Neurosurg Psychiatry* 2004; **75**(6):834–839.

41. Morrison CE, Borod JC, Perrine K et al, Neuropsychological functioning following bilateral subthalamic nucleus stimulation in Parkinson's disease. *Arch Clin Neuropsychol* 2004; **19**(2):165–181.

42. Daniele A, Albanese A, Contarino MF et al, Cognitive and behavioural effects of chronic stimulation of the subthalamic nucleus in patients with Parkinson's disease. *J Neurol Neurosurg Psychiatry* 2003; **74**(2):175–182.

43. Gironell A, Kulisevsky J, Rami L, Fortuny N, Garcia-Sanchez C, Pascual-Sedano B, Effects of pallidotomy and bilateral subthalamic stimulation on cognitive function in Parkinson disease. A controlled comparative study. *J Neurol* 2003; **250**(8):917–923.

44. Dujardin K, Defebvre L, Krystkowiak P, Blond S, Destee A, Influence of chronic bilateral stimulation of the subthalamic nucleus on cognitive function in Parkinson's disease. *J Neurol* 2001; **248**(7):603–611.

45. Fields JA, Troster AI, Wilkinson SB, Pahwa R, Koller WC, Cognitive outcome following staged bilateral pallidal stimulation for the treatment of Parkinson's disease. *Clin Neurol Neurosurg* 1999; **101**(3):182–188.

46. Carbon M, Ghilardi MF, Feigin A et al, Learning networks in health and Parkinson's disease: reproducibility and treatment effects. *Hum Brain Mapp* 2003; **19**(3):197–211.

47. Marini P, Ramat S, Ginestroni A, Paganini M, Deficit of short-term memory in newly diagnosed untreated parkinsonian patients: reversal after L-dopa therapy. *Neurol Sci* 2003; **24**(3):184–185.

48. Nieoullon A, Coquerel A, Dopamine: a key regulator to adapt action, emotion, motivation and cognition. *Curr Opin Neurol* 2003; **16**(Suppl 2):S3–S9.

49. Grossman M, Glosser G, Kalmanson J, Morris J, Stern MB, Hurtig HI, Dopamine supports sentence comprehension in Parkinson's disease. *J Neurol Sci* 2001; **184**(2):123–130.

50. Kulisevsky J, Role of dopamine in learning and memory: implications for the treatment of cognitive dysfunction in patients with Parkinson's disease. *Drugs Aging* 2000; **16**(5):365–379.

51. Growdon JH, Kieburtz K, McDermott MP, Panisset M, Friedman JH, Levodopa improves motor function without impairing cognition in mild non-demented Parkinson's disease patients. Parkinson Study Group. *Neurology* 1998; **50**(5): 1327–1331.

52. Cools R, Barker RA, Sahakian BJ, Robbins TW, L-dopa medication remediates cognitive inflexibility, but increases impulsivity in patients with Parkinson's disease. *Neuropsychologia* 2003; **41**(11):1431–1441.

53. Marjama-Lyons JM, Koller WC, Parkinson's disease. Update in diagnosis and symptom management. *Geriatrics* 2001; **56**(8):24–30, 33.

54. Brusa L, Bassi A, Stefani A et al, Pramipexole in comparison to L-dopa: a neuropsychological study. *J Neural Transm* 2003; **110**(4):373–380.

55. Abudi S, Bar-Tal Y, Ziv L, Fish M, Parkinson's disease symptoms – patients' perceptions. *J Adv Nurs* 1997; **25**:54–59.

56. Brod M, Mendelsohn GA, Roberts B, Patient's experiences of Parkinson's disease. *J Gerontol B Psychol Sci Soc Sci* 1998; **53**:P213–P222.

57. Lee KS, Merriman A, Owen A, Chew B, Tan TC, The medical, social and functional profile of Parkinson's disease patients. *Singapore Med J* 1994; **35**:265–268.

58. Hobson P, Holden A, Meara J, Measuring the impact of Parkinson's disease with the Parkinson's Disease Quality of Life Questionnaire. *Age Ageing* 1999; **28**:341–346.

59. Baron MS, Vitek JL, Bakay RA et al, Treatment of advanced Parkinson's disease by posterior GPi pallidotomy: 1-year results of a pilot study [see comments]. *Ann Neurol* 1996; **40**(3):355–366.

60. Block G, Liss C, Reines S, Irr J, Nibbelink D, Comparison of immediate-release and controlled release carbidopa/levodopa in Parkinson's disease. A multicenter 5-year study. The CR First Study Group. *Eur Neurol* 1997; **37**(1):23–27.

61. McRae C, O'Brien C, Freed C, Quality of life among persons receiving neural implant surgery for Parkinson's disease. *Mov Disord* 1996; **11**:605–606.

62. Wilson RS, Goetz CG, Stebbins GT, Neurologic illness. In: Spilker B (ed.) *Quality of Life and Pharmacoeconomics in Clinical Trials*. Lippincott-Raven: Philadelphia, 1996; 903–908.

63. Mahieux F, Michelet D, Manifacier MJ, Boller F, Fermanian J, Guillard A, Mini-Mental Parkinson: first validation study of a new bedside test contructed for Parkinson's disease. *Behav Neurol* 1995; **8**:15–22.

64. Jorm AF, A short form of the Informant Questionnaire on Cognitive Decline in the Elderly (IQCODE): development and cross-validation. *Psychol Med* 1994; **24**(1):145–153.

65. Farias ST, Mungas D, Reed B, Haan MN, Jagust WJ, Everyday functioning in relation to cognitive functioning and neuroimaging in community-dwelling Hispanic and non-Hispanic older adults. *J Int Neuropsychol Soc* 2004; **10**(3):342–354.

66. Pakrasi S, Mukaetova-Ladinska EB, McKeith IG, O'Brien JT, Clinical predictors of response to acetyl cholinesterase inhibitors: experience from routine clinical use in Newcastle. *Int J Geriatr Psychiatry* 2003; **18**(10):879–886.

67. Aarsland D, Laake K, Larsen JP, Janvin C, Donepezil for cognitive impairment in Parkinson's disease: a randomised controlled study. *J Neurol Neurosurg Psychiatry* 2002; **72**(6):708–712.

68. Leroi I, Brandt J, Reich SG et al, Randomized placebo-controlled trial of donepezil in cognitive impairment in Parkinson's disease. *Int J Geriatr Psychiatry* 2004; **19**(1):1–8.

69. Gabelli C, Rivastigmine: an update on therapeutic efficacy in Alzheimer's disease and other conditions. *Curr Med Res Opin* 2003; **19**(2):69–82.

70. Reading PJ, Luce AK, McKeith IG, Rivastigmine in the treatment of parkinsonian psychosis and cognitive impairment: preliminary findings from an open trial. *Mov Disord* 2001; **16**(6):1171–1174.

71. Bullock R, Cameron A, Rivastigmine for the treatment of dementia and visual hallucinations associated with Parkinson's disease: a case series. *Curr Med Res Opin* 2002; **18**(5):258–264.

72. Giladi N, Shabtai H, Gurevich T, Benbunan B, Anca M, Korczyn AD, Rivastigmine (Exelon) for dementia in patients with Parkinson's disease. *Acta Neurol Scand* 2003; **108**(5):368–373.

73. Aarsland D, Hutchinson M, Larsen JP, Cognitive, psychiatric and motor response to galantamine in Parkinson's disease with dementia. *Int J Geriatr Psychiatry* 2003; **18**(10):937–941.

74. Lemay S, Chouinard S, Blanchet P et al, Lack of efficacy of a nicotine transdermal treatment on motor and cognitive deficits in Parkinson's disease. *Prog Neuro-psychopharmacol Biol Psychiatry* 2004; **28**(1):31–39.

75. Turner DC, Clark L, Dowson J, Robbins TW, Sahakian BJ, Modafinil improves

cognition and response inhibition in adult attention-deficit/hyperactivity disorder. *Biol Psychiatry* 2004; **55**(10):1031–1040.

76. Bymaster FP, Katner JS, Nelson DL et al, Atomoxetine increases extracellular levels of norepinephrine and dopamine in prefrontal cortex of rat: a potential mechanism for efficacy in attention deficit/hyperactivity disorder. *Neuropsychopharmacology* 2002; **27**(5):699–711.

77. Simpson D, Plosker GL, Spotlight on atomoxetine in adults with attention-deficit hyperactivity disorder. *CNS Drugs* 2004; **18**(6):397–401.

78. Rabey JM, Nissipeanu P, Korczyn AD, Efficacy of memantine, an NMDA receptor antagonist, in the treatment of Parkinson's disease. *J Neural Transm Park Dis Dement Sect* 1992; **4**:277–282.

79. Merello M, Nouzeilles MI, Cammarota A, Leiguarda R, Effect of memantine (NMDA antagonist) on Parkinson's disease: a double-blind crossover randomized study. *Clin Neuropharmacol* 1999; **22**(5):273–276.

80. Jarvis B, Figgitt DP, Memantine. *Drugs Aging* 2003; **20**(6):465–476.

81. Lokk J, [Memantine can relieve certain symptoms in Parkinson disease. Improvement achieved in two out of three described cases with dyskinesia and cognitive failure]. *Lakartidningen* 2004; **101**(23):2003–2006.

82. Trend P, Kaye J, Gage H, Owen C, Wade D, Short-term effectiveness of intensive multidisciplinary rehabilitation for people with Parkinson's disease and their carers. *Clin Rehabil* 2002; **16**(7):717–725.

83. Wade DT, Gage H, Owen C, Trend P, Grossmith C, Kaye J, Multidisciplinary rehabilitation for people with Parkinson's disease: a randomised controlled study. *J Neurol Neurosurg Psychiatry* 2003; **74**(2):158–162.

84. Loewenstein DA, Acevedo A, Czaja SJ, Duara R, Cognitive rehabilitation of mildly impaired Alzheimer disease patients on cholinesterase inhibitors. *Am J Geriatr Psychiatry* 2004; **12**(4):395–402.

85. van Spaendonck KP, Berger HJ, Horstink MW, Borm GF, Cools AR, Memory performance under varying cueing conditions in patients with Parkinson's disease. *Neuropsychologia* 1996; **34**(12):1159–1164.

chapter 6

Dementia

Alexander I Tröster and Daniel I Kaufer

Introduction

Because Parkinson's disease (PD) is an extrapyramidal motor disorder, leading to rigidity, bradykinesia, tremor, and postural instability, the bulk of research on PD has focused on the movement disorder. Accompanying the increasing recognition that PD often involves a compromise of non-motor functions (such as cognition, affect, and sleep),[1] is research showing that non-motor dysfunction seriously detracts from patient and caregiver quality of life[2–4] and increases complexity and cost of treatment.[5] Consequently, there is great interest in understanding the mechanisms underlying the cognitive deficits and how such deficits might be detected and treated early.

After providing a definition of dementia, this chapter provides an overview of the epidemiology of dementia in PD, describes its cognitive clinical presentation, followed by diagnostic, assessment, and treatment issues. Though drawing heavily on empirical research for its conclusions, the chapter attends to broad clinical issues and its bibliography emphasizes recent reviews useful also to the non-specialist. The chapter only briefly mentions cognitive impairments in early PD and distinguishing Parkinson's disease with dementia (PDD) and dementia with Lewy bodies (DLB) because these areas are covered in Chapters 5 and 7, respectively.

Definition and detection of dementia

The term dementia has, for many persons, connotations of Alzheimer's disease (AD), rapid disease progression, irreversibility, and perhaps even death. However, the term is a general one that, in the absence of a known etiology, does not yield prognoses about progression or treatment response. This point, though obvious to the clinician, is frequently not obvious to the patient and bears emphasis when patients and family (or clinicians) initially voice concerns about a possible dementia. Early education is likely to reduce patient and family fears (and possibly ensuing avoidance of care) and enhance patient–physician collaboration in planning a systematic work-up and treatment plan.

The most recent Diagnostic and Statistical Manual of Mental Disorders (DSM-IV-TR)[6] defines dementia as an impairment of memory and at least one among aphasia, executive dysfunction, apraxia, and agnosia, sufficiently severe to interfere with occupational or social functioning. Diagnostic criteria for dementia due to PD, classified under Dementia Due to Other General Medical Conditions (Table 6.1), need to be applied cautiously given

---

Table 6.1 Diagnostic and statistical manual of mental disorders (DSM) criteria for the diagnosis of dementia in Parkinson's disease

1. Memory impairment
2. Impairment in one or more of
   a. Language
   b. Praxis (i.e., difficulty carrying out motor acts in the absence of motor impairment)
   c. Executive functions such as planning, abstraction, conceptualization, reasoning
   d. Gnosis (i.e., identification of objects or persons despite intact sensory functions)
3. "Each" of the cognitive impairments reflects a decline from a once higher level of functioning and is severe enough to impair occupational and/or social functioning
4. The cognitive impairments do not occur only during episodes of delirium (change in consciousness and cognition over a brief period of time)
5. There is evidence from laboratory and other diagnostic tests or the history that the dementia is a direct biological consequence of Parkinson's disease

Adapted from reference 6.

numerous concerns about these criteria. Specifically, in practice it is difficult to determine the extent to which functional (social or occupational) impairment in PD reflects motor disability as opposed to cognitive deficits. For this reason a careful interview of patients and those familiar with patients' functioning and symptom course is necessary. Questions about the following may be helpful in deciding whether occupational and social changes are related to dementia or another factor:

- reasons for poor occupational performance

    - was performance on tasks with motor demands (e.g., word processing, handwriting) slow? This might be suggestive of motor rather than cognitive dysfunction underlying poor performance
    - did the patient have new difficulty planning or sequencing activities, or with self-direction and goal prioritization such that deadlines were not met? This would be more suggestive of cognitive dysfunction

- reasons for social changes

    - is the patient less socially active because of embarrassment about motor signs (e.g., tremor, dyskinesias, spilling food?) or communication difficulty related to voice changes (e.g., hypophonia and dysarthria?)
    - is withdrawal preceded by a change in mood and affect, suggesting possible depression?
    - does the patient have unpredictable motor or non-motor fluctuations that might be associated with anxiety or panic, causing them to withdraw?
    - has the patient withdrawn from social interactions due to difficulty following conversations and remembering people's names?
    - is the patient less able to carry out hobbies and do-it-yourself tasks due to difficulty conceptualizing and understanding the steps involved rather than motor manipulation of objects?

Because motor symptoms are prone to disrupt performance of physical activities of daily living (i.e., those functions permitting independence within one's home, such as dressing, toileting), while cognitive symptoms are more likely to impact completion of instrumental activities of daily living (i.e., functions allowing independence within the community, such as housekeeping, financial and medication management),[7] patients should be questioned closely about the types of day-to-day activities for which they require assistance or have difficulty. Such questioning is also important because the decline in day-to-day functioning attributable to cognitive change (as required by DSM) may go unnoticed or be misattributed when persons have retired or when differential occupational and social performance expectations are held on the basis of age, gender, or co-morbid medical conditions.

The required presence of memory impairment for dementia diagnosis is also problematic given that disturbances in other areas of cognition often precede memory impairment in PDD. Furthermore, it is unclear whether the memory impairment must be primary or can be secondary to, for example, executive or attentional dysfunction. The concerns about whether memory and other functions are impaired are best addressed by formal neuropsychological evaluation (described later in more detail).

Nonetheless, given the fact that memory may not be impaired in PDD, Cummings and Benson[8] proposed alternate, less restrictive criteria for dementia. These criteria define dementia as an acquired, persistent impairment in at least three of five domains: (1) language, (2) memory, (3) complex cognition (executive functions), (4) visuospatial functions, and (5) personality or emotion. Occupational and social functioning need *not* be affected. However, the sensitivity, specificity, and validity of the DSM and Cummings and Benson criteria in diagnosing dementia in PD remain to be compared.

Epidemiology of dementia in Parkinson's disease

Dementia is rarely present early in PD and a dementia preceding or accompanying early motor symptoms should raise concern that cognitive symptoms might be better explained by Alzheimer's disease, diffuse Lewy body disease, depression, or iatrogenic factors. Indeed, recent consensus criteria[9] proposed that the clinical diagnostic term "PD with dementia" refer to the condition of individuals with a clinical diagnosis of PD who have had motor symptoms for 12 months or longer before developing cognitive and neuropsychiatric symptoms. Although dementia is not a typical feature of early PD, many individuals with PD will have mild cognitive changes characterized by one or more of the following: slowness of thought, inefficient learning and recall, diminished working memory, mild executive dysfunction, and mood disturbance.[10,11] Lieberman's[12] review revealed that an average of 19% of treated and untreated PD patients have *mild* cognitive dysfunction not meeting criteria for dementia. However, a recent study of a population-representative sample in the UK revealed that almost 40% of persons have cognitive impairments (especially of working memory and executive functions) detectable on neuropsychological testing at the time of disease diagnosis.[13]

Dementia prevalence (cases existing at a given time in the population of PD patients) varies from 8% to 93%, depending upon diagnostic criteria, sampling, and case ascertainment methods used, but the most commonly accepted proportions fall between 20% and 40%.[14] Because dementia increases risk of mortality, incidence (or the number of new cases per year in the population of interest) may be a more accurate "barometer" of dementia frequency. Dementia incidence is about 3% per year for persons with PD younger than 60 years and 15% or less for persons older than 80 years.[15-17] Several demographic and disease features, along with patterns of cognitive impairment, are risk factors for dementia in Parkinson's disease (see Table 6.2).

Clinical presentation and assessment

Neurobehavioral profile of dementia in Parkinson's disease

Cummings'[18] categorization of dementia as "cortical" and "subcortical" on the basis of neurobehavioral features has been criticized because most patients with dementia eventually evidence both cortical and subcortical pathology. Furthermore, there is heterogeneity in the cognitive profiles

Table 6.2 Risk factors for dementia in Parkinson's disease

Demographic variables	*Disease variables*	*Neurobehavioral variables*
Greater age	Later onset	Depression
Lower education	Disease duration	Diminished cognitive test
Lower socioeconomic status	Disease severity	performance:
Family history of Parkinson's	Susceptibility to levodopa-	(a) executive/attention
dementia	induced psychosis or	(b) verbal fluency
	confusion	(c) visuoperceptual
		(d) list learning

Adapted from reference 71.

among parkinsonians with mild cognitive impairments or dementia, with many persons demonstrating executive dysfunction, but others demonstrating memory problems or a combination thereof.[13] Even the qualitative nature of memory problems may differ among patients, with some showing deficits reminiscent of AD, and yet others showing those seen in subcortical dementias associated with, for example, progressive supranuclear palsy or Huntington's disease.[19] Despite the heterogeneity of the cognitive profile of dementia in PD (perhaps reflecting variability in neuropathological findings), at the group level, the neuropsychological deficits evident in PDD resemble those of the "subcortical" dementias. Perhaps the most striking features of the "subcortical" dementias, including PDD, are:[20]

- bradyphrenia (mental slowing)
- memory retrieval deficits (poor recall with relatively good performance on recognition testing)
- executive dysfunction
- diminished spontaneity
- depression.

Features of the "cortical" dementias such as Alzheimer's disease (e.g., aphasia, agnosia, and apraxia) are typically absent in PDD, sometimes even later in the course of dementia.

Attention and executive functions
Performance on complex attentional tasks requiring the self-allocation of attentional resources, divided attention, or selective attention, is impaired in PDD. As the disease progresses, patients with PDD may show difficulty even on those attentional tasks in which external cues are provided.[21,22]

Executive deficits are most readily observed on tasks that require patients to spontaneously or independently develop, initiate, and maintain efficient information-processing strategies. Difficulties performing tasks requiring coordination of complex mental and motor functions (e.g., operation of an automobile) may be related to defective execution of strategies to accomplish a task (e.g., turning a corner while driving).[23]

Language
Persons with PD often have motor speech abnormalities, but are not frankly aphasic. Nonetheless, some language changes do occur[24] and patients'

complaints of slowed and inefficient word production are probably not simply manifestations of motor speech problems. Instead, diminished performance on verbal fluency tasks requiring oral generation of words beginning with a given letter of the alphabet or belonging to a semantic category, such as items obtainable in a supermarket, probably reflect inefficient word retrieval strategies.[25-27] Impairment in visual confrontation naming, most often measured by the Boston Naming Test, is less pronounced in PDD than in Alzheimer's disease, if present at all,[28] and develops later in the course of the dementia.[29] Comprehension is grossly intact, though subtle impairments, perhaps secondary to strategic, attentional, and information-processing speed deficits, may be detected in syntactic comprehension on rigorous testing.[30] More recently it has been reported that patients with PD may show diminished conversational appropriateness, turn taking, and prosody.[31]

Memory
The memory deficit in early PDD is typically characterized by deficits in retrieval, rather than consolidation, meaning that patients with early PDD are able to retain information over time, but show deficits in retrieving information on free recall. However, unlike patients with Alzheimer's disease (AD), recall in PDD patients is typically aided by cues or recognition testing. As the dementia progresses, memory deficits include deficient encoding and consolidation that may be comparable to those of patients with AD.[32] While remote memory (recall of distant information) is typically preserved early on, deficits emerge as the dementia progresses.[33] However, the remote memory impairment is milder in PDD than AD, and in contrast to AD, in which the most remote memories are relatively preserved, PDD affects recall of information from the various decades of a patient's life to a similar extent.[34]

Visuoperceptual functions
Impaired visuospatial and visuoconstructive functions have been found consistently in PDD even when tasks minimize or eliminate motor demands.[35] Comparisons of the visuoperceptual deficits of PDD and AD are inconclusive, but DLB involves more prominent visuoconstructional and visuospatial disturbances than AD.[36]

Affect and emotion
Depression is common in PD, occurring in about 50% of patients. Though a meta-analysis reported a prevalence of 42% in studies using DSM,[37] the rate

is higher in research than community settings (about 50% vs 10%).[38] From the standpoint of dementia, depression is important because it exacerbates cognitive dysfunction in PD,[39] yet is poorly recognized by clinicians.[40] Okun and Watts[41] noted that depressed PD patients may spontaneously complain only of fatigue and low energy, and cautioned that such complaints should trigger a detailed interview about stressors and other possible symptoms of depression. The masked facies of PD (hypomimia) can easily be misconstrued as a depressed affect, necessitating specific inquiry into vegetative signs (e.g. insomnia, anorexia) and symptoms (e.g. sadness, crying, etc.) associated with depression.

Because depression in PD often co-occurs with other non-motor symptoms such as sleep disturbance, fatigue, anxiety, and sensory symptoms, the presence of any non-motor symptom should trigger questioning about other non-motor symptoms.[42] From a cognitive standpoint, it is especially important to inquire about anxiety, which is common in PD[43] and can exacerbate cognitive impairment,[44] and REM sleep behavior disorder, which is associated with dementia.[45]

Neurobehavioral evaluation

Given the high prevalence of cognitive changes in PD, every patient would ideally receive a baseline evaluation when first diagnosed with PD to facilitate the accurate detection and diagnosis of subsequent neurobehavioral changes and evaluation of treatment effects. In reality, this rarely occurs, probably primarily due to cost-effectiveness issues and the reluctance of many patients, and some physicians, to contemplate the threat of later, possibly significant, cognitive compromise. If a full neuropsychological evaluation is not indicated or cannot be achieved soon after diagnosis, screening should be carried out.

Cognitive screening

Screening examination's advantages include their brevity, simplicity of administration and scoring, patient acceptability, and limited expense. Such screening can be helpful in deciding whether a patient might require full neuropsychological evaluation. Possible disadvantages include the limited yield of information, use of cutoff scores that are not corrected for demographics and base rates, and limited sensitivity and specificity. Two commonly used screening instruments are the Mini Mental State Exam (MMSE)[46] and the Dementia Rating Scale (DRS).[47] Because the

MMSE does not readily capture deficits in working memory and executive functions, it might lack sensitivity to cognitive changes in PD. Indeed, a study comparing PD patients with and without mild cognitive impairment (defined by a neuropsychological test battery) found that the score of the mildly impaired group was only 1.5 points lower than that of the intact group, and in the normal range (mean 28.0).[48] Nonetheless, the MMSE probably has adequate sensitivity and specificity among patients with PD and unequivocal dementia (per DSM), as suggested by a study of 126 patients with PD that found a MMSE score cutoff for dementia of 23 or lower to have 98% sensitivity and 77% specificity.[49] Although the overall sensitivity and specificity of the DRS for detecting cognitive impairment in PD has not been reported, DRS subscale scores may help discriminate PDD and AD. For example, PDD is associated with lower initiation/perseveration and construction scores, but higher memory scores than AD.[50–52]

Neuropsychological evaluation

The components and length of a neuropsychological evaluation vary across clinical settings, but typically include:

- a clinical interview and review of records
- informal observations regarding patient behavior, cognition, and affect
- the administration of psychometric tests to measure intelligence, attention and executive functions, language, learning and memory, visuospatial perception, praxis, motor and sensory perception, mood state, quality of life, and personality/coping variables (Table 6.3 lists a sample of tests and the domains of functioning they evaluate)
- an integration of findings and recommendations into oral and/or written feedback that is provided to the patient, family, and healthcare providers.

A neuropsychological evaluation delineates the nature and extent of cognitive changes and provides a profile of relative neuropsychological strengths and weaknesses. Such knowledge is helpful in:

- determining the most probable etiology of cognitive changes
- developing and selecting strategies or treatments to limit the impact of cognitive deficits on functioning
- decision-making about the appropriateness and effectiveness of medical and neurosurgical interventions for a patient

Table 6.3 Commonly used neuropsychological tests by cognitive domain assessed

Cognitive domain	Test
Premorbid estimates	Barona Demographic Equations; North American Adult Reading Test (NAART); Wechsler Test of Adult Reading (WTAR); Wide Range Achievement Test (WRAT)
Neuropsychological screening	Mattis Dementia Rating Scale (DRS); Repeatable Battery for the Assessment of Neuropsychological Status (RBANS)
Intelligence	Kaufman Brief Intelligence Test (KBIT); Raven's Progressive Matrices; Wechsler Abbreviated Scale of Intelligence (WASI); Wechsler Adult Intelligence Scale (WAIS)
Attention and working memory	Auditory Consonant Trigrams (ACT); Brief Test of Attention (BTA); Continuous Performance Tests (CPT); Digit and Visual Spans; Paced Auditory Serial Addition Test (PASAT); Stroop Test[a]
Executive function	Cognitive Estimation Test (CET); Delis-Kaplan Executive Function Scale (DKEFS); Halstead Category Test; Trailmaking Test (TMT)[a]; Wisconsin Card Sorting Test (WCST);
Memory	Benton Visual Retention Test (BVRT-R); California Verbal Learning Test (CVLT); Rey Auditory Verbal Learning Test (RAVLT); Rey Complex Figure Test (RCFT)[a]; Wechsler Memory Scale (WMS)[a]
Language	Boston Naming Test (BNT); Controlled Oral Word Association Test (COWAT); Sentence Repetition; Token Test; Complex Ideational Material
Visuoperception	Benton Facial Recognition Test; Benton Judgment of Line Orientation (JLO); Hooper Visual Organization Test (VOT);
Motor and sensory perception	Finger Tapping[a]; Grooved Pegboard[a]; Hand Dynamometer[a]; Sensory-Perceptual Examination
Mood state and personality	Beck Anxiety Inventory (BAI); Beck Depression Inventory (BDI); Hamilton Depression Scale (HDS); Minnesota Multiphasic Personality Inventory (MMPI); Profile of Mood States (POMS); State-Trait Anxiety Inventory (STAI)
Quality of life, coping and stressors	Parkinson's Disease Questionnaire (PDQ); Coping Responses Inventory (CRI); Ways of Coping Questionnaire; Life Stressors and Social Resources Inventory (LISRES)

[a] Note: Tests may not be appropriate for patients with marked motor impairment.
Adapted from reference 72.

- guiding the patient and family in making and requesting adaptive changes in the patient's home, leisure, and work environments that enhance functioning and minimize handicap
- assessment of competence to consent to treatment[53]
- financial, legal, and placement planning.

A comprehensive neuropsychological evaluation that supplements screening should be strongly considered when:

- one suspects changes in the patient's ability to carry out activities of living that are unlikely to be related to motor signs
- there is concern about an evolving dementia
- the clinician suspects that screening tests are unlikely to be sufficiently sensitive
- a patient experiences occupational difficulties unrelated to motor symptoms and signs
- issues and questions arise regarding a person's competence
- the patient experiences emotional changes and/or is withdrawing from social roles
- a patient has experienced delirium or hallucinosis, given that such phenomena may be harbingers of dementia.

Prior to making a referral for neuropsychological evaluation, it is important to determine whether neuropsychological evaluation is appropriate to address the specific question the clinician or patient might have. This can be achieved by calling a neuropsychologist prior to making a referral. Of equal importance is that the referring clinician carefully articulates the referral question, which allows the neuropsychologist to tailor evaluative procedures accordingly, and that the neuropsychologist communicate findings (and their possible implications) to the referring clinician, patient, and family clearly while specifically addressing the referral question. It is very helpful to communicate to the neuropsychologist, at the time of referral, an estimate of the patient's disease severity (e.g., a Hoehn and Yahr stage) and any circumstances that need to be considered in planning a successful evaluation (e.g., existence of motor fluctuations or dyskinesias, times of optimal medication effect, any additional sensory or motor limitations, medications with potential cognitive side effects, co-morbidities). A general referral question (e.g., "organic vs functional?") will often yield a general report rather than one addressing practical and important issues. Given the detrimental impact of anticholinergic medications on memory and executive functions, especially in the elderly and those with cognitive compromise, if medically feasible, such medications should be tapered and withdrawn prior to neuropsychological evaluation.

Differential diagnosis

Dementia is a feature of many extrapyramidal disorders and forms of parkinsonism, and it is important to exclude those conditions. Table 6.4 lists conditions that produce parkinsonism and dementia, and some of their distinguishing features.

In addition to neuropsychological evaluation, several laboratory and clinical studies can be helpful in differential diagnosis. Structural imaging techniques (computed tomography (CT) and magnetic resonance imaging (MRI)) are useful in the evaluation and differential diagnosis of dementing disorders.[54] The diagnoses of vascular parkinsonism and normal-pressure hydrocephalus both rely on correlating the clinical syndrome with relevant lesions on CT or MRI imaging studies. Laboratory tests routinely obtained in a dementia work-up (vitamin B_{12}, thyroid stimulating hormone (TSH), and folate) should also be obtained when dealing with possible PDD as these may reveal that the cognitive deficits are potentially treatable or reversible. Historical information raising the possibility of a toxic heavy metal exposure (e.g. manganese) should prompt a 24-hour urine heavy metal screen. A strong family history of dementia may warrant genetic investigations in selected cases (for example, apolipoprotein E).

In addition to excluding other neurodegenerative and non-degenerative causes of parkinsonism and dementia, it is essential that possible iatrogenic causes of cognitive impairment be reviewed. In addition to reviewing patient medications, patients should be questioned about possible neurosurgical interventions they might have had for PD, as both types of therapy can have adverse cognitive effects.[55]

Treatment

Pharmacological

As noted, numerous medications and medical conditions can produce cognitive impairment. A first step in treating dementia, prior to adding any new medications, is to taper and withdraw any medications capable of causing

Table 6.4 Classification and salient features of parkinsonian dementia syndromes

Etiology	Distinguishing features
Degenerative (sporadic)	
Parkinson's disease with dementia (PDD)	Motor signs initially, later onset of dementia
Dementia with Lewy bodies (DLB)	Recurrent visual hallucinations; mental fluctuations
Progressive supranuclear palsy (PSP)	Early balance and bulbar deficits; down-gaze palsy
Corticobasal ganglionic degeneration (CBD)	Asymmetric limb signs (apraxia, myoclonus)
Multisystem atrophy (MSA):	"Parkinson-plus" syndromes
Olivopontocerebellar atrophy (OPCA)	Brainstem/cerebellar atrophy; ocular dismotility
Striatonigral degeneration (SND)	Pyramidal tract signs; laryngeal stridor
Shy–Drager syndrome	Marked orthostatic hypotension and dysautonomia
Degenerative (familial)	
Wilson's disease	Autosomal recessive; early-onset; impaired copper clearance
Hallevorden–Spatz disease	Autosomal recessive; early-onset; subcortical iron deposits
Idiopathic basal ganglia calcification (IBGC)	Autosomal dominant and recessive; subcortical calcium deposits
Machado–Joseph disease (cerebellar degeneration)	Autosomal dominant; ataxia and dysarthria; cerebellar atrophy
Progressive subcortical gliosis (PSG)	Autosomal dominant; white matter gliosis; frontal atrophy
Huntington's disease (HD)	Autosomal dominant; early-onset and end-stage parkinsonism
Neuroacanthocytosis	Autosomal dominant; HD-mimic; acanthocytic RBCs
Familial frontotemporal dementia (F-FTD)	Autosomal dominant; chromosome 17-linked; frontal atrophy

continued

Table 6.4 continued

Etiology	Distinguishing features
Miscellaneous	
Drug-induced encephalopathy/ parkinsonism	Relevant drug exposure (neuroleptic, anti-emetic)
Vascular parkinsonism	Multiple subcortical infarcts; may mimic PSP
Normal pressure hydrocephalus (NPH)	Prominent gait disturbance; urinary incontinence
Whipple's disease	May mimic PSP; GI symptoms prominent
Dementia pugilistica	Repetitive head trauma; cavum septum pellucidum

cognitive impairment.[56] If one is uncertain about the suspected medication's role in cognitive impairment, a brief neuropsychological evaluation can be obtained prior to tapering or withdrawing the medication(s), and then repeated after withdrawal. Similarly, if there is concern that cognitive impairment has been precipitated by deep brain stimulation (DBS) or an interaction of DBS and medication, referral to a neurologist with specific expertise in DBS is indicated. This specialist may then seek objective neuropsychological evaluation or screening while adjusting stimulation and medication parameters. If depression is suspected as causative, it is crucial to obtain neuropsychological evaluation before and after treatment with anti-depressants or psychotherapy. A single neuropsychological evaluation is less likely to differentiate dementia due to PD vs severe depression because the cognitive profiles associated with these two conditions overlap.

While cholinesterase inhibitors are widely used in the treatment of AD, they were initially used cautiously in PDD and DLB because they might exacerbate motor symptoms.[57] Recent studies, however, suggest that cholinesterase inhibitors, such as donepezil, rivastigmine, and galantamine can be safely used to ameliorate the neuropsychiatric and, to a lesser extent, the cognitive symptoms in PDD and DLB.[58-64] A recent study of more than 500 PDD patients after 24-week treatment with 3 to 12 mg rivastigmine, yielded modest benefit relative to placebo on the ADASCog measure. While improvement was observed in clinicians' global impression of change in almost 20% of rivastigmine-treated and 15% of placebo-treated persons, worsening was observed in about 13% of rivastigmine-treated and 23% of placebo-treated persons. Common side effects included nausea and vomiting, and tremor was observed in about 10% of the rivastigmine-treated group.[65]

Behavioral

Behavioral interventions have been and are being developed to reduce disruptive behaviors and the impact of cognitive deficits in dementia,[65-70] but such interventions have not been empirically evaluated specifically for PDD.

Conclusions and future directions

Many of the diagnostic criteria, diagnostic tools, therapies and interventions for dementia were developed for the prototypical "cortical" dementia, namely Alzheimer's disease (AD). Perhaps because of the lagging realization and appreciation of the widespread prevalence of cognitive impairment and dementia in PD, limited attention was paid to this facet of the movement disorder. Consequently, clinicians and researchers are often left to apply and extend the tools designed for AD to PDD. That this simplistic extension of tools to PDD has met with mixed success is hardly surprising, given that the dementia of PDD is of the "subcortical" type. This chapter has described succinctly some of the issues in the definition, detection, and treatment of PDD, and provided some practical recommendations. One hopes that a future edition of this work will allow a divulging of knowledge that is far more specific to PDD, a notion that belies the assumption that PDD is a distinct dementia. Before this hope can be realized, however, a significant challenge will have to be met. Specifically, one might more accurately refer to the "dementias" rather than the "dementia" of PD because PDD is clinically and neuropathologically heterogeneous, and, as the next chapter shows, differentiating among these dementias is complex and controversial. Only once we better understand the neurobiology and clinical manifestations of the dementias of PDD will it become clear whether PDD is a distinct condition requiring its own diagnostic criteria, tools, and therapies.

References

1. Marsh L, Neuropsychiatric aspects of Parkinson's disease. *Psychosomatics* 2000; **41**(1):15–23.
2. Karlsen KH, Larsen JP, Tandberg E, Maeland JG, Influence of clinical and demographic variables on quality of life in patients with Parkinson's disease. *J Neurol Neurosurg Psychiatry* 1999; **66**(4):431–435.

3. Schrag A, Jahanshahi M, Quinn N, What contributes to quality of life in patients with Parkinson's disease? *J Neurol Neurosurg Psychiatry* 2000; **69**(3):308–312.

4. Aarsland D, Larsen JP, Karlsen K, Lim NG, Tandberg E, Mental symptoms in Parkinson's disease are important contributors to caregiver distress. *Int J Geriatr Psychiatry* 1999; **14**(10):866–874.

5. Rubenstein LM, DeLeo A, Chrischilles EA, Economic and health-related quality of life considerations of new therapies in Parkinson's disease. *Pharmacoeconomics* 2001; **19**(7):729–752.

6. American Psychiatric Association, *Diagnostic and Statistical Manual of Mental Disorders*, Fourth Edition, Text Revision (DSM-IV-TR). American Psychiatric Association; Washington, DC, 2000.

7. Cahn DA, Sullivan EV, Shear PK, Pfefferbaum A, Heit G, Silverberg G, Differential contributions of cognitive and motor component processes to physical and instrumental activities of daily living in Parkinson's disease. *Arch Clin Neuropsychology* 1998; **13**:575–583.

8. Cummings JL, Benson DF, *Dementia: A Clinical Approach*, 2nd edn. Butterworth-Heinemann: Boston, MA, 1992.

9. McKeith IG, Galasko D, Kosaka K et al, Consensus guidelines for the clinical and pathologic diagnosis of dementia with Lewy bodies (DLB): report of the consortium on DLB international workshop. *Neurology* 1996; **47**(5):1113–1124.

10. Bondi MW, Tröster AI, Parkinson's disease: neurobehavioral consequences of basal ganglia dysfunction. In: Nussbaum PD (ed.) *Handbook of Neuropsychology and Aging*. Plenum: New York, 1997; 216–245.

11. Pillon B, Boller F, Levy R, Dubois B, Cognitive deficits and dementia in Parkinson's disease. In: Boller F, Cappa SF (eds) *Handbook of Neuropsychology*, 2nd edn. Elsevier: Amsterdam, 2001; 311–371.

12. Lieberman A, Managing the neuropsychiatric symptoms of Parkinson's disease. *Neurology* 1998; **50**(Suppl. 6):S33–S38.

13. Foltynie T, Brayne CE, Robbins TW, Barker RA, The cognitive ability of an incident cohort of Parkinson's patients in the UK. The CamPaIGN study. *Brain* 2004; **127**(Pt 3):550–560.

14. Mohr E, Mendis T, Grimes JD, Late cognitive changes in Parkinson's disease with an emphasis on dementia. *Adv Neurol* 1995; **65**:97–113.

15. Biggins CA, Boyd JL, Harrop FM et al, A controlled, longitudinal study of dementia in Parkinson's disease. *J Neurol Neurosurg Psychiatry* 1992; **55**(7):566–571.

16. Marder K, Tang MX, Cote L, Stern Y, Mayeux R, The frequency and associated risk factors for dementia in patients with Parkinson's disease. *Arch Neurol* 1995; **52**(7):695–701.

17. Mayeux R, Chen J, Mirabello E et al, An estimate of the incidence of dementia in idiopathic Parkinson's disease. *Neurology* 1990; **40**(10):1513–1517.

18. Cummings JL, Subcortical dementia. Neuropsychology, neuropsychiatry, and pathophysiology. *Br J Psychiatry* 1986; **149**:682–697.

19. Filoteo JV, Rilling LM, Cole B, Williams BJ, Davis JD, Roberts JW, Variable memory profiles in Parkinson's disease. *J Clin Exp Neuropsychol* 1997; **19**(6):878–888.

20. Kaufer DI, DeKosky ST, Diagnostic classifications: relationship to the neurobiology of dementias. In: Charney DS, Nestor JE (eds) *Neurobiology of Mental Illness*, 2nd edn. Oxford University Press: New York, 2004; 771–782.

21. Brown RG, Marsden CD, Internal versus external cues and the control of attention in Parkinson's disease. *Brain* 1988; **111**(Pt 2):323–345.

22. Wright MJ, Burns RJ, Geffen GM, Geffen LB, Covert orientation of visual attention

in Parkinson's disease: an impairment in the maintenance of attention. *Neuropsychologia* 1990; **28**(2):151–159.

23. Marsden CD, The mysterious motor function of the basal ganglia: the Robert Wartenberg Lecture. *Neurology* 1982; **32**(5):514–539.

24. Lewis FM, Lapointe LL, Murdoch BE, Language impairment in Parkinson's disease. *Aphasiology* 1998; **12**:193–206.

25. Randolph C, Braun AR, Goldberg TE, Chase TN, Semantic fluency in Alzheimer's, Parkinson's, and Huntington's disease: dissociation of storage and retrieval failures. *Neuropsychology* 1993; **7**(1):82–88.

26. Tröster AI, Fields JA, Testa JA et al, Cortical and subcortical influences on clustering and switching in the performance of verbal fluency tasks. *Neuropsychologia* 1998; **36**(4):295–304.

27. Troyer AK, Moscovitch M, Winocur G, Leach L, Freedman M, Clustering and switching on verbal fluency tests in Alzheimer's and Parkinson's disease. *J Int Neuropsychol Soc* 1998; **4**(2):137–143.

28. Tröster AI, Fields JA, Paolo AM, Pahwa R, Koller WC, Visual confrontation naming in Alzheimer's disease and Parkinson's disease with dementia [abstract]. *Neurology* 1996; **46**(Suppl):A292–A293.

29. Stern Y, Tang MX, Jacobs DM et al, Prospective comparative study of the evolution of probable Alzheimer's disease and Parkinson's disease dementia. *J Int Neuropsychol Soc* 1998; **4**(3):279–284.

30. Grossman M, Zurif E, Lee C et al, Information processing speed and sentence comprehension in Parkinson's disease. *Neuropsychology* 2002; **16**(2):174–181.

31. McNamara P, Durso R, Pragmatic communication skills in patients with Parkinson's disease. *Brain Lang* 2003; **84**(3):414–423.

32. Stern Y, Richards M, Sano M, Mayeux R, Comparison of cognitive changes in patients with Alzheimer's and Parkinson's disease. *Arch Neurol* 1993; **50**(10):1040–1045.

33. Huber SJ, Shuttleworth EC, Paulson GW, Dementia in Parkinson's disease. *Arch Neurol* 1986; **43**(10):987–990.

34. Paul RH, Graber JR, Bowlby DC, Testa JA, Harnish MJ, Beatty WW, Remote memory in neurodegenerative disease. In: Tröster AI (ed.) *Memory in Neurodegenerative Disease: Biological, Cognitive, and Clinical Perspectives.* Cambridge University Press: Cambridge, 1998; 184–196.

35. Huber SJ, Freidenberg DL, Shuttleworth EC, Paulson GW, Christy JA, Neuropsychological impairments associated with severity of Parkinson's disease. *J Neuropsychiat Clin Neurosci* 1989; **1**(2):154–158.

36. Walker Z, Allen RL, Shergill S, Katona CL, Neuropsychological performance in Lewy body dementia and Alzheimer's disease. *Br J Psychiatry* 1997; **170**:156–158.

37. Slaughter JR, Slaughter KA, Nichols D, Holmes SE, Martens MP, Prevalence, clinical manifestations, etiology, and treatment of depression in Parkinson's disease. *J Neuropsychiatry Clin Neurosci* 2001; **13**(2):187–196.

38. McDonald WM, Richard IH, DeLong MR, Prevalence, etiology, and treatment of depression in Parkinson's disease. *Biol Psychiatry* 2003; **54**(3):363–375.

39. Tröster AI, Letsch EA. Anxiety and depression. In: Pahwa R, Lyons KE, Koller WC (eds) *Therapy of Parkinson's Disease*, 3rd edn. Marcel Dekker: New York, 2004; 423–445.

40. Shulman LM, Taback RL, Rabinstein AA, Weiner WJ, Non-recognition of depression and other non-motor symptoms in Parkinson's disease. *Park Rel Disord* 2002; **8**:193–197.

41. Okun MS, Watts RL. Depression associated with Parkinson's disease: Clinical features and treatment. *Neurology* 2002; **58**(Suppl. 1):S63–S70.

42. Shulman LM, Taback RL, Bean J, Weiner WJ, Comorbidity of the nonmotor symptoms of Parkinson's disease. *Mov Disord* 2001; **16**(3):507–510.

43. Menza MA, Psychiatric aspects of Parkinson's disease. *Psychiatric Annals* 2002; **32**:99–104.

44. Ryder KA, Gontkovsky ST, McSwan KL, Scott JG, Bharucha KJ, Beatty WW, Cognitive function in Parkinson's disease: association with anxiety but not depression. *Aging Neuropsychol Cogn* 2002; **9**:77–84.

45. Boeve BF, Silber MH, Ferman TJ, REM sleep behavior disorder in Parkinson's disease and dementia with Lewy bodies. *J Geriatr Psychiatry Neurol* 2004; **17**(3):146–157.

46. Folstein MF, Folstein SE, Fanjiang G, MMSE: Mini-Mental State Examination Clinical Guide. Psychological Assessment Resources: Lutz, FL, 2002.

47. Mattis S. Dementia Rating Scale-2. Psychological Assessment Resources, Inc.: Lutz, FL, 2001.

48. Janvin C, Aarsland D, Larsen JP, Hugdahl K, Neuropsychological profile of patients with Parkinson's disease without dementia. *Dement Geriatr Cogn Disord* 2003; **15**(3):126–131.

49. Hobson P, Meara J, The detection of dementia and cognitive impairment in a community population of elderly people with Parkinson's disease by use of the CAMCOG neuropsychological test. *Age Ageing* 1999; **28**(1):39–43.

50. Brown GG, Rahill AA, Gorell JM et al, Validity of the Dementia Rating Scale in assessing cognitive function in Parkinson's disease. *J Geriatr Psychiatry Neurol* 1999; **12**(4):180–188.

51. Aarsland D, Litvan I, Salmon D, Galasko D, Wentzel-Larsen T, Larsen JP, Performance on the Dementia Rating Scale in Parkinson's disease with dementia and dementia with Lewy bodies: comparison with progressive supranuclear palsy and Alzheimer's disease. *J Neurol Neurosurg Psychiatry* 2003; **74**:1215–1220.

52. Paolo AM, Tröster AI, Glatt SL, Hubble JP, Koller WC, Differentiation of the dementias of Alzheimer's and Parkinson's disease with the Dementia Rating Scale. *J Geriatr Psychiatry Neurol* 1995; **8**(3):184–188.

53. Dymek MP, Atchison P, Harrell L, Marson DC, Competency to consent to medical treatment in cognitively impaired patients with Parkinson's disease. *Neurology* 2001; **56**(1):17–24.

54. Knopman DS, DeKosky ST, Cummings JL et al, Practice parameter: diagnosis of dementia (an evidence-based review). Report of the Quality Standards Subcommittee of the American Academy of Neurology. *Neurology* 2001; **56**(9):1143–1153.

55. Burn DJ, Tröster AI, Neuropsychiatric complications of medical and surgical therapies for Parkinson's disease. *J Geriatr Psychiatry Neurol* 2004; **17**(3):172–180.

56. Hanagasi HA, Emre M, Management of the neuropsychiatric and cognitive symptoms in Parkinson's disease. *Practical Neurol* 2002; **2**:94–102.

57. Richard IH, Justus AW, Greig NH, Marshall F, Kurlan R, Worsening of motor function and mood in a patient with Parkinson's disease after pharmacologic challenge with oral rivastigmine. *Clin Neuropharmacol* 2002; **25**(6):296–299.

58. Bullock R, Cameron A, Rivastigmine for the treatment of dementia and visual hallucinations associated with Parkinson's disease: a case series. *Curr Med Res Opin* 2002; **18**(5):258–264.

59. Kaufer DI, Pharmacologic therapy of dementia with Lewy bodies. *J Geriatr Psychiatry Neurol* 2002; **15**(4):224–232.

60. McKeith I, Del Ser T, Spano P et al, Efficacy of rivastigmine in dementia with Lewy bodies: a randomised, double-blind, placebo-controlled international study. *Lancet* 2000; **356**(9247):2031–2036.

61. Reading PJ, Luce AK, McKeith IG, Rivastigmine in the treatment of parkinsonian

psychosis and cognitive impairment: preliminary findings from an open trial. *Mov Disord* 2001; **16**(6):1171–1174.

62. Aarsland D, Laake K, Larsen JP, Janvin C, Donepezil for cognitive impairment in Parkinson's disease: a randomised controlled study. *J Neurol Neurosurg Psychiatry* 2002; **72**(6):708–712.

63. Aarsland D, Mosimann UP, McKeith IG, Role of cholinesterase inhibitors in Parkinson's disease and dementia with Lewy bodies. *J Geriatr Psychiatry Neurol* 2004; **17**(3):164–171.

64. Leroi I, Brandt J, Reich SG et al, Randomized placebo-controlled trial of donepezil in cognitive impairment in Parkinson's disease. *Int J Geriatr Psychiatry* 2004; **19**(1):1–8.

65. Emre M, Aarsland D, Albanese A, et al, Rivastigime for dementia associated with Parkinson's disease. *New Engl J Med* 2004; **351**(24): 2509–2518.

66. Bayles KA, Kim ES, Improving the functioning of individuals with Alzheimer's disease: emergence of behavioral interventions. *J Commun Disord* 2003; **36**(5):327–343.

67. Loewenstein DA, Acevedo A, Czaja SJ, Duara R, Cognitive rehabilitation of mildly impaired Alzheimer disease patients on cholinesterase inhibitors. *Am J Geriatr Psychiatry* 2004; **12**(4):395–402.

68. Tarnanas I, A virtual environment for the assessment and the rehabilitation of the visuo-constructional ability in dementia patients. *Stud Health Technol Inform* 2000; **70**:341–343.

69. McCurry SM, Logsdon RG, Vitiello MV, Teri L, Treatment of sleep and nighttime disturbances in Alzheimer's disease: a behavior management approach. *Sleep Med* 2004; **5**(4):373–377.

70. Teri L, Gibbons LE, McCurry SM et al, Exercise plus behavioral management in patients with Alzheimer disease: a randomized controlled trial. *JAMA* 2003; **290**(15):2015–2022.

71. Alm N, Astell A, Ellis M, Dye R, Gowans G, Campbell J, A cognitive prosthesis and communication support for people with dementia. *Neuropsychol Rehabil* 2004; **14**:117–134.

72. Tröster AI, Woods SP, Neuropsychological aspects of Parkinson's disease and parkinsonian syndromes. In: Pahwa R, Lyons KE, Koller WC (eds) *Handbook of Parkinson's Disease*, 3rd edn. Marcel Dekker: New York, 2003; 127–157.

73. Tröster AI, Fields JA, The role of neuropsychological evaluation in the neuro-surgical treatment of movement disorders. in Tarsy D, Vitek JL, Lozano AM (eds) *Surgical Treatment of Parkinson's Disease and other Movement Disorders*. Humana Press: Totowa, New Jersey, 2003; 213–240.

chapter 7

Dementia secondary to Parkinson's disease versus dementia with Lewy bodies

Laura Marsh and Dag Aarsland

Introduction

Dementia with Lewy bodies (DLB) is an increasingly recognized diagnostic entity among neurodegenerative disorders. Clinically, DLB is distinguished as a global dementia syndrome that is accompanied by cognitive fluctuations, parkinsonism, and visual hallucinations. Neuropathologically, DLB is characterized by the presence of neuronal inclusions called Lewy bodies in various brain regions.[1] Thus, patients with DLB and patients with Parkinson's disease (PD) and dementia (PDD) share common clinical and neuropathological features: both are parkinsonian dementia syndromes that involve neurodegeneration and abnormal aggregation of the α-synuclein protein, the major constituent of Lewy bodies. However, it is controversial whether DLB and PDD represent different diseases or syndromic variants of the same underlying disease process, one commencing initially with motor dysfunction and the other with cognitive dysfunction.[2,3] The relative importance of concomitant Alzheimer's disease (AD) neuropathological changes in both DLB and PDD is also debated. In the absence of a resolution of these controversies, the perspective of serving patients should be given priority. To that end, it is important to understand the basis of the controversy and its impact on clinical care. This chapter reviews the clinical and neurobiological features of DLB and PDD and provides practical guidelines on the management of patients who present with DLB relative to patients with PD who later develop a global dementia syndrome.

DLB and PDD: What are the controversial issues?

Once thought to be a rare condition, DLB is now regarded as a common cause of dementia in the elderly.[4] Several terms and diagnostic criteria were proposed in initial descriptions of the dementia syndrome associated with Lewy bodies.[5,6] Improvements in pathologic staining methods increased recognition of the syndrome as a frequent cause of dementia. Following a consensus conference in 1995, the term DLB was introduced and clinical and pathological inclusion and exclusion criteria were defined (Table 7.1).[1] On the basis of validation studies with autopsy findings, these criteria were maintained following their review at subsequent consensus conferences in 1998[7] and 2003.[4]

As the original DLB diagnostic criteria were developed primarily to distinguish DLB from AD, the issue of distinctions and commonalities between DLB and PDD were not a prominent focus until the 2003 consensus conference.[4] At that time, it was agreed that the initial clinical and pathological criteria should continue to be regarded as the most appropriate working standards for research studies. However, shortcomings of the consensus criteria were also recognized, such as the need for operationalized clinical features and prospective longitudinal and imaging studies to validate the clinical criteria with neuropathological findings, especially for comparisons of patients with PDD versus DLB.

Table 7.1 Consensus criteria for clinical diagnosis of probable and possible DLB[1]

Dementia
Core features ≥ 2 = Diagnosis of probable DLB; 1 = Possible DLB:
– Fluctuating cognition (varying attention/arousal/alertness)
– Recurrent visual hallucinations
– Spontaneous motor features of parkinsonism.

Other supportive features
– Repeated falls   – Neuroleptic sensitivity
– Syncope   – Systematized delusions
– Transient loss of consciousness   – Other hallucinations

A diagnosis of DLB is less likely in the presence of: Stroke disease, evident as focal neurologic signs or on brain imaging; evidence on physical examination and investigation of any physical illness or other brain disorder sufficient to account for the clinical picture.

A particular difficulty with the existing clinical diagnostic criteria for DLB is the stipulation that the dementia syndrome must occur before or within 1 year of onset of parkinsonism[1] and that the diagnosis of PDD should be used when the dementia syndrome becomes evident more than one year after the onset of parkinsonism.[8] Distinguishing DLB from PDD in terms of the temporal course of these features is often not difficult; in most patients with idiopathic PD, dementia occurs as a later stage complication, at least 8–10 years after the onset of motor symptoms.[9,10] However, some patients with apparent idiopathic PD develop prominent dementia syndromes with psychosis earlier in the course of their motor syndrome, but not within its first year. Such cases highlight how the "one-year rule" for distinguishing DLB and PDD is arbitrary in the absence of its empiric validation. Furthermore, from a clinical management perspective, it would be important to know whether the temporal course of dementia versus parkinsonism has an impact on treatment decisions in patients with PDD or DLB. Whereas cross-sectional studies estimate 30% dementia prevalence in PD,[11] longitudinal studies of PD patients show that the cumulative prevalence of dementia approaches 80% in PD patients an average of 10 years after the onset of motor symptoms.[12] At that point, the common features of dementia plus parkinsonism and/or psychosis in PDD and DLB suggest that similar treatments could be employed.

Efforts to understand the clinicopathological relationships between DLB and PDD are further confounded by the absence of formal clinical or pathological criteria for PDD and the heterogeneity of PD itself. Since PDD may comprise several types of dementia syndromes, as discussed in Chapter 6, it might be difficult to develop universal criteria for PDD that are analogous to those used for DLB. However, an international consortium of researchers in this area is working to develop operational criteria for PDD in order to facilitate comparison studies of PDD and DLB. Similarly, in contrast to DLB, there are no accepted neuropathological criteria for either PDD or idiopathic PD.[13] While it is generally thought that the pathological diagnosis of PD requires identification of both Lewy bodies and neurodegeneration in the substantia nigra pars compacta (SNpc),[13] studies of various genetic forms of PD provide evidence that the clinical syndrome of PD is associated with considerable clinical, genetic, and neuropathological heterogeneity. This includes, at times, the absence of Lewy bodies, which are regarded as the *sine qua non* for PD, yet are also known to occur in a number of diverse disorders.

Dementia with Lewy bodies

Epidemiology

Prevalence estimates for DLB from clinical and community-based studies have been as high as 20–25% of all demented cases over the age of 65.[14,15] Other studies report a lower prevalence of DLB, but this may be accounted for by methodological differences in studies, particularly with respect to the criteria used and the study population.[16] As rates of vascular dementia tend to be similar to those for DLB, DLB is generally regarded as the second most common neurodegenerative dementia syndrome after AD. The onset of DLB appears to increase with age, usually beginning after age 50. Symptom progression and survival rates for DLB appear comparable to AD,[4] but some patients have a relatively rapid course of decline. It is not known whether prevalence is affected by significant age and gender effects and no specific risk factors have been identified.

Neuropathological features

Lewy body pathology occurs in a number of neurological disorders. However, for DLB, the only essential pathological feature is Lewy bodies, which are neuronal inclusions containing abnormally phosphorylated neural filament proteins aggregated with ubiquitin and α-synuclein. Based on the number and regional distribution of Lewy bodies that immunoreact to ubiquitin, the 1996 Consensus guidelines for neuropathological diagnosis of DLB defined three pathological subtypes: brainstem predominant type, limbic (transitional) type, and neocortical type. How these three categories correspond to different clinical profiles is not established.[4] In many cases of DLB, associated pathological features include cortical β-amyloid deposits, neurofibrillary tangles, Lewy neurites, regional neuronal loss, in particular of medial temporal and frontal cortices, and spongiform changes. AD pathological changes, particularly senile plaques, are evident in as many as 75% of patients with DLB. Neocortical neurofibrillary tangles are less common in DLB compared to AD, but may influence the clinical presentation.[17,18] In neurochemical studies of DLB, there are prominent nigrostriatal dopaminergic deficits, similar to PD, although substantia nigral neuronal loss is less than in PD.[19] The other important change is atrophy of cholinergic neurons in the basal forebrain, leading to reduced cortical cholinergic markers and a cholinergic deficit that is more severe in DLB compared to AD.[20]

It is important to appreciate that the neuropathological characterization of DLB and related disorders continues to evolve. Whereas brainstem Lewy bodies typically appear as spherical eosinophilic inclusions with a dense core and surrounding halo, cortical Lewy bodies are less well-defined depositions that were difficult to detect until the development of anti-ubiquitin immunocytochemical staining techniques in the 1980s. The more recent development of α-synuclein antibodies enables greater detection of intraneuronal inclusions and Lewy neurites in cortical and limbic areas.

Clinical features

In addition to evidence for a progressive dementia syndrome on initial presentation, at least two of the three core features of DLB, i.e., parkinsonism, hallucinations, and cognitive fluctuations, are required for a diagnosis of probable DLB (Table 7.1).[1] The diagnosis of "possible" DLB requires presence of one additional feature. These criteria have high levels of specificity (>90%)[21] but sensitivity has been as low as 50% in some studies.[7]

Cognitive features

Progressive cognitive impairment of sufficient severity to interfere with normal social or occupational function (i.e., dementia) is typically the presenting feature of DLB. The neuropsychological profile of the dementia syndrome in DLB is characterized by prominent attentional dysfunction along with executive, visuospatial, and memory deficits, which are most likely related to a combination of fronto-subcortical deficits superimposed on cortical and hippocampal pathologies. Compared to patients with AD, DLB patients in the earlier stages have relatively less impairments involving orientation, memory, and naming abilities, but greater deficits in verbal fluency, set-shifting, and response inhibition. The visuospatial deficits can be especially prominent whereas memory impairments become more evident with progression. As patients with DLB advance and the deficits become more global, a distinctive profile is less evident.

Fluctuations in cognitive functioning, secondary to fluctuating attention and consciousness, are a key feature of the cognitive profile of DLB and are seen in 80–90% of patients.[1] Clinically, distinguishing the dementia syndrome of DLB from delirium can be difficult. However, in DLB, patients are observed to have *spontaneous* periods of extreme confusion, impaired awareness, or decreased consciousness with reduced arousability that alternate with periods of increased lucidity and functional capabilities.[22] These fluctuations can occur on a day-to-day basis, but the duration and frequency of the episodes varies and contributes to greater variability in cognitive test performance in patients with DLB. By contrast, cognitive fluctuations in AD patients tend to occur in response to the cognitive demands of the environment.[23] Fluctuating cognitive abilities in DLB have also been objectively measured in terms of reaction times, and linked to variations in cortical arousal as measured electrophysiologically.[24] Overall, the phenomenon of fluctuating cognition has been notoriously difficult to reach agreement upon, resulting in misdiagnosis of DLB in validation studies. Scales developed to improve consistency across clinicians in the assessment of cognitive fluctuations in patients with dementia include the "Clinician Assessment of Fluctuations" and the "One Day Fluctuation Assessment Scale".[25] The "Mayo Fluctuations Questionnaire," an informant-completed scale, is also available.[26]

Psychiatric features

A variety of psychiatric symptoms commonly occur in DLB. Visual hallucinations, a core clinical feature of DLB, are frequently present and occur in up to 70% of patient samples.[26,27] The visual hallucinations are typically vivid and well-formed, involving people, animals, or complex scenes. Patients frequently describe them in great detail and may even attempt to interact with them, such as providing food and drink or becoming aggressive when the hallucination seems to threaten the spouse. In a 1-year follow-up study, visual hallucinations were more likely to be chronic and persistent in DLB, as compared to AD.[28] Other psychiatric phenomena in DLB include other non-visual hallucinations, delusions, delusional misidentification syndromes, such as the Capgras syndrome (i.e. the patient believes that the person, usually the spouse, has been replaced by an imposter), depression[18] and rapid eye movement (REM) sleep behavior disorder (RBD). In contrast to AD or typical PD, the psychiatric disturbances such as visual and auditory hallucinations, delusions, delusional misidentification, and depression are more likely to be present in early stages of DLB.[27] In addition, the presence of auditory or visual hallucinations in patients with Mini-Mental State[29] scores greater than 20 is highly suggestive of DLB. Although neither hallucinations nor parkinsonism are required for the diagnosis of DLB, presence of dementia or psychosis before onset of parkinsonian signs or early in the course after onset of motor signs suggests an alternative diagnosis to idiopathic PD, such as DLB, Alzheimer's disease, or pre-existing psychopathology.[30] The diagnosis of DLB should also be strongly considered when hallucinations, especially non-visual hallucinations, occur before initiation of antiparkinsonian treatment. RBD, a parasomnia, involves the loss of normal sleep muscle atonia during REM sleep in association with prominent dreaming, vocalizations, and/or physical activity that can range from simple calm pantomiming behaviors to complex and violent behaviors.[31] It can be present in 72% of patients.[26] When seen with dementia, the presence of RBD and dementia may represent an early manifestation of DLB, preceding development of parkinsonism or hallucinations.[32]

Motor features/L-dopa response

Parkinsonism is present in at least two-thirds of patients with DLB,[33] although the incidence of spontaneous parkinsonism over the course of DLB is unclear. High rates of psychiatric and behavioral disturbances in DLB increase the likelihood of antipsychotic use, which is also associated with drug-induced parkinsonism. Since primary and drug-induced parkinsonism are difficult to distinguish in patients taking antipsychotic agents, it is important to clarify medication status at the time of onset of parkinsonism. The pattern of motor symptoms varies in DLB, with lower rates of resting tremor and asymmetric motor signs and greater occurrence of rigidity and postural and gait impairment in DLB compared to PD patients without dementia.[34] In autopsy-proven cases, occurrence of any one of four clinical features (myoclonus, absence of rest tremor, no response to levodopa, or no perceived need to treat with levodopa) was ten times more likely to represent the diagnosis of DLB than PD.[35] However, while the parkinsonism of DLB is typically associated with a diminished response to levodopa, it is important to recognize that some patients with DLB, nonetheless, clearly benefit from levodopa therapy. Accordingly, a levodopa therapy trial should be attempted in every patient.[36]

Autonomic dysfunction

Autonomic dysfunction is another common feature of parkinsonian disorders that is also present in DLB. Dysautonomia tends to be a late complication, but there are exceptions when autonomic failure is the presenting symptom of DLB.[37] The actual frequency of dysautonomia in DLB is unclear, but the symptoms tends to be less severe and prominent in comparison with multiple system atrophy (MSA) and most often include orthostatic hypotension, urinary symptoms, and sweat loss.[38] Falls may also be a feature of autonomic nervous system pathology. In the first DLB workshop in 1995, syncopal events associated with DLB were described in which patients have episodes of extreme loss of tone. Also described were transient episodes of loss of responsiveness that may represent the consequence of extreme attentional fluctuations and the up-regulation of muscarinic receptors and subsequent effects on the peripheral nervous system.[27]

Neuroleptic sensitivity

Neuroleptic sensitivity is a significant concern in the assessment and management of DLB, especially given the high rates of disruptive psychiatric symptoms. The response to neuroleptics can vary, involving enhanced parkinsonism, extreme sedation with difficulties maintaining adequate fluid and water intake, and even more severe and catastrophic reactions resembling the neuroleptic malignant syndrome. The latter can include symptoms such as severe rigidity, impaired consciousness, pyrexia, postural hypotension, increased confusion, cardiovascular collapse, and rapid progression to death.[39] Neuroleptic sensitivity is more likely to develop after administration of typical neuroleptics, but DLB patients frequently have poor tolerance of many of the atypical antipsychotics, including risperidone, olanzapine, and clozapine. The phenomenon may be related to either a failure to up-regulate D2 receptors in response to neuroleptic blocking or reduced dopaminergic innervation.[40] The profound cholinergic deficit in DLB along with the anticholinergic properties of many neuroleptics, especially clozapine, is also likely to play a role. The use of neuroleptics in managing psychosis in DLB is discussed below as well as in Chapter 10.

How are the clinical symptoms of DLB and PDD related? Comparative studies of DLB and PDD

With the exception of dementia occurring early in DLB and later in PDD in relation to parkinsonism, the cross-sectional clinical profiles of DLB and PDD in individual patients are frequently indistinct. As many of the initial studies of DLB focused on comparisons to AD, there is still a need for prospective longitudinal studies aimed at characterizing the similarities and differences in the profile and course of cognitive deficits in DLB relative to PDD. This section highlights clinical issues relevant to patient assessment and reviews results from studies comparing DLB and PDD.

Cognition

As mentioned above, until data are available from longitudinal studies on the course and treatment response of cognitive deficits in autopsy-confirmed cases of DLB and PDD, it is unclear whether the timing of the onset of dementia and parkinsonism is a meaningful distinction between DLB and PDD that influences their respective clinical presentations and treatments. Until then, from a clinical standpoint, several factors confound the clinical delineation of DLB versus PDD. First, while all patients with DLB have a progressive dementia syndrome, by definition, PD is not exclusively associated with development of dementia after the onset of motor symptoms. However, cognitive impairment is present to some degree in nearly all patients with idiopathic PD, even early in its course. Thus, it can be difficult to decide when cognitive impairment is sufficiently severe to warrant classification as a dementia syndrome,[11] an issue also discussed in Chapters 5 and 6. Second, the exact time of onset of parkinsonism relative to the onset of dementia cannot always be identified in patients with established dementia and parkinsonism, especially if a reliable proxy is not available. Likewise, a reliable history of medication trials for parkinsonism or psychosis is not always obtainable. Finally, the cognitive profile of PDD is heterogeneous, which adds to the complexity of its diagnosis. A subset of patients with PDD develops prominent cognitive deficits (either selective or global) early in the course after onset of motor symptoms, and those symptoms are more likely to resemble the cognitive features that characterize DLB. However, some clinical features of DLB, as well as in PDD, will also overlap with symptoms in AD, along with a host of other conditions that cause parkinsonism and dementia.[41] Even in recently diagnosed PD, subgroups of patients demonstrate different patterns of cognitive impairment that may reflect neuropathological changes ultimately related to the development of dementia.[42] Some have a more prominent executive-visuospatial disturbance suggestive of striatal and frontal Lewy-body pathology, whereas others manifest a more amnestic-dominant profile that may be related to Alzheimer-like brain changes.

Once dementia is evident in PD, patients with PDD, like DLB, characteristically present with prominent visuospatial, attentional and executive impairments and relatively less memory impairment. Cross-sectional studies directly comparing clinical features of DLB and PDD tend to show overlapping cognitive profiles that are distinct from patients with AD, even when all groups with dementia are matched for overall level of cognitive deficits.[43] Fluctuating attention was found in both DLB and PDD, but not in patients with AD or PD without dementia.[24] An additional study comparing pentagon copying in patients with DLB and PDD suggested a similar severity of impairment in the two conditions, and a pattern of errors indicating executive dysfunction.[44] Thus, the cognitive profile in both PDD and DLB appears to be intermediate between a subcortical pattern, similar to that observed in patients with progressive supranuclear palsy, and the profile of cortical deficits evident in patients with AD.[45]

However, there are also subtle differences between PDD and DLB that may not be apparent clinically. In the context of mild dementia, patients with DLB had more pronounced executive impairment than PD patients.[45] Thus, there may be more marked executive dysfunction early in the course in DLB than in PDD.[45] Differences in clinical profiles between individual patients may be related to the relative density of the different neuropathological abnormalities in different brain regions over the course of the disease.

Psychiatric symptoms

A characteristic psychiatric profile has also been reported in both DLB and PDD. Visual hallucinations are more common in DLB (70%) and PDD (25–40%) than in patients with AD.[46] Another distinguishing feature of the Lewy-body dementia syndromes is the high frequency of REM-sleep behavioral disorders, which are suggestive of Lewy-body diseases.[31] Other symptoms commonly reported, such as depression, apathy and anxiety, are common in other dementias as well, although a higher frequency of depression and apathy may occur in DLB and PDD than in other dementias.[27]

Motor symptoms

Parkinsonism, occurring spontaneously and unrelated to previous use of neuroleptic drugs, occurs in the majority of DLB patients. While it is frequently stated that parkinsonism is mild in DLB, comparative studies indicate that motor symptoms in DLB can be at least as severe as in PDD[47] and that severe neuroleptic sensitivity occurs in DLB as well as PD with or without dementia.[48] There is some evidence that gait and postural disturbances, symptoms considered to be mediated by transmitter deficits other than dopaminergic changes, are more severe in DLB than in PD,[34] and are possibly more symmetrical than in PD. However, interestingly, the pattern of motor symptoms in patients with PDD tends to resemble that in DLB patients, but differs from non-demented PD patients. This observation is consistent with the higher risk of dementia in PD patients who have greater gait and postural disturbances compared to those with tremor dominant parkinsonism.[49]

How are the brain changes in DLB and PDD related? Comparative clinico-pathologic studies

Pathological changes

Both DLB and PDD have limited cortical atrophy compared with other dementia syndromes. There is no substantial subcortical atrophy in pathologically confirmed cases, but mild frontal and medial temporal lobe atrophy are consistent features.[50] Both conditions also have significant but similar atrophy and pathology in the amygdala.[51] In contrast, hippocampal pyramidal neurons innervating frontal cortex selectively degenerate in DLB,[52] with potential relevance for the observed subtle differences in executive functioning reported above.

Lewy bodies are a common feature of both PDD and DLB and the amount of Lewy body pathology tends to be similar in DLB, PDD, and PD across cortical regions.[53] However, the relationship between Lewy body pathology and dementia is not straightforward. For example, cortical Lewy bodies can be present in PD, regardless of the presence or absence of dementia.[54] Yet, in PDD patients, limbic and cortical Lewy body disease was associated with dementia.[55] Potential differences in the underlying disease processes of DLB and PDD are also suggested by differences in regional Lewy body pathology. In DLB, a greater number of temporal lobe Lewy bodies correlated with the early occurrence of visual hallucinations[56] whereas increasing Lewy body densities in limbic and frontal cortices correlated with the severity of dementia in PDD.[57]

The relationship between Alzheimer pathology and cognitive impairment in DLB and PDD is also inconsistent. Most cases of DLB can be differentiated from those with PDD by the substantial deposition of cortical β-amyloid even in the absence of significant neurofibrillary tangle formation.[53,58] While the amount of β-amyloid deposition and cortical Lewy bodies correlates with dementia severity in DLB, the relative contribution of AD changes and Lewy body pathology to PDD is not clear. In one series, up to one-third of cases with PD at autopsy had prominent dementia, and the degree of cognitive impairment was significantly correlated with Alzheimer's pathology.[59] Thus, while there is overlapping pathology among some patients with DLB and PDD, there may also be distinct processes in that the density of β-amyloid-positive plaques in some patients with DLB can be equivalent to that found in AD.

Neurochemical changes in PDD and DLB

Striatal cell and dopamine loss is pronounced in both DLB and PD with differences in the symmetry and rostrocaudal gradient of dopamine loss in DLB and PDD related to the presentation of parkinsonian symptoms.[19] The degree of nigral loss is also correlated with disease duration, which is usually longer in PDD than in DLB. Greater loss of striatal dopamine is therefore observed in PD compared with DLB,[19] with more abundant residual neuritic pathology observed in DLB than in PD.[60] In PD, but not DLB, there is also a compensatory increase in striatal D2 receptors and dopamine turn-over,[19] with PDD patients having intermediate D2 binding between DLB and PD.[61] For DLB, these differences may underlie the relatively diminished responsiveness to levodopa and the high risk of severe neuroleptic sensitivity reactions relative to PDD. The striatal dopaminergic deficit in DLB is being translated into a useful clinical imaging tool for differentiating DLB from Alzheimer's disease and other dementia syndromes.[62]

Neurochemical studies consistently find marked cortical cholinergic deficits in both PDD and DLB.[20] However, differential involvement of the cholinergic system in DLB and PD has also been reported. Cholinergic markers are reduced in the striatum in patients with DLB, but not PD.[63] In DLB, there is a correlation between visual hallucinations and cholinergic deficits in the temporal cortex, but this has not been found in PDD.[64]

The impact on cortical cholinergic receptors is similar in PDD and DLB with both showing increased muscarinic binding[65] and a considerable reduction in nicotinic binding, although in the insular cortex the reductions were more marked in PDD than DLB.[66] In a study comparing muscarinic receptor binding within the striatum in DLB and PD patients, M1 receptors were significantly reduced in DLB but not PD. However, the three PD patients with dementia had binding levels intermediate between PD and DLB.[61] In both DLB and PD, there is a similar reduction in striatal nicotinic binding consistent with these receptors being located on dopaminergic terminals.[63]

Neuroimaging

Compared to AD, volumetric imaging methods showed relative preservation of medial temporal lobe structural volumes[67] and greater volume deficits in the basal forebrain[68] in patients with DLB. Functional neuroimaging studies show occipital hypoperfusion and a marked decrease in striatal binding in DLB compared to controls and AD patients.[69]

Clinical course

Few prospective studies of DLB exist, and studies directly comparing the course of DLB and PDD have not been reported. The rate of progression of parkinsonism, once identified, appears to be similar in DLB and PD.[70,71] However, the relative rates of cognitive decline in DLB and PDD have not been compared directly. Although the mortality rate in PD does not seem to be significantly different from non-PD subjects, dementia has been shown to negatively affect mortality in PD.[72] While PD patients frequently need to be placed in nursing homes, and dementia is recognized as an independent predictor of nursing home placement in PD,[73] this aspect of care has not been explicitly studied in DLB.

Management and treatment

In the absence of disease-modifying therapies or a valid classification system or biomarker that distinguishes DLB from PDD, clinical care focuses on symptomatic approaches. With a few exceptions, the ongoing management of DLB is relatively similar to that for PDD. By contrast, it is clear that DLB patients should be managed differently from patients with AD, and the presence of dementia in PD requires different management compared to that of non-demented PD patients. Therefore, a major task for the clinician is to distinguish the Lewy body dementia syndrome, i.e. either DLB or PDD, from AD and other dementias and to identify cognitive impairment and dementia when it occurs in PD patients. Once identified, such patients should be followed thoroughly, carefully balancing the potential benefit of treatment of parkinsonism, hallucinations and dementia with the risk of adverse neuropsychiatric effects of dopaminergic drugs and neuroleptic sensitivity reactions.

The management of PDD and DLB is especially challenging because of the interplay between motor, cognitive, and psychiatric symptoms in DLB and PDD, the potential adverse effects of medications on each of these domains, and the general frailty of these patients. Pharmacological therapies for the symptomatic treatment of DLB are few and largely consist of acetyl-cholinesterase inhibitors. No guidelines exist regarding poor response or intolerability with such medications. As with other dementia syndromes, treatment also includes careful monitoring for medical conditions or medications that can cause delirium or have adverse effects on the mental state, the use of behavioral strategies that maximize function and limit distress, such as redirection, reduced stimulation, or increased activity via the use of daycare programs, and attention to caregivers, including illness teaching, counselling, or referral for their specific care.

Cholinesterase inhibitors

Currently available cholinesterase inhibitors include donepezil, rivastigmine, and galantamine. The prominent cholinergic deficit in DLB and PDD and its association with cognitive deficits supports an important role for cholinesterase inhibitors, which have been shown to have a favorable effect on cognitive deficits, psychosis, and behavioral disturbances in various dementia populations.[74] In addition to several open label studies and case reports, controlled clinical trials of cholinesterase inhibitors include one large randomized trial[75] and one small double-blind crossover study[76] in DLB and one large multi-site and two small single-site controlled trails in PDD patients.[77-79] In the only study comparing treatment effects of a cholinesterase inhibitor (donepezil) across diseases,[80] there were similar improvements in both cognitive and psychiatric symptoms on donepezil in DLB and PDD patients, and no change in parkinsonism in both groups. However, PDD patients showed a greater worsening of psychiatric symptoms after withdrawal of donepezil.

At this point, there is no obvious advantage of one cholinesterase inhibitor over another, though a patient with side-effects to one type may tolerate another type. In general, cholinesterase inhibitors are well-tolerated, though increasing the imbalance between acetylcholine and dopamine can enhance parkinsonism in some patients.[81] Cholinergic effects can also lead to a variety of other side-effects, including intolerable gastrointestinal complaints such as diarrhea and stomach cramps and cardiac syncope from vagal effects.[82] Starting at a lower dose than the recommended starting dosages and a slower titration to the recommended dose seems to limit adverse effects. Given the high risk of severe sensitivity reactions and increased risk of cerebrovascular incidents during treatment with neuroleptics, further clinical trials of cholinesterase inhibitors are encouraged to establish their role in DLB and PDD. At this point, there is little evidence on which to base a conclusion regarding the differential treatment response in DLB versus PDD.

Neuroleptics

Neuroleptic sensitivity, especially to typical neuroleptics, occurs in DLB and PDD.[48,83] These reactions are characterized by a sudden onset of sedation, increased confusion, rigidity and immobility, and may even substantially reduce survival.[39] While the symptoms of severe sensitivity reactions experienced by the respective groups of patients are similar, neuroleptic intolerance may not be as severe in patients with PDD, who may also be less likely to die within a few months of neuroleptic exposure. Use of antipsychotic agents in PDD is reviewed in Chapter 10 and similar caveats hold in DLB, for the most part. The one exception is clozapine, which is regarded as the gold standard for treatment of psychosis in PD patients, including in the setting of dementia.[84] However, studies of clozapine for treatment of PD-related psychosis have included patients with mild to moderate degrees of dementia, and there has not been formal study of the effects or safety of clozapine in patients with more advanced dementia syndromes and psychosis. In DLB patients, clozapine can be very poorly tolerated, presumably because of greater sensitivity to its anticholinergic effects.[85] Recent reports of higher mortality rates and risk of cerebrovascular incidents in elderly patients with dementia associated with risperidone and olanzapine underscore the potential high risk of these agents. Given preliminary evidence that cholinesterase inhibitors may improve hallucinations both in DLB[75] and PDD,[86] these agents should be considered as initial treatment for psychosis in DLB and PDD. When symptoms are more acute and disruptive, however, low dose quetiapine (e.g., 12.5–25 mg) is the most appropriate starting agent, with upward titration as indicated and tolerated.

Levodopa

Controlled treatment trials of levodopa therapy are needed in DLB to provide guidelines on its use in this population. In the one study published to date, DLB, PDD, and PD patients showed a positive response on the L-dopa test, indicating a potential for clinical benefit during treatment. However, the proportion of good responders was highest in PD, somewhat less in PDD, and lowest in DLB patients.[36] However, a range of side-effects may occur during treatment with these agents, including neuropsychiatric disturbances. Although there is no clear evidence, our clinical experience suggests that both PDD and DLB patients are at a particular high risk of adverse effects during dopaminergic therapy, but DLB patients with psychosis suffer adverse cognitive and psychiatric effects of levodopa at much lower doses than PD patients with dementia and psychosis. Some DLB patients may not tolerate dopaminergic agents at all because of enhanced confusion, sedation, and/or hypotension. In others, a low dose of 25/100 Sinemet three times daily, or less, can result in sufficient motor improvement that substantially reduces caregiver burden. With PDD patients, there is always an ongoing need for assessment of the antiparkinsonian regimen. The presence of dementia indicates a need to consider the therapeutic utility of anticholinergics, selegeline, amantadine, and dopamine agonists in the regimen. Gradual elimination of such agents and restricted use of L-dopa (Sinemet) can be helpful to the mental state without compromising motor function. We strongly recommend discontinuation of anticholinergic medications in PD patients who develop dementia, and, given their potential for adverse cognitive effects, advise their judicious use, if at all, earlier in the course of PD.

Conclusions

Differentiating DLB from PDD on clinical grounds alone is often challenging, if not impossible. This difficulty impacts care, since clinicians rely on accurate diagnoses for treatment planning. Per definition, the most obvious difference is the early onset of dementia in DLB, whereas dementia usually occurs after 8–10 years of motor symptoms in PDD. However, some patients may present with a more equivocal history. With them, and in patients with established PDD, there is considerable overlap in the clinical, neurochemical and pathological features of DLB and PDD. Shared pathophysiological processes are suggested by the similarities of parkinsonism and visual hallucinations, cognitive deficits, patterns of atrophy, Lewy body pathology, and cholinergic and dopaminergic deficits that appear amenable to similar treatments. However, severity of executive dysfunction, frequency of visual hallucinations and delusions, and relative predominance of postural instability/gait disorders are significantly greater in DLB than in PDD. While neurochemical and pathological differences are likely to subserve these differences, the few existing studies do not clearly show a different course or treatment response in DLB and PDD, once dementia has developed. At this point, further research remains needed to clarify the nosological relationship between PDD and DLB, the clinicopathological correlates of Lewy body-related α-synuclein pathology in these conditions, and the appropriate treatments.[87]

References

1. McKeith IG, Galasko D, Kosaka K et al, Consensus guidelines for the clinical and pathologic diagnosis of dementia with Lewy bodies (DLB): Report of the consortium on DLB international workshop. *Neurology* 1996; **47**(5):1113–1124.
2. Richard IH, Papka M, Rubio A, Kurlan R, Parkinson's disease and dementia with Lewy bodies: One disease or two? *Mov Disord* 2002; **17**(6):1161–1165.
3. McKeith IG, Spectrum of Parkinson's disease, Parkinson's dementia, and Lewy body dementia. *Neurol Clin* 2000; **18**(4):865–902.
4. McKeith IG, Mintzer J, Aarsland D et al, Dementia with Lewy bodies. *The Lancet Neurology* 2004; **3**:19–28.
5. Okasaki H, Lipkin LE, Aronson SM, Diffuse intracytoplasmic inclusions (Lewy type) associated with progressive dementia and quadriparesis in flexion. *J Neuropathol Exp Neurol* 1961; **20**:237–244.
6. Kosaka K, Yoshimura M, Ikeda K, Budka H, Diffuse type of Lewy body disease. Progressive dementia with abundant cortical Lewy bodies and senile changes of varying degree – a new disease? *Clin Neuropathol* 1984; **3**:185–192.
7. McKeith IG, Perry EK, Perry RH, Report of the second dementia with Lewy body international workshop: diagnosis and treatment. Consortium on Dementia with Lewy Bodies. *Neurology* 1999; **53**(5):902–905.
8. Gelb DJ, Oliver E, Gilman S, Diagnostic criteria for Parkinson disease. *Arch Neurol* 1999; **56**(1):33–39.
9. Hobson P, Meara J, Risk and incidence of dementia in a cohort of older subjects with Parkinson's disease in the United Kingdom. *Mov Disord* 2004; **19**(9):1043–1049.
10. Hughes TA, Ross HF, Musa S et al, A 10-year study of the incidence of and factors predicting dementia in Parkinson's disease. *Neurology* 2000; **54**:1596–1602.
11. Emre M, Dementia associated with Parkinson's disease. *The Lancet Neurology* 2003; **2**(4):1–16.
12. Aarsland D, Andersen K, Larsen JP, Lolk A, Kragh-Sørensen P, Prevalence and characteristics of dementia in Parkinson disease. *Arch Neurol* 2003; **60**:387–392.
13. Calne DB, Mizuno Y, The neuromythology of Parkinson's disease. *Parkinsonism Relat Disord* 2004; **10**(5):319–322.
14. Rahkonen T, Eloniemi-Sulkava U, Rissanen S, Vatanen A, Viramo P, Sulkava R, Dementia with Lewy bodies according to the consensus criteria in a general population aged 75 years or older. *J Neurol Neurosurg Psychiatry* 2003; **74**(6):720–724.
15. Stevens T, Livingston G, Kitchen G, Manela M, Walker Z, Katona C, Islington study of dementia subtypes in the community. *Br J Psychiatry* 2002; **180**:270–276.
16. Barker RA, Foltynie T, How common is dementia with Lewy bodies? *J Neurol Neurosurg Psychiatry* 2003; **74**(6):697–698.
17. Merdes AR, Hansen LA, Jeste DV et al, Influence of Alzheimer pathology on clinical diagnostic accuracy in dementia with Lewy bodies. *Neurology* 2003; **60**(10):1586–1590.
18. Ballard CG, Jacoby R, Del Ser T et al, Neuropathological substrates of psychiatric

symptoms in prospectively studied patients with autopsy-confirmed dementia with Lewy bodies. *Am J Psychiatry* 2004; **161**(5):843–849.

19. Piggott MA, Marshall EF, Thomas N et al, Striatal dopaminergic markers in dementia with Lewy bodies, Alzheimer's, and Parkinson's diseases: rostrocaudal distribution. *Brain* 1999; **122**:1449–1468.

20. Tiraboschi P, Hansen LA, Alford M et al, Cholinergic dysfunction in diseases with Lewy bodies. *Neurology* 2000; **54**(2):407–411.

21. McKeith IG, Ballard CG, Perry RH et al, Prospective validation of consensus criteria for the diagnosis of dementia with Lewy bodies. *Neurology* 2000; **54**(5):1050–1058.

22. Walker MP, Ayre GA, Cummings JL et al, Quantifying fluctuation in dementia with Lewy bodies, Alzheimer's disease, and vascular dementia. *Neurology* 2000; **54**(8):1616–1625.

23. Bradshaw J, Saling M, Hopwood M, Anderson V, Brodtmann A, Fluctuating cognition in dementia with Lewy bodies and Alzheimer's disease is qualitatively distinct. *J Neurol Neurosurg Psychiatry* 2004; **75**(3):382–387.

24. Ballard CG, Aarsland D, McKeith IG et al, Fluctuations in attention. PD dementia vs DLB with parkinsonism. *Neurology* 2002; **59**:1714–1720.

25. Walker MP, Ayre GA, Cummings JL et al, The Clinician Assessment of Fluctuation and the One Day Fluctuation Assessment Scale. Two methods to assess fluctuating confusion in dementia. *Br J Psychiatry* 2000; **177**:252–256.

26. Ferman TJ, Smith GE, Boeve BF et al, DLB fluctuations: specific features that reliably differentiate DLB from AD and normal aging. *Neurology* 2004; **62**(2):181–187.

27. Ballard C, Holmes C, McKeith I et al, Psychiatric morbidity in dementia with Lewy bodies: a prospective clinical and neuropathological comparative study with Alzheimer's disease. *Am J Psychiatry* 1999; **156**(7):1039–1045.

28. Ballard CG, O'Brien JT, Swann AG, Thompson P, Neill D, McKeith IG, The natural history of psychosis and depression in dementia with Lewy bodies and Alzheimer's disease: persistence and new cases over 1 year of follow-up. *J Clin Psychiatry* 2001; **62**(1):46–49.

29. Folstein MF, Folstein SE, McHugh PR, "Mini-mental state." A practical method for grading the cognitive state of patients for the clinician. *J Psychiatr Res* 1975; **12**(3):189–198.

30. Goetz CG, Vogel C, Tanner CM, Stebbins GT, Early dopaminergic drug-induced hallucinations in parkinsonian patients. *Neurology* 1998; **51**:811–814.

31. Boeve BF, Silber MH, Ferman TJ, REM sleep behavior disorder in Parkinson's disease and dementia with Lewy bodies. *J Geriatr Psychiatry Neurol* 2004; **17**(3):146–157.

32. Ferman TJ, Boeve BF, Smith GE et al, Dementia with Lewy bodies may present as dementia and REM sleep behavior disorder without parkinsonism or hallucinations. *J Int Neuropsychol Soc* 2002; **8**:907–914.

33. Serby M, Samuels SC, Diagnostic criteria for dementia with Lewy bodies reconsidered. *Am J Geriatr Psychiatry* 2001; **9**(3):212–216.

34. Burn DJ, Rowan EN, Minett T et al, Extrapyramidal features in Parkinson's disease with and without dementia and dementia with Lewy bodies: a cross-sectional comparative study. *Mov Disord* 2003; **18**(8):884–889.

35. Louis ED, Klatka LA, Liu Y, Fahn S, Comparison of extrapyramidal features in 31 pathologically confirmed cases of diffuse Lewy body disease and 34 pathologically confirmed cases of Parkinson's disease. *Neurology* 1997; **48**(2):376–380.

36. Bonelli SB, Ransmayr G, Steffelbauer M, Lukas T, Lampl C, Deibl M, L-dopa responsiveness in dementia with Lewy bodies, Parkinson disease with and without dementia. *Neurology* 2004; **63**(2):376–378.

37. Kaufmann H, Nahm K, Purohit D, Wolfe D, Autonomic failure as the initial presentation of Parkinson disease and dementia with Lewy bodies. *Neurology* 2004; **63**(6):1093–1095.

38. Thaisetthawatkul P, Boeve BF, Benarroch EE et al, Autonomic dysfunction in dementia with Lewy bodies. *Neurology* 2004; **62**(10):1804–1809.

39. McKeith I, Fairbairn A, Perry R, Thompson P, Perry E, Neuroleptic sensitivity in patients with senile dementia of Lewy body type. *BMJ* 1992; **305**(6855):673–678.

40. Piggott MA, Perry EK, Marshall EF et al, Nigrostriatal dopaminergic activities in dementia with Lewy bodies in relation to neuroleptic sensitivity: comparisons with Parkinson's disease. *Biol Psychiatry* 1998; **44**(8):765–774.

41. Burn DJ, O'Brien JT, Use of functional imaging in parkinsonism and dementia. *Mov Disord* 2003; **18**(Suppl 6):S88–S95.

42. Foltynie T, Brayne CEG, Robbins TW, Barker RA, The cognitive ability of an incident cohort of Parkinson's patients in the UK. The CamPaIGN study. *Brain* 2004; **127**:550–560.

43. Noe E, Marder K, Bell KL, Jacobs DM, Manly JJ, Stern Y, Comparison of dementia with Lewy bodies to Alzheimer's disease and Parkinson's disease with dementia. *Mov Disord* 2004; **19**(1):60–67.

44. Cormack F, Aarsland D, Ballard C, Tovee MJ, Pentagon drawing and neuropsychological performance in dementia with Lewy bodies, Alzheimer's disease, Parkinson's disease and Parkinson's disease with dementia. *Int J Geriatr Psychiatry* 2004; **19**(4):371–377.

45. Aarsland D, Litvan I, Salmon D, Galasko D, Wentzel-Larsen T, Larsen JP, Performance on the dementia rating scale in Parkinson's disease with dementia and dementia with Lewy bodies: comparison with progressive supranuclear palsy and Alzheimer's disease. *J Neurol Neurosurg Psychiatry* 2003; **74**:1215–1220.

46. Aarsland D, Cummings JL, Psychiatric aspects of Parkinson's disease, Parkinson's disease with dementia, and dementia with Lewy bodies. *J Geriatr Psychiatry Neurol* 2004; **17**(3):111.

47. Aarsland D, Ballard C, McKeith I, Perry RH, Larsen JP, Comparison of extrapyramidal signs in dementia with Lewy bodies and Parkinson's disease. *J Neuropsychiatry Clin Neurosci* 2001; **13**(3):374–379.

48. Aarsland D, Perry R, Larsen JP et al, Neuroleptic sensitivity in Parkinson's disease and parkinsonian dementias. *J Clin Psychiatry* 2005; **66**:633–637.

49. Levy G, Tang M-X, Louis ED et al, The association of incident dementia with mortality in PD. *Neurology* 2002; **59**:1708–1713.

50. Burton EJ, McKeith IG, Burn DJ, Williams ED, O'Brien JT, Cerebral atrophy in Parkinson's disease with and without dementia: a comparison with Alzheimer's disease, dementia with Lewy bodies and controls. *Brain* 2004; **127**(Pt 4): 791–800.

51. Cordato NJ, Halliday GM, Harding AJ, Hely MA, Morris JG, Regional brain atrophy in progressive supranuclear palsy and Lewy body disease. *Ann Neurol* 2000; **47**:718–728.

52. Harding AJ, Lakay B, Halliday GM, Selective hippocampal neuron loss in dementia with Lewy bodies. *Ann Neurol* 2002; **51**:125–128.

53. Harding AJ, Halliday GM, Cortical Lewy body pathology in the diagnosis of dementia. *Acta Neuropathol (Berl)* 2001; **102**:355.

54. Colosimo C, Hughes AJ, Kilford L, Lees AJ, Lewy body cortical involvement may not always predict dementia in Parkinson's disease. *J Neurol Neurosurg Psychiatry* 2003; **74**(7):852–856.

55. Apaydin H, Ahlskog JE, Parisi JE, Boeve BF, Dickson DW, Parkinson disease

neuropathology: later-developing dementia and loss of the levodopa response. *Arch Neurol* 2002; **59**(1):102–112.

56. Harding AJ, Broe GA, Halliday GM, Visual hallucinations in Lewy body disease relate to Lewy bodies in the temporal lobe. *Brain* 2002; **125**(Pt 2):391–403.

57. Kovari E, Gold G, Herrmann FR et al, Lewy body densities in the entorhinal and anterior cingulate cortex predict cognitive deficits in Parkinson's disease. *Acta Neuropathol (Berl)* 2003; **106**(1):83–88.

58. Mastaglia FL, Johnsen RD, Byrnes ML, Kakulas BA, Prevalence of amyloid-beta deposition in the cerebral cortex in Parkinson's disease. *Mov Disord* 2003; **18**:81–86.

59. Jellinger KA, Seppi K, Wenning GK et al, Impact of coexistent Alzheimer pathology on the natural history of Parkinson's disease. *J Neural Transm* 2002; **109**:329–339.

60. Duda JE, Pathology and neurotransmitter abnormalities of dementia with Lewy bodies. *Dement Geriatr Cogn Disord* 2004; **17**(Suppl 1):3–14.

61. Piggott MA, Owens J, O'Brien J et al, Muscarinic receptors in basal ganglia in dementia with Lewy bodies, Parkinson's disease, and Alzheimer's disease. *J Chem Neuroanat* 2003; **25**:161–173.

62. O'Brien JT, Colloby S, Fenwick J et al, Dopamine transporter loss visualized with FP-CIT SPECT in the differential diagnosis of dementia with Lewy bodies. *Arch Neurol* 2004; **61**(6):919–925.

63. Court JA, Piggott MA, Lloyd S et al, Nicotine binding in human striatum: elevation in schizophrenia and reductions in dementia with Lewy bodies, Parkinson's disease, and Alzheimer's disease in relation to neuroleptic medication. *Neuroscience* 2000; **98**:78–87.

64. Ballard C, Piggott MA, Johnson M et al, Delusions associated with elevated muscarinic binding in dementia with Lewy bodies. *Ann Neurol* 2000; **48**:868–876.

65. Perry EK, Irving D, Kerwin JM et al, Cholinergic transmitter and neurotrophic activities in Lewy body dementia: similarity to Parkinson's disease and distinction from Alzheimer's disease. *Alzheimer Dis Assoc Disord* 1993; **7**(2):69–79.

66. Pimlott SL, Piggott MA, Johnson M et al, Nicotinic acetylcholine receptor distribution in Alzheimer's disease, dementia with Lewy bodies, Parkinson's disease, and vascular dementia: in vitro binding study using 5–[(125)i]-a-85380. *Neuropsychopharmacology* 2004; **29**:108–116.

67. Barber R, Ballard C, McKeith IG, Gholkar A, O'Brien JT, MRI volumetric study of dementia with Lewy bodies: a comparison with AD and vascular dementia. *Neurology* 2000; **54**(6):1304–1309.

68. Brenneis C, Wenning GK, Egger KE et al, Basal forebrain atrophy is a distinctive pattern in dementia with Lewy bodies. *Neuroreport* 2004; **15**(11):1711–1714.

69. Gilman S, Koeppe RA, Little R et al, Striatal monoamine terminals in Lewy body dementia and Alzheimer's disease. *Ann Neurol* 2004; **55**:774–780.

70. Ballard C, O'Brien J, Swann A et al, One year follow-up of parkinsonism in dementia with Lewy bodies: A cross-sectional comparison study. *Dement Geriatr Cogn Disord* 2000; **11**:219–222.

71. Poewe WH, Wenning GK, The natural history of Parkinson's disease. *Neurology* 1996; **47**(Suppl 3):S146–S152.

72. Levy G, Tang M-X, Cote LJ et al, Motor impairment in PD. Relationship to incident dementia and age. *Neurology* 2000; **55**:539–544.

73. Aarsland D, Larsen JP, Tandberg E et al, Predictors of nursing home placement in Parkinson's disease: a population-based prospective study. *J Am Ger Soc* 2000; **48**:938–942.

74. Simard M, van Reekum R, The acetylcholinesterase inhibitors for treatment of

cognitive and behavioral symptoms in dementia with Lewy bodies. *J Neuropsychiatry Clin Neurosci* 2004; **16**(4):409–425.

75. McKeith IG, Del Ser T, Spano P et al, Efficacy of rivastigmine in dementia with Lewy bodies: a randomized, double-blind, placebo-controlled international study. *Lancet* 2000; **356**:2031–2036.

76. Beversdorf DQ, Warner JL, Davis RA, Sharma UK, Nagaraja HN, Scharre DW, Donepezil in the treatment of dementia with Lewy bodies. *Am J Geriatr Psychiatry* 2004; **12**(5):542–544.

77. Emre M, Aarsland D, Albanese A et al, Rivastigmine for dementia associated with Parkinson's disease. *New Engl J Med* 2004; **351**(24):2509–2518.

78. Aarsland D, Laake K, Larsen JP, Janvin C, Donepezil for cognitive impairment in Parkinson's disease: a randomized controlled study. *J Neurol Neurosurg Psychiatry* 2002; **72**:708–712.

79. Leroi I, Brandt J, Reich SG et al, Randomized placebo controlled trial of donepezil in cognitive impairment in Parkinson's disease. *Int J Geriatr Psychiatry* 2004; **19**(1):1–8.

80. Minett TS, Thomas A, Wilkinson LM et al, What happens when donepezil is suddenly withdrawn? An open label trial in dementia with Lewy bodies and Parkinson's disease with dementia. *Int J Geriatr Psychiatry* 2003; **18**(11):988–993.

81. Kaufer DI, Pharmacologic treatment expectations in the management of dementia with Lewy bodies. *Dement Geriatr Cogn Disord* 2004; **17**:32–39.

82. Newby VJ, Kenny RA, McKeith IG, Donepezil and cardiac syncope: case report (letter). *Int J Geriatr Psychiatry* 2004; **19**:1110–1112.

83. Ballard C, Grace J, McKeith I et al, Neuroleptic sensitivity in dementia with Lewy bodies and Alzheimer's disease (letter). *Lancet* 1998; **351**:1032–1033.

84. Friedman JH, Lannon MC, Factor SA et al, Low dose clozapine for the treatment of drug-induced psychosis (DIP) in idiopathic Parkinson's disease (PD): results of the double-blind, placebo-controlled PSYCLOPS trial. *Neurology* 1998; **50**:70.

85. Burn DJ, McKeith IG, Current treatment of dementia with Lewy bodies and dementia associated with Parkinson's disease. *Mov Disord* 2003; **18**(6):S72–S79.

86. Aarsland D, Mosimann UP, McKeith IG, Role of cholinesterase inhibitors in Parkinson's disease and dementia with Lewy bodies. *J Geriatr Psychiatry Neurol* 2004; **17**(3):164–171.

87. Collins B, Constant J, Kaba S, Barclay CL, Mohr E, Dementia with Lewy bodies. Implications for clinical trials. *Clin Neuropharmacol* 2004; **27**(6):281–292.

chapter 8

Depression

Daniel Weintraub, Paul E Holtzheimer III and William M McDonald

Introduction

Parkinson's disease (PD) is the second most common degenerative neurological disorder, affecting approximately one million individuals in the US. Although PD is primarily a movement disorder, the high prevalence of psychiatric complications suggests that PD could more accurately be conceptualized as a neuropsychiatric disease. Affective and cognitive dysfunctions, though receiving less attention than motor aspects of the disease, have long been recognized as a part of PD. In first describing the clinical profile of PD in his 1817 monograph, James Parkinson acknowledged depression as a cardinal feature of the illness, stating of one patient, "A more melancholy object I never beheld."[1]

Although depression is common in PD, occurring in up to one-half of patients,[2] there is an incomplete understanding of its clinical presentation, its neuropathophysiology, and how best to treat it. Reports on the frequency of depression have varied depending on the research setting, the type of depression being studied, and the diagnostic criteria that are used; appropriate criteria for a diagnosis of depression in PD (dPD) are confounded by symptom overlap such as insomnia, psychomotor changes, and fatigue. In addition, depression frequently co-occurs with other non-motor symptoms, including anxiety, psychosis, and cognitive impairment.

The neurobiological and neuroanatomical changes that occur in PD suggest a pathophysiological basis for the psychiatric symptoms, although "reactive depression" can also occur. Antidepressants are regularly prescribed in PD, even though their efficacy and effectiveness have not been adequately assessed, and their possible impact on parkinsonism is unknown.

Depression in PD has been associated with excess disability, poorer outcomes, and caregiver distress. Therefore, it is important to identify and address current impediments to the diagnosis and treatment of depression in this population, particularly as it appears to be underrecognized and undertreated in clinical practice.[3,4]

This chapter is an overview of the prevalence of mood disorders in PD and their impact on disability, quality of life, and outcomes. The etiology and pathophysiology of dPD will be reviewed, focusing primarily on the contribution of disease-specific neurobiological changes. Clinical correlates and co-morbid non-motor symptoms will be covered, as well as a review of existing knowledge on the treatment of dPD.

Epidemiology

The majority of epidemiological studies on dPD report prevalence rates between 20–40%, with estimates varying from less than 5% to as high as 75%.[5-8] This variation reflects methodological differences between the studies, including sampling methods, survey sites, and assessment tools both to define depression and to quantify the severity of depressive symptoms. More recent studies using community samples and formal diagnostic criteria (e.g., Diagnostic and Statistical Manual of Mental Disorders[9] [DSM-IV] criteria) have reported that *major* depression may occur in 5–10% of PD patients, with an additional 10–30% experiencing either *minor* or *subsyndromal* depression.[7,10-13] Although the typical depression case may be non-severe, the evidence in total suggests that dPD is common.

Impact and course of depression in PD

The presence of dPD is associated with excess disability,[13,14] worse quality of life,[15] and increased caregiver distress,[16] and it exacerbates the physical and emotional burden that PD places on patients and their caregivers. In a survey of PD patients, caregivers, and clinicians in six countries, depressive symptoms were the single most important factor in patient quality of life ratings, even ranking ahead of disease severity.[17]

Preliminary longitudinal research indicates that dPD is associated with impairment in fine motor skills,[18] more rapid progression of motor impairment and disability,[19] and the development of psychosis.[20] Depression may also be a risk factor for global cognitive impairment[19,21,22] or dementia.[23,24] Future studies need to determine whether successful treatment of depression can ameliorate such secondary impairments.

Little is known about the long-term course of dPD. It has been reported to be a chronic illness,[19] and one naturalistic study found that only one-third of patients with depression at baseline showed an improvement in their symptoms over a 9-year period.[25]

Etiology and pathophysiology

Theories related to the etiology of dPD argue that depression either (1) is "reactive" and secondary to the psychosocial stress of a chronic disease, or (2) results from neurodegenerative changes that occur in PD. These two theories are not mutually exclusive and are discussed below.

It was once thought that depression occurred primarily in the early and late stages of PD, with patients in the middle stages typically unaffected. These findings supported the hypothesis that dPD could be subdivided into "psychological" and "biological" subtypes: the diagnosis of a chronic, progressive, and disabling illness was presumed to effect a psychological depression in early PD, while advanced neurodegeneration (i.e., cell death, dysfunction in neural pathways, and neurotransmitter depletion) in late PD was said to underlie a biological depression.

PD patients and their families clearly have to adjust to managing a chronic illness that may result in significant impairment in physical, occupational, interpersonal, social, sexual, and recreational domains. They are acutely aware that there is no cure for the disease and that existing treatments are palliative and lose effectiveness over time. In many patients there are symptoms of a reactive depression, particularly at the time of initial diagnosis. Findings from studies that reported an association between depression and early-onset PD[12,26] suggest that younger patients may experience more significant career, family, and financial disruptions.[27]

However, the high rates of dPD are not completely explained as a reaction to the stress of the illness. Some researchers have found that PD patients have more depressive symptoms than patients with other chronic disabling diseases.[28,29] In addition, recent research on the association between severity of depression and stage or severity of PD has been equivocal.[5,21,28,29]

Interesting findings suggesting a biological basis for dPD comes from case-control studies and prospective studies using large case registries. This research has found that PD patients have a higher lifetime prevalence of anxiety and depressive disorders,[30] than non-PD controls patients with depression are at higher risk of subsequently developing PD.[31] These findings implicate depression as a potential risk factor for or a prodromal symptom of PD in some patients.

From a biological standpoint, the high frequency of dPD has been explained by dysfunction in the following brain regions, pathways, and neurotransmitters: (1) subcortical nuclei and the frontal lobes; (2) basal ganglia-thalamic-frontal cortex circuit and the basotemporal limbic circuit; and (3) brainstem monoamine and indolamine systems (i.e., dopamine, serotonin, and norepinephrine (noradrenaline)).

One previous PET study in PD found an association between depressive symptoms and altered basal ganglia metabolism.[32] Another region implicated in depression is the limbic system, and in PD depressed patients were found to have reduced basal limbic system echogenicity using structural neuroimaging.[33] Functional brain imaging studies have reported simultaneous frontal cortex and basal ganglia hypometabolism in PD patients with depression, changes which are presumed to reflect neurodegeneration of the cortical-striatal-thalamo-cortical circuits.[32,34]

Regarding neurotransmitters, a disproportionate degeneration of dopamine neurons in the ventral tegmental area (VTA) has been reported in patients with a history of dPD.[35] Other monoaminergic neurotransmitter systems (e.g., serotonin and norepinephrine) are also significantly affected in PD. Imaging studies have found both a decrease in signal intensity of the pontomesencephalic midline structures, which contain neural pathways originating in monoaminergic brainstem nuclei, in depressed PD patients,[33] and a negative correlation between UPDRS depression items and dorsal midbrain binding ratios, which reflect regional serotonin transporter densities.[36] In addition, preliminary research has demonstrated associations between dPD and a functional polymorphism (the short allele) in the promoter region of the serotonin transporter (5-HT)[37,38] and reduced CSF levels of the serotonin metabolite 5-hydroxyindolacetic acid (5-HIAA).[39]

If the combination of pan-neurotransmitter deficits and the disruption in cortico-subcortical pathways contributes to the high prevalence of dPD, then this characteristic and perhaps unique combination of neurobiological changes may dictate different depression treatment strategies than those commonly employed for depression in the non-PD population. For instance, depressed PD patients do not demonstrate the euphoric response to psycho-stimulant medication seen in non-PD depressed patients,[40] which suggests that structurally related antidepressants (e.g., bupropion) may not be as effective in this population.

Clinical correlates

Some epidemiological studies have found that dPD is associated with being female,[10] having a personal history of depression,[5] early-onset PD (i.e., before age 55),[12,26] right-sided (left brain) predominant motor symptoms,[5] and atypical parkinsonism (e.g., prominent akinesia-rigidity or extensive vascular disease).[11,21] However, non-confirmatory results mean that consensus has not been reached on clinical correlates of dPD.

Patients with long-standing exposure to levodopa frequently develop motor fluctuations, including dyskinesias during "on" periods and worsening parkinsonism during "off" periods. In some patients, "off" periods are associated with temporary dysphoria and anxiety[41] which may be relieved by levodopa administration,[42] but in others there does not appear to be an association between either "off" states and worsening mood or "on" states and improved mood.[43] While such brief mood changes may not meet criteria for existing affective disorders, they can be debilitating and distressing to patients. In addition, patients with mood fluctuations in the context of motor fluctuations are more likely to also have dPD and other neuropsychiatric complications.[44]

Surgery has become increasingly common as a treatment for PD. Pallidotomy and thalamotomy are well-established ablative surgical treatments, and in general neither is thought to have significant cognitive or psychiatric sequelae.[45] Non-ablative deep brain stimulation (DBS), usually of the sub-thalamic nucleus (STN), has become the most common surgical treatment for PD. However, the impact of DBS on psychiatric symptoms and cognition appears varied. A number of psychiatric side-effects have been reported with STN DBS, including depression, mania, psychosis, and delirium,[46–48] but there is research reporting both improvement and worsening in mental status post-DBS.[49] The STN has a heterogeneous organization that includes connections to limbic regions, which may explain the reported association with mood changes in some patients.

Common co-morbid non-motor symptoms in depression

Psychosis,[50,51] anxiety,[52] apathy,[53] fatigue,[54] and insomnia[55] have all been associated with dPD. Research suggests not only a significant association between psychosis and depressive disorders, but that depressed patients non-responsive to antidepressant treatment are more likely to have co-morbid psychosis.[4] The majority of patients with a depression diagnosis also meet criteria for an anxiety disorder, and vice versa.[52] Although apathy is thought to be a distinct psychiatric syndrome associated with frontal lobe impairment,[56] there is extensive overlap between depression and apathy in PD.[53] It is unclear to what extent these co-morbid psychiatric symptoms either are secondary to or lead to depression, are associated with underlying cognitive impairment and not independently associated with depression, are core features of PD, or are secondary to the pharmacologic treatment of PD (i.e., dopamine toxicity).

Cognitive impairment is a common non-motor complication of PD that is made worse by depression.[22,57] Depressive symptoms early in the course of PD are related to a more rapid cognitive decline[19] and an increased risk of developing dementia.[58] Conversely, cognitive impairment has been associated with an increased risk of developing depression in some studies,[21] and the combination of dementia and depression is correlated with lower levels of CSF 5-HIAA in PD than either dementia or depression alone.[59] Interestingly, PD patients with major depression have significantly greater cognitive decline and decline in functional ability than patients with minor depression when followed over time, suggesting qualitative differences between different types of depression in this population.[19]

Among common cognitive changes that occur in PD, executive impairment in particular has been associated with depression.[60–62] These frontal system deficits may be due to the additive effects of PD and depression.[22] Non-PD elderly patients with major depression have been reported to demonstrate significant impairment in executive functioning compared with elderly controls, and non-responders to antidepressant treatment had more executive dysfunction than responders.[63] The exact nature of the association in PD between executive dysfunction and depression, its potential to confound depression by presenting with co-morbid apathy, its impact on the outcome of antidepressant treatment, and its reversibility with successful antidepressant treatment all remain in question. It has been argued that D_2/D_3 dopamine agonists (e.g., pramipexole and ropinirole) might be appropriate for the depression-executive dysfunction syndrome of late life.[64]

Relationship of co-morbid medical disorders to depression

Hypothyroidism, testosterone deficiency, elevated plasma homocysteine, and vitamin B_{12} deficiency levels have all been associated with depression in non-PD populations, although research linking these disorders to dPD has been sparse. These disorders may go unrecognized, as their clinical symptoms overlap with PD, particularly PD complicated by depression.

Homocysteine is a by-product in the metabolic pathway of levodopa, and increased homocysteine levels are correlated with long-term treatment with levodopa/carbidopa, a complication that can be managed with folic acid supplementation. A recent study found that PD patients with elevated homocysteine levels were more depressed than patients with normal homo-cysteine levels.[65] Administration of 800–3600 mg per day of S-adenosyl-methionine (SAM), which plays a role in the metabolism of homocysteine, has improved dPD in a preliminary study.[66]

Depression is a common complication of hypothyroidism, and the incidence of hypothyroidism in PD is increased.[67] However, hypothyroidism may be difficult to diagnose clinically in this population because the symptoms of poor concentration, fatigue, flat affect, and bradykinesia overlap with PD symptoms. In addition, certain PD medications (e.g., levo-dopa) may inhibit thyroid-stimulating hormone (TSH) in patients with primary hypothyroidism and mask the laboratory diagnosis early in the disease.[67] Therefore, to screen for hypothyroidism in PD it is also necessary to check T_3 and T_4 levels.

Testosterone levels decline progressively with age, and approximately 20–25% of males >60 years of age show signs of clinical hypogonadism. Many symptoms of testosterone deficiency are non-specific and overlap with non-motor symptoms of PD, such as decreased enjoyment of life, lack of energy, sexual dysfunction, and depression. In a preliminary open-label study, testosterone-deficient men with PD who were administered testosterone replacement therapy showed a suggestion of improvement in anxiety scores, verbal fluency, and part I of the UPDRS, which covers psychosis, depression, and cognitive impairment.[68]

Vitamin B_{12} deficiency is associated with a variety of neuropsychiatric symptoms, including depression,[69] and is relatively common in older patients. Therefore, an evaluation of B_{12} status should be included in the workup of PD patients presenting with mood symptoms.

Presentation, assessment and diagnosis of depression

Assessing dPD is challenging, partly as a result of symptom overlap with core PD symptoms (e.g., insomnia, psychomotor slowing, difficulty concentrating, and fatigue). In addition, PD patients may withdraw from social activities not only as a result of depression, but if they are uncomfortable being in public when experiencing tremors or dyskinesias. Even the appearance of a patient with PD (e.g., bradykinetic movements and flat facies) can be mistaken for that of someone with severe, melancholic depression.

Non-somatic symptoms of depression (e.g., suicide ideation, anhedonia, feelings of guilt, and psychic anxiety) are more likely to indicate the presence of a depressive disorder in PD than are somatic symptoms (e.g., sleep and appetite changes, low energy, and psychomotor retardation).[70] There is also evidence that depressed PD patients have a different symptom profile than depressed patients without PD. This profile includes higher rates of anxiety, pessimism, irrationality, suicide ideation without suicide behavior, and less guilt and self-reproach.[8,71]

Also complicating the diagnostic process is the common occurrence of other affective disturbances that can confound depression. For instance, PD patients can experience brief episodes of tearfulness, variably termed affective lability, "pseudobulbar" affect, emotionalism, or "emotional incontinence." The tearfulness is typically mood-incongruent or regarded as excessive and not necessarily associated with an underlying depressive disorder. In addition, PD patients frequently experience apathy, which can give the appearance of depression. Since dPD is frequently co-morbid with other non-motor symptoms (such as psychosis and cognitive impairment), it may be difficult to categorize syndromes for which depressive symptoms are but one component.

When depression is suspected, the clinician should begin with a careful history and physical examination. A past history of depression is a predictor of future depression. Recent changes in mood and behavior should be assessed within the context of the patient's current PD treatment (e.g., potential on-off phenomena or recent surgery). The DSM-IV recommends using an exclusive or disease-etiologic approach (i.e., not considering a specific criterion to be met if its presence is better explained by PD rather than depression).[72,73] However, this approach is difficult to put into practice, due to symptom overlap between PD and depression.

We recommend that the clinician focus on symptoms of depressed mood and/or anhedonia (loss of interest and pleasure), questioning both the patient and available family members about changes from baseline. If the clinician notes a significant change in mood, loss of interest or pleasure in activities, increased crying spells, guilt, or a sense of despair or hopelessness, then a more focused interview on depressive symptoms should ensue. At this point, the clinician should inquire about the presence of vegetative symptoms (e.g., sleep, appetite, energy, and concentration), without regard to etiology, in order to determine if the patient meets criteria for major depression. Patients with PD can also have other clinically significant depressive disturbances that do not meet criteria for major depression. These include disorders such as minor depression, dysthymia, subsyndromal depression, and adjustment disorders.

Case example 1

A 65-year-old man with PD presents with a worsening of his motor symptoms. He has become increasingly withdrawn because he is concerned that he may become "frozen" (i.e., unable to move) when in public. His sleep is erratic because he cannot turn over in bed and he has to get up to urinate several times a night. He has little energy when he is off, but says he feels pretty good when his medication "kicks in." He is pleasant and cooperative on interview and says that he would love to get a medication that could "help me get out and play golf again."

This man has a number of symptoms of depression (withdrawal, insomnia, and fatigue), but would not meet formal criteria for a depressive disorder. His withdrawal is not due to a lack of interest but an understandable concern about his worsening motor symptoms. He would in fact enjoy playing golf and the interaction with him in the office shows that his mood is quite good, all things considered.

Case example 2

Compare that case with a second patient who has similar symptoms, but with a clear depressive component. A 65-year-old man with PD presents with a worsening of his PD motor symptoms. He has become increasingly withdrawn because he is concerned that he may become "frozen" in public. His sleep is erratic because he cannot turn over in bed and he has to get up to urinate several times a night. He has little energy when he is off but says he feels pretty good when his medication "kicks in." He is quiet and evasive when you talk with him in your office. His wife expresses concern that he is no longer interested in the grandchildren when they come over, and in fact goes to his bedroom when he hears the doorbell ring. He refuses to answer the phone. He used to be an avid golfer, but when asked about playing or perhaps accompanying his son on a golf outing, he says that he knows he will never play again and there is no use in trying.

The second patient has similar symptoms but a very different tone to the interview. His withdrawal is not simply due to a concern over being "frozen," but also to a loss of interest. He no longer wants to play golf and thinks he can never play again. He is clearly depressed in his interaction with the physician and shows the typical pessimism and lack of interaction that would be expected of a depressed patient. This patient should probably be offered treatment for depression.

The high prevalence of dPD necessitates that all patients be screened for depression on a regular basis. Depression screening tools can be useful, though they have not been comprehensively evaluated in PD. One commonly used instrument, the Geriatric Depression Scale (GDS) uses a "yes/no" format, is self-administered, and emphasizes the cognitive symptoms of depression. There are 30- and 15-item versions of the GDS, and a cut-off score of 5 on the 15-item GDS demonstrated high sensitivity and low specificity for a diagnosis of depression in a primary care setting.[74] Thus, a more detailed evaluation for depression should occur with a score >4 on the 15-item GDS (or >9 on the 30-item version).

The Beck Depression Inventory (BDI) is another self-rated instrument that is more strongly weighted to assess cognitive symptoms of depression (e.g., guilt and loss of pleasure). Research with the BDI has determined optimal cutoff scores of 13/14 for distinguishing PD patients with and without a DSM-IV depression diagnosis and 8/9 for depression screening.[73]

The Hamilton Depression Rating Scale (HDRS) is used primarily in clinical research. The Montgomery Asberg Depression Rating Scale (MADRS) is also used in research settings but can be used in clinical practice to monitor the course of depression. Unlike the GDS and BDI, both the HDRS and MADRS are administered by a trained rater. A cutoff score of 14/15 on the MADRS was found to be optimal both for discriminating PD patients with and without a DSM-IV depression diagnosis and for depression screening.[75]

It is important to involve a patient's caregiver or significant other in the assessment and treatment process, even with non-demented patients, both to provide collateral information and to enhance treatment compliance. PD patients are often perceived as withdrawn and depressed by observers, even when they do not endorse depressed mood.[76] This suggests that others may be misinterpreting non-depressive symptoms in the patient with PD. However, this could also indicate that the patient may lack insight into their mood disturbance.

The impact of depression on caregiver well-being and health should also be considered. Addressing relevant psychosocial concerns (e.g., support in the home, cost of medications and assistive devices, transportation issues, and changes in lifestyle) may help improve overall quality of life for both the caregiver and patient.

Consultation with a geriatric psychiatrist or neuropsychiatrist should be considered in difficult cases. These cases would include patients in which there is diagnostic uncertainty or those with treatment-resistant depression, suicide ideation, psychosis, and co-morbid conditions, including panic disorder and mania. Treatment-resistant depression is usually defined as a patient who has failed three or more antidepressant trials when the trials were of sufficient length (e.g., at least 8 weeks) and dosage. In clinical practice, patients frequently do not tolerate medications, cannot afford them, or simply do not finish a course of medication because they are not convinced that they are depressed, or, at least, have a depressive disturbance warranting specific treatment. Consultation with a psychiatrist and close follow-up and counseling may increase treatment adherence. "Watchful waiting" with a follow-up appointment within 2–4 weeks to monitor the patient's status can also be a useful strategy when the diagnosis is unclear.

PD depression with co-morbid psychosis is complicated. The antiparkinsonian medications are associated with the development of psychosis, and certain conditions including mania and depression are also associated with psychosis. The etiology of the psychosis should inform the decision of whether to treat the psychosis by decreasing the PD medication or by adding another medication (e.g., an antipsychotic). Similarly, panic disorder can be a co-morbid condition or simply anxiety related to a fear of going "off." A psychiatrist can often help clarify these diagnostic issues.

The presence of suicide ideation or mania suggests a complex psychiatric problem and should also trigger a referral to a psychiatrist. Generally, PD patients do not express suicide ideation, though some describe having a plan to end their life if they became so disabled that they could no longer function. Suicide ideation should prompt an immediate referral for further evaluation. Manic depressive illness or bipolar disorder can also be very difficult to manage in PD. The anti-PD medications can make mania worse, and the medications used to treat mania (e.g., lithium, valproic acid, and atypical antipsychotics) can worsen parkinsonism. Again, a referral to a psychiatrist familiar with PD may help with the assessment, formulation, and treatment of these patients.

Treatment of depression in PD

The results of numerous open-label trials using selective serotonin reuptake inhibitors (SSRIs) and other newer antidepressants in PD suggest a positive effect and reasonable tolerability for active treatment.[77–81] However, efficacy can only be established through the conduct of placebo-controlled studies, and at the time of this submission there have been only three published, placebo-controlled antidepressant treatment studies for depression in PD.[82–84] One study showed efficacy for a tricyclic antidepressant (nortriptyline). However, tricyclic antidepressants can be difficult for PD patients to tolerate because they can aggravate PD-associated orthostatic hypotension, constipation, dry mouth, and cognitive problems. The other two studies evaluated SSRIs and showed no difference between the two; however, these studies were underpowered and reported large effect sizes for both active treatment and placebo condition. There is some concern about SSRIs worsening parkinsonism,[85,86] perhaps by increasing serotonin-mediated inhibition from the raphe nucleus and decreasing dopamine release from the nigrostriatal pathway.[87] However, clinical experience and the results of two placebo-controlled studies and numerous open-label studies suggest that most PD patients are able to tolerate SSRI treatment without clinically significant worsening of their parkinsonism.[77–81] Notwithstanding, it is important that the safety and tolerability of antidepressants in PD be tested in the context of placebo-controlled trials.

Examining the experience of patients receiving routine clinical care, it was reported that half of PD patients currently taking an antidepressant at an adequate dosage[88] still met DSM-IV criteria for a depressive disorder.[4] This finding may partly have been due to under-treatment, as only 11% (1/9) of patients taking an antidepressant and still meeting criteria for depression were taking an antidepressant dosage within the highest recommended range, and only 33% (3/9) had received more than one antidepressant trial. This research also found that the overwhelming majority of PD patients in clinical practice are treated primarily and solely with an SSRI, yet a recent review found insufficient data supporting the effectiveness and safety of this class of medications in PD to recommend their use.[89]

Several PD medications have been used in the treatment of depression. Levodopa is not thought to have a consistent mood-elevating or -depressing effect, although there have been case reports of patients using levodopa for its stimulating effects. Preliminary studies have reported the effectiveness of the dopamine agonist pramipexole as an antidepressant in both non-PD and PD populations.[90] It is important to determine whether the combination of a dopamine agonist and an antidepressant is superior to either alone, and if dopamine agonists offer prophylaxis against the development of depression in PD. In addition, selegiline, a selective monoamine oxidase B (MAO-B) inhibitor at lower dosages, has been reported to have antidepressant properties, although it is not commonly used either as an antidepressant or a PD medication. There also has been concern that the combination of selegiline and SSRIs might lead to serotonin syndrome, although clinical experience suggests that the combination is safe.[91]

Many questions remain concerning the pharmacologic treatment of dPD. For instance, it is unclear if the altered neural substrate (e.g., impairment of neural pathways servicing the frontal lobe and multiple monoaminergic deficits) means PD patients will experience a more limited or variable response to standard antidepressant treatment than that reported in other populations. Also, the appropriate dosing titration schedules and final therapeutic ranges for antidepressant use in PD have yet to be established. Likewise, the duration of antidepressant treatment for PD patients is not clear, including as to whether chronic antidepressant therapy is indicated for select patients or in general.

Concerning non-pharmacologic approaches, electroconvulsive therapy (ECT) can successfully treat both depression and the motor symptoms associated with PD, although the motor benefits wear off once treatment is discontinued.[92] Two open trials of transcranial magnetic stimulation (TMS) for dPD reported a moderate improvement in both mood and motor symptoms.[93,94]

It is unclear whether there is a place for psychotherapy (e.g., cognitive behavioral therapy (CBT) or problem-solving therapy (PST)) in the treatment of dPD, either as an alternative first-line treatment or as an approach to rehabilitation for those with partial medication response. Anecdotally, however, there are many PD patients who prefer psychotherapy, do not respond to pharmacotherapy, or are reluctant to take another medication, for fear of side-effects or to avoid adding to an already complex medication regimen, so psychotherapy may be an important alternative. When using psychotherapy in PD, we have often found it helpful to involve significant others in the psychotherapeutic process.

Given the available evidence, it is reasonable to begin treatment of depression in PD with an SSRI. While the safety and efficacy of SSRIs have not been firmly established in dPD, the potential risks and benefits of using these medications must be weighed against the risks of an untreated depressive episode. If an SSRI is not completely effective, there are very little data to guide clinical practice, though we would suggest substituting or adding a "newer" antidepressant with a different pharmacological profile. These medications might include antidepressants that affect both serotonin and norepinephrine (noradrenaline), such as venlafaxine, duloxetine, or mirtazapine, or a medication such as the unicyclic aminoketone, bupropion, a norepinephrine reuptake inhibitor and relatively weak dopamine reuptake inhibitor. If the patient has failed two adequate trials of antidepressant therapy, consultation with a psychiatrist may help resolve any diagnostic issues and provide additional guidance on appropriate somatic treatments (including the use of tricyclic antidepressants and ECT).

The addition of psychotherapy may be beneficial, especially in patients without significant cognitive impairment or psychosis. Although not a specific treatment for depression, it is believed that regular exercise optimizes both physical and mental health in PD. Other non-motor symptoms, such as insomnia, daytime fatigue, and pain, may contribute to depression, so it is important to diagnose and treat these symptoms when they are present. Finally, assessment and treatment of any contributing co-morbid medical conditions (e.g., hypothyroidism, B_{12} deficiency, etc.) is important.

Conclusion

Depression occurs in approximately half of PD patients, increases both motor and cognitive disability, and is a primary source of both patient and caregiver distress. The high prevalence of depression in PD cannot be explained solely as a reaction to psychosocial stress and is due in part to neurodegeneration affecting neurons in the basal ganglia, disruption in cortico-striatal and basotemporal limbic circuit pathways, and pan-monoamine deficiencies. There is great interindividual variability in the presentation of depression in PD, and consistent clinical and biological correlates have not been established. Diagnosing depression in PD is challenging, primarily due to frequent co-morbid non-motor conditions, cognitive impairment, and symptom overlap between depression and PD itself. Although uncontrolled studies and clinical experience suggest that antidepressant treatment overall is well-tolerated and beneficial to many patients, efficacy and tolerability has yet to be demonstrated in a double-blind, placebo-controlled trial. There is a pressing need for additional research in PD depression to validate diagnostic criteria, to develop sensitive and specific instruments for screening and measuring severity of depression, to better understand its neurobiological basis, to establish efficacious and effective forms of treatment, and to determine moderators and mediators of treatment response.

References

1. Parkinson J, *An Essay on the Shaking Palsy*. Sherwood, Neely and Jones: London, 1817.
2. Dooneief G, Mirabello E, Bell K, Marder K, Stern Y, Mayeux R, An estimate of the incidence of depression in idiopathic Parkinson's disease. *Arch Neurol* 1992; **49**:305–307.
3. Shulman LM, Taback RL, Rabinstein AA et al, Non-recognition of depression and other non-motor symptoms in Parkinson's disease. *Parkinsonism Relat Disord* 2002; **8**:193–197.
4. Weintraub D, Moberg PJ, Duda JE et al, Recognition and treatment of depression in Parkinson's disease. *J Geriatr Psychiatry Neurol* 2003; **16**:178–183.
5. Starkstein SE, Preziosi TJ, Bolduc PL et al, Depression in Parkinson's disease. *J Nervous Mental Dis* 1990; **178**:27–31.
6. Allain H, Schuck S, Manduit N, Depression in Parkinson's disease. *BMJ* 2000; **320**:1287–1288.

7. Hantz P, Caradoc-Davies G, Caradoc-Davies T et al, Depression in Parkinson's disease. *Am J Psychiatry* 1994; **151**:1010–1014.

8. Cummings JL, Depression and Parkinson's disease: a review. *Am J Psychiatry* 1992; **149**:443–454.

9. First MB, Spitzer RL, Gibbon M et al, *Structured Clinical Interview for DSM-IV Axis I Disorders (SCID), Clinician Version.* American Psychiatric Press: Washington, DC, 1996.

10. Tandberg E, Larsen JP, Aarsland D et al, The occurrence of depression in Parkinson's disease. A community-based study. *Arch Neurol* 1996; **53**:175–179.

11. Starkstein SE, Petracca G, Chemerinski E et al, Depression in classic versus akinetic-rigid Parkinson's disease. *Mov Disord* 1998; **13**:29–33.

12. Cole SA, Woodard JL, Juncos JL et al, Depression and disability in Parkinson's disease. *J Neuropsychiat Clin Neurosci* 1996; **8**:20–25.

13. Liu CY, Wang SJ, Fuh JL et al, The correlation of depression with functional activity in Parkinson's disease. *J Neurol* 1997; **244**:493–498.

14. Weintraub D, Moberg PJ, Duda JE et al, Impact of psychiatric and other non-motor symptoms on disability in Parkinson's disease. *J Am Geriatr Soc* 2004; **52**:784–788.

15. Schrag A, Jahanshahi M, Quinn N, What contributes to quality of life in patients with Parkinson's disease. *J Neurol Neurosurg Psychiatry* 2000; **69**:308–312.

16. Aarsland D, Larsen JP, Tandberg E, Laake K, Predictors of nursing home placement in Parkinson's disease: a population-based, prospective study. *J Am Geriatr Soc* 2000; **48**:938–942.

17. Global Parkinson's Disease Study Steering Committee, Factors impacting on quality of life in Parkinson's disease: results from an international survey. *Mov Disord* 2002; **17**:60–67.

18. Kuhn W, Heye N, Müller Th et al, The motor performance test series in Parkinson's disease is influenced by depression. *J Neural Trans* 1996; **103**:349–354.

19. Starkstein SE, Mayberg HS, Leiguarda R, Preziosi TJ, Robinson RG, A prospective longitudinal study of depression, cognitive decline, and physical impairments in patients with Parkinson's disease. *J Neurol Neurosurg Psychiatry* 1992; **55**:377–382.

20. Giladi N, Treves TA, Paleacu D et al, Risk factors for dementia, depression and psychosis in long-standing Parkinson's disease. *J Neurol Trans* 2000; **107**:59–71.

21. Tandberg E, Larsen JP, Aarsland D et al, Risk factors for depression in Parkinson disease. *Arch Neurol* 1997; **54**:625–630.

22. Tröster AI, Stalp LD, Paolo AM, Fields JA, Koller WC, Neuropsychological impairment in Parkinson's disease with and without depression. *Arch Neurol* 1995; **52**:1164–1169.

23. Marder K, Tang M-X, Cote L et al, The frequency and associated risk factors for dementia in patients with Parkinson's disease. *Arch Neurol* 1995; **52**:695–701.

24. Stern Y, Marder K, Tang M-X et al, Antecedent clinical features associated with dementia in Parkinson's disease. *Neurology* 1993; **43**:1690–1692.

25. Rojo A, Aguilar M, Garolera MT et al, Depression in Parkinson's disease: clinical correlates and outcome. *Parkinsonism Relat Disord* 2003; **10**:23–28.

26. Kostic VS, Filipovic SR, Lecic D et al, Effect of age at onset of frequency of depression in Parkinson's disease. *J Neurol Neurosurg Psychiat* 1994; **57**:1265–1267.

27. Brown RG, Maccarthy B, Gotham A-M et al, Depression and disability in Parkinson's disease: a follow-up of 132 cases. *Psychol Med* 1988; **18**:49–55.

28. Ehmann TS, Beninger RJ, Gawel MJ et al, Depressive symptoms in Parkinson's disease: a comparison with disabled control subjects. *J Geriatr Psychiat Neurol* 1989; **2**:3–9.

29. Menza MA, Mark MH, Parkinson's disease and depression: the relationship to disability and personality. *J Neuropsychiat Clin Neurosci* 1994; **6**:165–169.

30. Shiba M, Bower JH, Maraganore DM et al, Anxiety disorders and depressive disorders preceding Parkinson's disease: a case-control study. *Mov Disord* 2000; **15**:669–677.
31. Schuurman AG, van den Akker, M, Ensinck KTJL et al, Increased risk of Parkinson's disease after depression. *Neurology* 2002; **58**:1501–1504.
32. Mentis MJ, McIntosh AR, Perrine K et al, Relationships among the metabolic patterns that correlate with mnemonic, visuospatial, and mood symptoms in Parkinson's disease. *Am J Psychiatry* 2002; **159**:746–754.
33. Berg D, Supprian T, Hofmann E et al, Depression in Parkinson's disease: brainstem midline alteration on transcranial sonography and magnetic imaging. *J Neurol* 1999; **246**:1186–1193.
34. Mayberg HS, Starkstein SE, Sadzot B et al, Selective hypometabolism in the inferior frontal lobe in depressed patients with Parkinson's disease. *Ann Neurol* 1990; **28**:57–64.
35. Brown AS, Gershon S, Dopamine and depression. *J Neurol Trans* 1993; **91**:75–109.
36. Murai T, Muller U, Werheid K et al, In vivo evidence for differential association of striatal dopamine and midbrain serotonin systems with neuropsychiatric symptoms in Parkinson's disease. *J Neuropsychiat Clin Neurosci* 2001; **13**:222–228.
37. Mössner R, Henneberg A, Schmitt A et al, Allelic variation of serotonin transporter expression is associated with depression in Parkinson's disease. *Mol Psychiat* 2001; **6**:350–352.
38. Menza MA, Palermo B, DiPaola R et al, Depression and anxiety in Parkinson's disease: possible effect of genetic variation in the serotonin transporter. *J Geriatr Psychiat Neurol* 1999; **12**:49–52.
39. Mayeux R, Stern Y, Sano M et al, The relationship of serotonin to depression in Parkinson's disease. *Mov Disord* 1998; **3**:237–244.
40. Cantello R, Aguggia M, Gilli M et al, Major depression in Parkinson's disease and the mood response to intravenous methylphenidate: possible role of the "hedonic" dopamine synapse. *J Neurol Neurosurg Psychiat* 1989; **52**:724–731.
41. Menza MA, Sage J, Marshall E et al, Mood changes and "on-off" phenomena in Parkinson's disease. *Mov Disord* 1990; **5**:148–151.
42. Maricle RA, Nutt JG, Valentine RJ et al, Dose–response relationship of levodopa with mood and anxiety in fluctuating Parkinson's disease: a double-blind, placebo-controlled study. *Neurology* 1995; **45**:1757–1760.
43. Richard IH, Justus AW, Kurlan R, Relationship between mood and motor fluctuations in Parkinson's disease. *J Neuropsychiat Clin Neurosci* 2001; **13**:35–41.
44. Racette BA, Hartlein JM, Hershey T et al, Clinical features and comorbidity of mood fluctuations in Parkinson's disease. *J Neuropsychiat Clin Neurosci* 2002; **14**:438–442.
45. Green J, McDonald WM, Vitek JL et al, Neuropsychological and psychiatric sequelae of pallidotomy for PD: Clinical trial findings. *Neurology* 2002; **58**:858–865.
46. Bejjani BP, Damier P, Arnulf I et al, Transient acute depression induced by high-frequency deep-brain stimulation. *New Engl J Med* 1999; **340**:1476–1480.
47. Herzog J, Volkmann J, Krack P et al, Two-year follow-up of subthalamic deep brain stimulation in Parkinson's disease. *Mov Disord* 2003; **18**:1332–1337.
48. Berney A, Vingerhoets F, Perrin A et al, Effect on mood of subthalmic DBS for Parkinson's disease: A consecutive series of 24 patients [comment]. *Neurology* 2002; **59**:1427–1429.
49. Houeto JL, Mesnage V, Mallet L et al, Behavioral disorders, Parkinson's disease and subthalamic stimulation. *J Neurol Neurosurg Psychiat* 2002; **72**:701–707.
50. Aarsland D, Larsen JP, Cummings JL et al, Prevalence and clinical correlates of psychotic symptoms in Parkinson disease. *Arch Neurol* 1999; **56**:595–601.

51. Marsh L, Williams JR, Rocco M et al, Psychiatric comorbidities in patients with Parkinson disease and psychosis. *Neurology* 2004; **63**:293–300.
52. Menza MA, Robertson-Hoffman DE, Bonapace AS, Parkinson's disease and anxiety: comorbidity with depression. *Biol Psychiat* 1993; **34**:465–470.
53. Starkstein SE, Mayberg HS, Preziosi TJ, Andrezejewski P, Leiguarda R, Robinson RG, Reliability, validity, and clinical correlates of apathy in Parkinson's disease. *J Neuropsychiat Clin Neurosci* 1992; **4**:134–139.
54. Lou J-S, Kearns G, Oken B et al, Exacerbated physical fatigue and mental fatigue in Parkinson's disease. *Mov Disord* 2001; **16**:190–196.
55. Caap-Ahlgren M, Dehlin O, Insomnia and depressive symptoms in patients with Parkinson's disease. Relationship to health-related quality of life. An interview of patients living at home. *Arch Gerontol Geriatr* 2001; **32**:23–33.
56. Pluck GC, Brown RG, Apathy in Parkinson's disease. *J Neurol Neurosurg Psychiat* 2002; **73**:636–642.
57. Norman S, Tröster AI, Fields JA, Brooks R, Effects of depression and Parkinson's disease on cognitive functioning. *J Neuropsychiat Clin Neurosci* 2002; **14**:31–36.
58. Hughes TA, Ross HF, Musa S et al, A 10-year study of the incidence of and factors predicting dementia in Parkinson's disease. *Neurology* 2000; **54**:1596–1602.
59. Sano M, Stern Y, Williams J et al, Coexisting dementia and depression in Parkinson's disease. *Arch Neurol* 1989; **46**:1284–1286.
60. Kuzis G, Sabe L, Tiberti C, Leiguarda R, Starkstein SE, Cognitive functions in major depression and Parkinson disease. *Arch Neurol* 1997; **54**:982–986.
61. Wertman E, Speedie L, Shemesh Z et al, Cognitive disturbances in Parkinsonian patients with depression. *J Neuropsychiat Neuropsychol Behav Neurol* 1993; **6**:31–37.
62. Anguenot A, Loll PY, Neau JP et al, Depression and Parkinson's disease: study of a series of 135 Parkinson's patients. *Can J Neurol Sci* 2002; **29**:139–146.
63. Kalayam B, Alexopolous GS, Prefrontal dysfunction and treatment response in geriatric depression. *Arch Gen Psychiat* 1999; **56**:713–718.
64. Alexopolous GS, "The Depression-Executive Dysfunction Syndrome of Late Life": A specific target for D_3 agonists? *Am J Geriatr Psychiat* 2001; **9**:22–29.
65. O'Suilleabhain PE, Sung V, Hernandez C et al, Elevated homocysteine plasma level in patients with Parkinson disease: Mood, affective, and cognitive associations. *Arch Neurol* 2004; **61**:865–868.
66. Di Rocco A, Rogers JD, Brown R et al, S-adenosyl-methionine improves depression in patients with Parkinson's disease in an open-label clinical trial. *Mov Disord* 2000; **15**:1225–1229.
67. Tandeter HB, Shvartzman P, Parkinson's disease camouflaging early signs of hypothyroidism [comment]. *Postgrad Med* 1993; **94**:187–190.
68. Okun MS, Walter BL, McDonald WM et al, Beneficial effects of testosterone replacement for the nonmotor symptoms of Parkinson disease. *Arch Neurol* 2002; **59**:1750–1753.
69. Lindenbaum J, Healton EB, Savage DG et al, Neuropsychiatric disorders caused by cobalamin deficiency in the absence of anemia or macrocytosis. *New Engl J Med* 1988; **318**:1720–1728.
70. Leentjens AF, Marinus J, Van Hilten JJ et al, The contribution of somatic symptoms to the diagnosis of depression in Parkinson's disease: a discriminant analytic approach. *J Neuropsychiat Clin Neurosci* 2003; **15**:74–77.
71. Slaughter JR, Slaughter KA, Nichols D et al, Prevalence, clinical manifestations, etiology, and treatment of depression in Parkinson's disease. *J Neuropsychiat Clin Neurosci* 2001; **13**:187–196.
72. Hoogendijk WJ, Sommer IEC, Tissingh G et al, Depression in Parkinson's disease: the impact of symptom overlap on prevalence. *Psychosomatics* 1998; **39**:416–421.

73. Leentjens AF, Verhey FRJ, Luijckz G-J et al, The validity of the Beck Depression Inventory as a screening and diagnostic instrument for depression in patients with Parkinson's disease. *Mov Disord* 2000; **15**:1221–1224.

74. D'Ath P, Katona P, Mullan E et al, Screening detection and management of depression in elderly primary care attenders. I: The acceptability and performance of the 15 item Geriatric Depression Scale (GDS15) and the development of short versions. *Fam Pract* 1994; **11**:260–266.

75. Leentjens AF, Verhey FRJ, Lousberg R, Spitsbergen H, Wilmink FW, The validity of the Hamilton and Montgomery-Åsberg Depression Rating Scales as screening and diagnostic tools for depression in Parkinson's disease. *Intern J Geriatr Psychiat* 2000; **15**:644–649.

76. Pitcairn TK, Clemie S, Gray JM, Pentland B, Impressions of parkinsonian patients from their recorded voices. *Br J Disord Commun* 1990; **25**:85–92.

77. Dell'Agnello G, Ceravolo R, Nuti A et al, SSRIs do not worsen Parkinson's disease: evidence from an open-label, prospective study. *Clin Neuropharmacol* 2001; **24**:221–227.

78. Ceravolo R, Nuti A, Piccinni A et al, Paroxetine in Parkinson's disease: effects on motor and depressive symptoms. *Neurology* 2000; **55**:1216–1218.

79. Hauser RA, Zesiewicz TA, Sertraline for the treatment of depression in Parkinson's disease. *Mov Disord* 1997; **12**:756–759.

80. Rampello L, Chiechio S, Raffaele R et al, The SSRI, citalopram, improves bradykinesia in patients with Parkinson's disease treated with L-dopa. *Clin Neuropharmacol* 2002; **25**:21–24.

81. Tesei S, Antonini A, Canesi M et al, Tolerability of paroxetine in Parkinson's disease: a prospective study. *Mov Disord* 2000; **15**:986–989.

82. Wermuth L, Sørensen PS, Timm S et al, Depression in idiopathic Parkinson's disease treated with citalopram: a placebo-controlled trial. *Nordic J Psychiat* 1998; **52**:163–169.

83. Leentjens AF, Vreeling FW, Luijckx GJ et al, SSRIs in the treatment of depression in Parkinson's disease. *Intern J Geriatr Psychiat* 2003; **18**:552–554.

84. Andersen J, Aabro E, Gulmann N et al, Anti-depressive treatment in Parkinson's disease: a controlled trial of the effect of nortriptyline in patients with Parkinson's disease treated with L-dopa. *Acta Neurol Scand* 1980; **62**:210–219.

85. van de Vijver DA, Roos RA, Jansen PA et al, Start of a selective serotonin reuptake inhibitor (SSRI) and increase of antiparkinsonian drug treatment in patients on levodopa. *Br J Clin Pharmacol* 2003; **54**:168–170.

86. Richard IH, Kurlan R, Parkinson Study Group, A survey of antidepressant use in Parkinson's disease. *Neurology* 1997; **49**:1168–1170.

87. Jimenez-Jimenez FJ, Tejeiro J, Martinez-Junquera G et al, Parkinsonism exacerbated by paroxetine. *Neurology* 1994; **44**:2406.

88. Alexopolous GS, Katz IR, Reynolds CF III et al, The expert consensus guideline series: pharmacotherapy of depressive disorders in older patients. *Postgrad Med Special Rep* 2001 October; 1–86.

89. Treatment of depression in idiopathic Parkinson's disease. *Mov Disord* 2002; **17**(Suppl. 4):S112–S119.

90. Rektorova I, Rektor I, Bares M et al, Pramipexole and pergolide in the treatment of depression in Parkinson's disease: a national multicentre prospective randomized study. *Eur J Neurol* 2003; **10**:399–406.

91. Richard IH, Kurlan R, Tanner C et al, Serotonin syndrome and the combined use of deprenyl and an antidepressant in Parkinson's disease. *Neurology* 1997; **48**:1070–1077.

92. Moellentine C, Rummans T, Ahlskog JE et al, Effectiveness of ECT in patients with parkinsonism. *J Neuropsychiat Clin Neurosci* 1998; **10**:187–193.
93. Dragasevic N, Potrebi A, Damjanovi A et al, Therapeutic efficacy of bilateral prefrontal slow repetitive transcranial magnetic stimulation in depressed patients with Parkinson's disease: an open study. *Mov Disord* 2004; **17**:528–532.
94. Fregni F, Santos CM, Myczkowski ML et al, Repetitive transcranial magnetic stimulation is as effective as fluoxetine in the treatment of depression in patients with Parkinson's disease. *J Neurol Neurosurg Psychiat* 2004; **75**:1171–1174.

chapter 9

Anxiety

Matthew Menza and Roseanne DeFronzo Dobkin

Introduction

Anxiety as a psychiatric complication of Parkinson's disease (PD) has received relatively little attention from the research community.[1] Nonetheless, it is a common and very disabling complication with which patients and clinicians struggle. The diagnosis of anxiety is often missed and the suffering associated with anxiety is often minimized. Nonetheless, anxiety is a treatable aspect of PD, and treatment can significantly improve the quality of an individual's life.

It is perhaps not surprising that individuals with PD have difficulty with anxiety, as anxiety disorders are common in the elderly.[2,3] However, anxiety appears to be even more of a problem for patients with PD than it is for the general population of a similar age.[4,5] Anxiety also affects quality of life in PD.[6,7] Yet, since anxiety is often intertwined with the motor aspects of the illness and depression, it may take an experienced clinician to tease apart the disorders.

This chapter reviews issues relevant to the practicing clinician who is treating anxiety in patients with PD and issues relevant to the individual living with PD. In doing so, we hope to help clinicians and patients identify and treat anxiety. These issues include the prevalence of anxiety, how to recognize anxiety in the context of PD, and the impact of anxiety on the quality of one's life. We also discuss relationships between motor fluctuations and anxiety as well as between depression and anxiety. Lastly, we review recommendations on treatment, including medications and non-pharmacologic therapies which may be of help.

Prevalence of anxiety disorders in Parkinson's disease

It is interesting that anxiety, like depression, is often present before patients develop motor symptoms and receive a diagnosis of PD. In a large case-control study, for example, the odds of having had an anxiety disorder 5, 10, and 20 years prior to the onset of the movement disorder was over twice that for those individuals who went on to develop PD compared to matched controls.[8] A number of other authors examining smaller groups of patients have found similar results.[9–11]

In fact, anxiety itself may be a risk factor for developing PD or a pro-dromal symptom of the illness itself. In the prospective Health Professionals Follow Study, a cohort of 35 815 US male health professionals, the risk of developing PD at 12 year follow up was one and a half times greater in men with high levels of anxiety compared to men with the lowest level of anxiety at baseline.[12]

Several studies have assessed prevalence and severity of anxiety symptoms after the patient has a confirmed PD diagnosis. In one of our studies, for example, 28% of patients with PD had a DSM-III-R anxiety disorder diagnosis and another 40% had anxiety symptoms but no formal diagnosis. Only 5% of the age- and disability-matched osteoarthritis control subjects had an anxiety disorder diagnosis.[5] In a questionnaire study from our group, 104 patients with PD rated themselves significantly higher on anxiety scales compared to age- and disability-matched controls.[13] These studies have con-sistently found PD patients to have more severe anxiety symptoms and a higher prevalence of anxiety disorders compared to matched controls and population estimates in the elderly. A number of other investigators, using a variety of methodologies, have reported similar results, with prevalence rates ranging from 24% to 75%.[2–4,13–18]

So, it appears that there is little debate that patients with PD have an increased prevalence of anxiety symptoms and anxiety disorders, compared to age- and illness-matched controls. These data are also consistent with our clinical experience that many of these patients have been worriers over most of their life. As one recent woman described it, "I worry for the ducks going barefoot."

The clinical nature of anxiety in PD

What is the clinical nature of the anxiety that one sees in patients with PD? Research studies, as well as our own clinical experience, indicate that the symptomatology of anxiety is sometimes difficult to classify within our current diagnostic categories. The typical symptoms of anxiety include excessive worry, fatigue, concentration problems, sleep disturbance, restlessness, increased tremor and worsening motor function. Obviously, many of these symptoms, such as sleep disturbance, concentration problems, fatigue, tremor, and restlessness may be attributable directly to the PD. Unfortunately, this overlap of symptoms has not been critically studied.

A variety of other issues may also complicate the diagnosis of anxiety in individuals with PD. For instance, many individuals with PD report excessive worry, but it fluctuates greatly from day to day, as well as from hour to hour. Furthermore, they may attribute the anxiety directly to the problems they face in daily life from the motor symptoms of the illness.

Despite the difficulties of the overlap and variability of symptoms, researchers have been able to characterize the clinical symptoms of anxiety seen in these patients. For instance, in one study we observed that 12% of our patients had panic disorder, 12% had generalized anxiety disorder (GAD), 2% had phobic disorders, 2% had anxiety disorder not otherwise specified, and 40% had anxiety symptoms without meeting criteria for a diagnosis.[5] Most studies are consistent with these results, showing a mix of GAD, social phobia, panic disorder,[18–20] and occasionally obsessive compulsive disorder.[11]

Recognizing anxiety in patients with PD

Anxiety is frequently not recognized in patients with PD.[21] For example, in a cross sectional study, Shulman et al.[22] found that while 39% of patients endorsed significant anxiety on standardized testing, only 19% had been identified by their treating neurologist; thus half had gone undetected.

The lack of recognition is likely the result of a variety of factors. Patients are often hesitant to discuss their worries and physicians may overlook the importance of these disorders. In addition, as discussed above, there is considerable overlap between the symptoms of anxiety and those of PD itself. This may lead many patients and physicians to misattribute the symptoms of anxiety to PD. Further complicating the picture, the most commonly used rating scale for anxiety, the Hamilton Anxiety Scale (HAM-A),[23] rates insomnia, difficulty in concentration, constipation, sweating, and pains as symptoms of anxiety even though all of these may be part of uncomplicated PD. For example, Berrios et al.[24] point out that autonomic dysfunction, including flushing, dizziness, and urinary frequency, is often seen in patients with PD and should not be mistaken for anxiety.

While this has not been carefully studied, the key to resolving this conundrum is to focus on excessive worrying. If this cognitive symptom is present then the other symptoms, even if related primarily to PD, should be used to evaluate the severity of the anxiety disturbance. This approach, referred to as an inclusive one, meaning symptoms are included regardless of etiology, has been validated in PD-related depression,[25] in which there is also considerable symptom overlap.

Information on anxiety can usually be easily elicited by asking patients if they have considered themselves "worriers" over their lifetime and if these worries have gotten worse since they developed PD. This is a clinical recommendation that we have found useful in our experience and given the importance of anxiety in affecting quality of life, we believe that it is important to take this inclusive approach.

Importance of anxiety in PD

Quality of life

Health-related quality of life (HRQL) is a term frequently used that refers to the psychosocial consequences of the physical, mental, and social aspects of a medical illness.[26] It has been documented that anxiety exerts a deleterious effect on the HRQL of patients with PD and elderly patients with medical illnesses other than PD. In these non-PD populations, anxiety has been found to be related to decreases in HRQL, increased healthcare costs, and decrements in physical health, as well as increased healthcare utilization and dissatisfaction with those services.[27,28]

While the majority of HRQL research in PD focuses on depression,[29] limited research also suggests a relationship between anxiety and overall quality of life in the PD population.[30,31] Anxiety has been connected with increased disability (e.g., problems with mobility, ADL, stigma, isolation)[31] and a lowered sense of emotional well-being in PD patients,[30] thus negatively impacting HRQL. In another study, anxiety was a stronger predictor of HRQL in the areas of quality of interpersonal interaction, health satisfaction, and overall well being (bodily pain, mental health) than either physical symptoms or depression.[7]

Cognitive functioning

A relationship between anxiety and cognitive impairment has been noted in both the non-PD and PD elderly.[2,6,32] For example, in a longitudinal study of the non-PD elderly with no depression or cognitive impairment at baseline, only anxiety was found to be a significant predictor of future cognitive decline.[32] In a PD population, Ryder et al.[6] found that anxiety accounted for a greater proportion of variance on a standardized cognitive performance battery than either depression or neurological variables. Thus, anxiety is an important variable to consider when assessing cognitive functioning in PD patients.

Relationship of anxiety to motor symptoms

Most studies have not identified a relationship between severity of motor symptoms and severity of anxiety.[19] That is, it does not appear that, in general, patients are reacting to the burden of the illness by becoming anxious. However, there are data to suggest that anxiety is associated with motor fluctuations.

Motor fluctuations are rapid changes in rigidity and tremor that occur commonly in patients with PD and increase as the illness progresses. The fluctuations are referred to as "on-off" or "wearing off" phenomena and most commonly appear at the end of levodopa dose schedules when the symptoms of the illness return. Less frequently, the fluctuations have little apparent relationship to dosing schedule and may appear at any time.[33] In some cases the fluctuations are severe, with abrupt freezing with little warning.

It is less well recognized that mood and anxiety symptoms may also fluctuate rapidly in these patients. These changes in mood and anxiety usually parallel the changes in the motor function, such that when the patient is off they are more anxious and more depressed.[34–37] While these studies have generally found that patients are more anxious during off periods, there is not always a strict temporal relationship between the fluctuations and mood changes.[33] Because changes in anxiety and mood often accompany the motor fluctuations, it is imperative that this relationship be explored in individual patients – the information may be crucial in the patient's treatment.

A relationship between anxiety and the clinical symptoms of PD may also be seen when patients are stressed and anxiety increases. It is widely believed that stress and anxiety are associated with a transient increase in tremor and motor dysfunction. This phenomenon has not been studied closely but is widely endorsed by patients and experienced clinicians.

Relationship between depression and anxiety

Comorbidity between depressive and anxiety symptoms is common in the non-PD elderly,[38,39] and has been linked with quality of life and treatment response.[40] For example, co-morbid major depression and generalized anxiety disorder are incrementally associated with substantial impairments in work, increased disability, diminished well-being, and increased healthcare utilization.[27,41]

A number of groups have also found high rates of comorbidity between depression and anxiety in patients with PD. Henderson et al.,[42] for example, found depression and anxiety to be highly comorbid compared to a matched control group and Schiffer et al.[14] reported that anxiety syndromes were present in 75% of patients with PD and a depressive disorder. In a study from our group,[5] 42 patients with PD and 21 matched medical controls were evaluated using DSM-III-R criteria and a variety of psychiatric rating scales. Of the 12 patients with PD who had an anxiety disorder diagnosis, 11 (92%) had a co-morbid depressive disorder diagnosis. Of the 18 patients with a depressive disorder, 12 (67%) also had an anxiety disorder diagnosis.

The impact of co-morbid anxiety and depression on the course and treatment of the illness is unclear. However, some speculate that co-morbid depression and anxiety in PD may be linked with greater chronicity, treatment resistance, and poorer prognosis.[43] For example, Shulman et al.[22,44] found the increased co-morbidity of non-motor symptoms (e.g., depression and anxiety) to be linked with greater PD severity.

There are obvious clinical implications to these data. Finding symptoms of either depression or anxiety should alert us to the potential presence of the other. One then needs to do a careful inventory of all of the relevant diagnostic criteria before proceeding with treatment.

The etiology of anxiety in Parkinson's disease

There are a variety of hypotheses as to why there should be an association between PD and anxiety. Certainly, this is an illness that interferes with an individual's functioning and ability to cope with the stresses of life. The majority of studies, however, suggest that there is little relationship between severity of motor disability and severity of anxiety.[45] Despite these findings, it is plausible that for some individuals the affective consequences of increased physical disability include excessive worry and a sense of lack of control.

It is likely that the anxiety one sees in these patients is at least in part related to neurochemical changes in the brain that accompany PD. Many of the neurotransmitters that have been implicated in anxiety (norepinephrine (noradrenaline), serotonin, dopamine, and GABA) are also damaged, variably, in PD.[46,47] There is evidence linking adrenergic changes to the anxiety seen in PD[48] and PD patients are reportedly unusually susceptible to yohmbine-induced panic attacks.[49] Serotonin has been postulated to play a central role in anxiety and numerous indices of serotonin are altered in PD.[50] These changes include a loss of serotonin neurons in the median and dorsal raphe, decreased concentration of serotonin throughout the brain and decreases in serotonin reuptake sites.

Anxiety in PD could also be more directly related to dopaminergic deficits or interactions between dopaminergic deficits and the variable deficits in norepinephrine and serotonin. It seems less likely that dopamine deficits alone drive the anxiety as no difference between anxious and non-anxious PD patients in disability ratings (which correlate with the degree of dopaminergic deficit) has been found.[23]

Genetic factors are known to play an important role in predisposition to anxiety-related disorders.[51] A polymorphism of the serotonin transporter, which plays an important role in regulating serotonergic tone, is of particular interest as it has been associated with the anxiety in humans,[52] especially in the presence of stress.[53] A relationship between anxiety (and depression) and genetic alleles of the serotonin transporter has also been found in PD patients.[54] In this study from our group, 50% of the patients with a short allele (indicative of high synaptic serotonin) had significant anxiety while none of the patients with the homozygous long allele had significant anxiety.

A relationship between cognitive impairment and anxiety has also been noted by Marsh et al.,[55] who suggest that some of the behavioral manifestations characteristic of anxiety, including perseverative thinking and difficulty switching set may be related to functional cognitive deficits in the frontal lobe. They further hypothesize that patients with cognitive impairment are vulnerable to anxiety because the executive dysfunction leads to difficulties with problem-solving and the inability to resolve anxiogenic situations.

Others have suggested that some of the anxiety seen in these patients may be secondary to Parkinson's medications[18] and weak correlations between levodopa dose and anxiety have been found.[5] The question of the relationship between dopaminergic drugs and anxiety remains open. In our clinical experience, there are some patients who do experience these drugs as anxiogenic.

Treatment of anxiety in Parkinson's disease

Unfortunately, there are few research data from which to derive treatment recommendations for these patients. To our knowledge, there has been no controlled trial examining the treatment of anxiety in PD. Nonetheless, one can, based on clinical experience and controlled data in the geriatric non-PD population, develop some general principles and make some recommendations on treating anxiety in PD.

First, it is extremely important that maximal control of the motor aspects of PD is obtained. As previously discussed, motor fluctuations are strongly correlated with mood and anxiety problems, and attempts to treat anxiety in the presence of uncontrolled fluctuations are not likely to be adequately successful. This will necessitate coordination of treatment between different providers, a process that is not always easy in today's healthcare climate.

Next, treat any co-occurring depression. In a small, open-label study of citalopram in patients with depression and anxiety, anxiety did improve on citalopram.[56] This study suggested that anxiety symptoms may respond to an SSRI and that anxiety is particularly responsive if the depression also improves. Furthermore, anxiety, co-morbid with depression, is effectively treated in non-PD patients with antidepressants and this treatment can improve these long-term outcomes.[57]

One should also refer to clinical practice guidelines and select an empirically validated treatment for anxiety. As there is a paucity of research regarding the treatment of anxiety in PD, one can look to experience with the non-PD geriatric population as informative. Current guidelines and research regarding medication management, cognitive-behavioral treatment, and other interventions in the non-PD and PD elderly are further reviewed below.

Pharmacotherapy

The current recommendations for the treatment of anxiety in geriatric patients without PD are to use an SSRI or venlafaxine as first-line pharmacotherapy, despite the limited evidence base.[58] It is prudent to begin at lower doses than normal as elderly patients are susceptible to side-effects. Furthermore, SSRIs will sometimes increase the tremor and rigidity of PD. We do not find this worsening, when it occurs, to be limiting in treatment. It is generally possible to lower the SSRI dose or to increase the dopaminergic treatment slightly and regain adequate motor control. Mirtazepine and the tricyclic antidepressants, with appropriate attention to side-effects and cardiac issues, may also be of use.

The atypical antipsychotic quetiapine, which is useful in psychotic and disinhibited conditions in PD, is also sometimes useful for anxiety symptoms. Clozapine, another atypical antipsychotic, though cumbersome to use because of the required CBC testing, may be considered in refractory cases. Gabapentin, useful in non-PD patients, may also be tried. There are no controlled data on the use of these medications for anxiety in PD, so all must be used cautiously. Because of the potential for adverse effects on motor and cognitive function, starting doses are much lower, e.g., quetiapine or clozapine 6.25–12.5 mg, gabapentin 100 mg, upward titration is slower, and maintenance doses may also be lower.

A safety issue relevant to the SSRIs and other antidepressants involves the use of selegiline (deprenyl), a monoamine oxidase inhibitor (MAOI), which has a mild therapeutic effect on motor symptoms and may slow the progression of PD. Unlike the MAOIs traditionally used as antidepressants, which inhibit both the A and B form of the enzyme, deprenyl is a selective MAO-B inhibitor when given in doses of up to 10 mg per day. While hypertensive effects are unusual and the normal MAOI dietary precautions are not needed, there are reports of adverse interactions with fluoxetine.[59,60] Because of these reports, the manufacturers of all SSRIs recommend against their concurrent administration with deprenyl. Despite these warnings, the SSRIs and deprenyl are widely used together by PD specialists, though one must only do this with adequate patient education and clinical monitoring.

Two studies of buspirone, an anxiolytic medication, both designed to examine motor effects and not anxiety, found that it was well tolerated in the typical dosing range in PD.[61,62] As the patients were not selected for anxiety, there were no anti-anxiety effects found in either study. Buspirone is an effective treatment for anxiety in non-PD patients[63] and can be considered for patients with PD, though given the high rate of co-morbidity with depression, it would not be a first-line drug.

Benzodiazepines are typically the first-line treatments in primary care clinics for anxiety in the elderly.[64] However, benzodiazepines are problematic in the elderly as they increase risk for fall and fractures by 50% or more.[65] In addition, benzodiazepines are associated with a risk of cognitive impairment in this age group.[66] Nonetheless, when used carefully with appropriate caution they may be helpful.

Cognitive-behavioral treatment

There are some data suggesting the efficacy of cognitive-behavior therapy (CBT) in anxiety disorders in the elderly, particularly in the areas of generalized anxiety and panic disorders.[40] CBT has generally followed protocols with documented efficacy in younger populations, incorporating core techniques such as psychoeducation, relaxation training, cognitive-restructuring, exposure, problem-solving, and sleep hygiene.[67] However, certain adjustments have been made to better meet the needs of older individuals. These include progressing at a slower pace, assigning less-intensive homework, using audiotapes to reinforce material covered in treatment sessions, and utilizing enlarged/simplified forms.[68]

For example, in a manual adapted for primary care, Stanley et al.[68] suggested increasing the amount of information provided about the nature of anxiety and its management, using written/visual aids (e.g., writing on a white board in-session, summary sheets, graphing symptom changes) to adjust for variation in learning and sensory function, assigning weekly readings to reinforce material covered in session, and making weekly reminder and trouble-shooting phone calls. This group allowed additional sessions for patients with learning difficulties or in time of crisis. It was also recommended that coping statements and thought-stopping techniques be emphasized in lieu of cognitive restructuring techniques for patients with cognitive limitations.

Overall, meaningful improvements in worry, anxiety, co-morbid depression, and quality of life have been noted following CBT for the treatment of anxiety disorders in the elderly in randomized clinical trials and have been maintained over substantial follow-up periods (6 months–1 year).[69,70]

To date, no trials examining the efficacy or applicability of CBT for the treatment of anxiety in PD have been conducted and we can only generalize from the above-referenced studies that this treatment modality may be effective in the Parkinson's population. Additional research is needed to further elucidate this area.

Additional interventions

Exercise, which is useful in non-PD patients for the alleviation of depression and anxiety may also be useful for patients with PD.[71] In a small open-label study of exercise in PD patients, Battile et al.[72] suggested that a moderate-intensity exercise intervention was related to improvements in overall quality of life. This pilot study is the only published study of exercise in PD patients, but is consistent with our clinical experience that exercise has an overall salutary effect on their quality of life. Based on this experience, we routinely recommend exercise for our patients.

Small studies have also suggested that anxiety may improve after surgical interventions for PD. Higginson et al.[73] reported that scores on the Beck Anxiety Inventory improved significantly after surgical intervention in 39 patients, with improvement unrelated to improvement in the movement disorder. Martinez-Martin et al.[74] also found a significant pre–post improvement on the Hospital Anxiety and Depression Scale in 17 patients receiving deep brain stimulation. Therefore, it is possible that the development of new, innovative interventions may help relieve anxiety in the PD population.

Conclusions

Anxiety is common in patients with PD and is associated with a variety of poor outcomes, including poor quality of life. Despite this, the diagnosis is often overlooked or its impact minimized. Nearly all of the DSM-IV categories of anxiety may be found in these patients, but the symptoms tend to cluster in GAD, panic, and social phobia categories. There is a considerable overlap between the symptoms of anxiety disorders and the symptoms of PD itself, but a diagnosis can be made by focusing on the cognitive symptoms of anxiety. Anxiety in patients with PD is likely to be partially related to the neurochemical and degenerative changes that accompany PD, but the development of increasing disability may also worsen anxiety symptoms.

The treatment of anxiety in PD is largely unstudied but recommendations based on clinical experience and data derived from geriatric populations can be made. The first step in treatment is to optimize the management of other co-occurring clinical conditions, including PD. The second step involves treating the depression that is often found in patients with anxiety. Further treatment will usually involve some combination of the SSRIs, other newer antidepressants, CBT, exercise, and occasionally benzodiazepines and atypical antipsychotics. This is an aspect of PD that warrants attention if we are to improve the quality of life for individuals with this illness.

Acknowledgment

This work was supported by R01NS43144-01A1 from NINDS.

References

1. Marsh L, Anxiety disorders in Parkinson's disease. *Int Rev Psychiatry* 2000; **12**:307–318.
2. Beekman AT, Bremmer MA, Deeg DJ et al, Anxiety disorders in later life: a report from the Longitudinal Aging Study Amsterdam. *Int J Geriatr Psychiatry* 1998; **13**:717–726.
3. Regier DA, Boyd JH, Burke JD et al, One-month prevalence of mental disorders in the United States. Based on five Epidemiologic Catchment Area sites. *Arch Gen Psychiatry* 1988; **45**:977–986.
4. Stein MS, Heuser IJ, Juncos JL et al, Anxiety disorders in patients with Parkinson's disease. *Am J Psychiatry* 1990; **147**(2):217–220.
5. Menza MA, Robertson-Hoffmann DE, Bonapace AS, Parkinson's disease and anxiety: comorbidity with depression. *Biol Psychiat* 1993; **34**:465–470.
6. Ryder KA, Gontkovsky ST, McSwan KL et al, Cognitive function in Parkinson's disease: association with anxiety but not depression. *Aging Neuropsychol Cognit* 2002; **9**(2):77–84.
7. Chrischilles EA, Rubenstein LM, Voelker MD, Wallace RB, Rodnitzky RL, Linking clinical variables to health-related quality of life in Parkinson's disease. *Parkinsonism Relat Disord* 2002; **8**:199–209.
8. Shiba M, Bower JH, Maraganore DM et al, Anxiety disorders and depressive disorders preceding Parkinson's disease: a case control study. *Mov Disord* 2000 **15**(4):669–677.
9. Gonera EG, van't Hom M, Gerger JC et al, Symptoms and duration of the prodromal phase in Parkinson's disease. *Mov Disord* 1997; **12**:871–876.
10. Henderson R, Kurlan R, Kersun JM, Como P, Preliminary examination of the comorbidity of anxiety and depression in Parkinson's disease. *J Neuropsch Clin Neurosci* 1992; **4**:257–264.
11. Lauterbach EC, Duvoisin RC, Anxiety disorders in familial Parkinsonism. *Am J Psychiat* 1992; **148**:274.
12. Weisskopf MG, Chen H, Schwarzschild MA, Kawachi I, Ascherio A, Prospective study of phobic anxiety and risk of Parkinson's disease. *Mov Disord* 2003; 18; 6; 46–51.
13. Menza M, Mark M, Parkinson's disease and depression: The relationship to disability and personality. *J Neuropsych Clin Neurosci* 1994; **6**:165–169.

14. Schiffer RB, Kurlan R, Rubin A et al, Evidence of atypical depression in Parkinson's disease. *Am J Psychiat* 1988; **145**:1020–1022.

15. Myers JK, Weissman MM, Tischcler GL et al, Six-month prevalence of psychiatric disorders in three communities. *Arch Gen Psychiat* 1984; **41**:959–967.

16. Wells KB, Golding JM, Burnam MA, Psychiatric disorder in a sample of the general population with and without chronic medical conditions *Am J Psychiat* 1988; **145**:976–981.

17. Brown RG, MacCarthy B, Psychiatric morbidity in patients with Parkinson's disease. *Psychol Med* 1990; **20**:77–87.

18. Vasquez A, Jimenez-Jimenez FJ, Garcia-Ruiz P et al, "Panic attacks" in Parkinson's disease: a long-term complication of levodopa therapy. *Acta Neurol Scand* 1993; **87**:14–18.

19. Richard IH, Schiffer RB, Kurlan R, Anxiety and Parkinson's disease. *J Neuropsych Clin Neurosci* 1996; **8**:383–392.

20. Rubin AJ, Kurlan R, Miller C, Shoulson I, Atypical depression and Parkinson's disease. *Ann Neurol* 1986; **20**:150.

21. Marsh L, Solvasson B, Cahn DA et al, Psychiatric outcome after pallidotomy for Parkinson's disease. *Biol Psych* 1997; **41**:107S.

22. Shulman LM, Taback RL, Rabinstein AA, Weiner WJ, Non-recognition of depression and other non-motor symptoms in Parkinson's disease. *Parkinsonism Relat Disord* 2002; **8**(3):193–197.

23. Hamilton M, The assessment of anxiety status by rating. *Br J Med Psychol* 1959; **32**:50–55.

24. Berrios GE, Campbell C, Politynska BE, Autonomic failure, depression and anxiety in Parkinson's disease. *Br J Psychiatry* 1995; **166**:789–792.

25. Leentjens AF, Verhey FR, Lousberg R, Spitsbergen H, Wilmink FW, The validity of the Hamilton and Montgomery-Asbury depression rating scales as screening and diagnostic tools for depression in Parkinson's disease. *Int J Geriat Psychiat* 2000; **15**:644–649.

26. Bowling A, *Health related quality of life: a discussion of the concept, its use, and measurement. Measuring Disease.* Open University Press: Buckingham, 1995; 1–19.

27. Debeurs E, Beekman ATF, van Balkom AJLM et al, Consequences of anxiety in older persons: its effect on disability, well-being, and use of health services. *Psychol Med* 1999; **29**:583–593.

28. Creed F, Morgan R, Fiddler M et al, Depression and anxiety impair health-related quality of life and are associated with increased costs in general medical inpatients. *Psychosomatics* 2002; **43**:302–309.

29. Schrag A, Selai C, Medical and psychosocial determinants of quality of life in Parkinson's disease. *Mental and Behavioral Dysfunction in Movement Disorders.* Humana Press Inc: Totowa, NJ, 2003, 501–526.

30. Marinus M, Leentjens AFG, Visser M, Stiggelbout AM, van Hilten JJ, Evaluation of the hospital anxiety and depression scale in patients with Parkinson's disease. *Clin Neuropharmacol* 2002; **25**(6):318–324.

31. Marinus J, Visser M, Martinez-Martin P, van Hilten JJ, Stiggelbout AM, A short psychosocial questionnaire for patients with Parkinson's disease: the SCOPA-PS. *J Clin Epidemiol* 2003; **56**:61–67.

32. Sinoff G, Werner P, Anxiety disorder and accompanying subjective memory loss in the elderly as a predictor of future cognitive decline. *Int J Geriatr Psychiatry* 2003; **18**:951–959.

33. Richard IH, Justus AW, Kurlan R, Relationship between mood and motor fluctuations in Parkinson's disease. *J Neuropsychiatry Clin Neurosci* 2001; **13**:35–41.

34. Maricle RA, Nutt JG, Valentine RJ, Carter JH, Dose–response relationship of

levodopa with mood and anxiety in fluctuating Parkinson's disease: A double-blind, placebo-controlled study. *Neurology* 1995; **45**(9):1757–1760.

35. Nissenbaum H, Quinn NP, Brown RG, Toone B, Gotham AM, Marsden CD, Mood swings associated with the "on-off" phenomenon in Parkinson's disease. *Psychol Med* 1987; **17**:899–904.

36. Menza MA, Sage J, Marshall E, Cody R, Duvoisin R, Mood changes and "on-off" phenomena in Parkinson's disease. *Mov Disord* 1990; **5**:148–151.

37. Siemers ER, Shekhar A, Quaid K, Dickson H, Anxiety and motor performance in Parkinson's disease. *Mov Disord* 1993; **8**(4):501–506.

38. Flint AJ, Epidemiology and comorbidity of anxiety disorders in the elderly. *Am J Psychiat* 1994; **151**:640–649.

39. Clayton PJ, The comorbidity factor: Establishing the primary diagnosis in patients with mixed symptoms of anxiety and depression. *J Clin Psychiatry* 1990; **51**(11 Suppl):35–39.

40. Lauderdale SA, Sheikh JI, Anxiety disorders in older adults. *Clin Geriatr Med* 2003; **19**(4):721–741.

41. Kessler RC, DuPont RL, Berglund P, Wittchen HU, Impairment in pure and comorbid generalized anxiety disorder and major depression at 12 months in two national surveys. *Am J Psychiat* 1999; **156**:1915–1923.

42. Henderson R, Kurlan R, Kersun JM, Como P, Preliminary examination of the comorbidity of anxiety and depression in Parkinson's disease. *J Neuropsychiat Clin Neurosci* 1992; **4**:257–264.).

43. Brooks DJ, Doder M, Depression in Parkinson's disease. *Curr Opin Neurol* 2001; **14**(4):465–470.

44. Shulman LM, Taback RL, Bean J, Weiner WJ, Comorbidity of the non-motor symptoms of Parkinson's disease. *Mov Dis* 2001; **16**(3):507–510.

45. Cummings JL, Depression and Parkinson's disease. *Am J Psychiat* 1992; **149**:443–454.

46. Hornykiewicz O, Kish SJ, Biochemical pathophysiology of Parkinson's disease. *Adv Neurol* 1986; **45**:19–34.

47. Agid Y, Cervera P, Hirsch E et al, Biochemistry of Parkinson's disease 28 years later: a critical review. *Mov Disord* 1989; **4**(Suppl 1):S126–S144.

48. Schiffer RB, Anxiety disorders in Parkinson's disease: Insights into the neurobiology of neurosis. *J Psychosom Res* 1999; **47**(6):506–508.

49. Kurlan R, Lichter D, Schiffer RB, Panic/anxiety in Parkinson's disease: Yohimbine Challenge (abst). *Neurology* 1989; **39**:421.

50. Mayeux R, Williams Y, Clinical and biochemical features of depression in Parkinson's disease. *Am J Psychiatry* 1986; **143**:756–759.

51. Plomin R, Owen MJ, McGuffin P, The genetic basis of complex human behaviors. *Science* 1994; **264**:1733–1739.

52. Lesch KP, Bengal D, Heils A, Association of anxiety-related traits with a polymorphism in the serotonin transporter gene regulatory region. *Science* 1996; **274**:1527–1531.

53. Caspi A, Sugden K, Moffitt TE et al, Influence of life stress on depression: moderation by a polymorphism in the 5-HTT gene. *Science* 2003; **301**(5631):386–389.

54. Menza MA, Palermo B, DiPaola R, Sage JI, Ricketts MH, Depression and anxiety in Parkinson's disease: possible effect of genetic variation in the serotonin transporter. *J Geriatr Psychiatry Neurol* 1999; **12**:49–52.

55. Marsh L, Vaughan C, Schretlen D, Brandt J, Mandir AS, Psychomotor aspects of mood disorders in Parkinson's disease. *Biol Psych* 2000; **47**:165S.

56. Menza MA, Marin H, Kaufman K, Mark M, Lauritano M, Citalopram treatment of

depression in Parkinson's disease: The impact on anxiety, disability, and cognition. *J Neuropsychiat Clin Neurosci* 2004; **16**(3):315–319.

57. Russell JM, Koran LM, Rush J et al, Effect of concurrent anxiety on response to sertraline and imipramine in patients with chronic depression. *Depress Anxiety* 2001; **13**(1):18–27.

58. Lenze EJ, Pollock BG, Shear MK et al, Treatment considerations for anxiety in the elderly. *CNS Spectrums* 2003; **8**(Suppl 3):6–13.

59. Suchowersky O, de Vries JD, Interaction of fluoxetine and selegiline. *Can J Psychiat* 1990; **35**:571–572.

60. Jermain DM, Hughes PL, Follender AB. Potential fluoxetine–selegiline interaction. *Ann Pharmacother* 1992; **26**:1300.

61. Ludwig CL, Weingerger DR, Bruno G et al, Buspirone, Parkinson's disease, and the locus ceruleus. *Clin Neuropharmacol* 1986; **9**:373–378.

62. Bonifati V, Fabrizio E, Cipriani R et al, Buspirone in levodopa-induced dyskinesias. *Clin Neuropharmacol* 1994; **17**:73–82.

63. Gorman JM, Treating generalized anxiety disorder. *J Clin Psychiatry* 2003; **64**(Suppl 2):24–29.

64. Gleason PP, Schulz R, Smith NL et al, Correlates and prevalence of benzodiazepine use in community-dwelling elderly. *J Gen Intern Med* 1998; **13**:243–250.

65. Wang PS, Bohn RL, Glynn RJ et al, Hazardous benzodiazepine regimens in the elderly: effects of half-life, dosage, and duration on risk of hip fracture. *Am J Psychiat* 2001; **158**:892–898.

66. Hanlon JT, Horner RD, Schmader KE et al, Benzodiazepine use and cognitive function among community-dwelling elderly. *Clin Pharmacol Ther* 1998; **64**:684–692.

67. Stanley MA, Averill PM, *Strategies for treating generalized anxiety in the elderly. Handbook of Psychotherapy and Counseling with Older Adults.* John Wiley & Sons: New York, 1997, 511–525.

68. Stanley MA, Diefenbach GJ, Hopko DR, Cognitive behavioral treatment for older adults with generalized anxiety disorder. A therapist manual for primary care settings. *Behav Modif* 2004; **28**(1):73–117.

69. Barrowclough C, King P, Colville J, Russell E, Burns A, Tarrier N, A randomized trial of the effectiveness of cognitive-behavioral therapy and supportive counseling for anxiety symptoms in older adults. *J Consul Clin Psychol* 2001; **69**(5):756–762.

70. Wetherell JL, Gatz M, Craske MG, Treatment of generalized anxiety in older adults. *J Consult Clin Psychol* 2003; **71**(1):31–40.

71. Dunn AL, Trivedi MH, O'Neal HA, Physical activity dose-response effects on outcomes of depression and anxiety. *Med Sci Sports Exerc* 2001 **33**(6 Suppl):S587–S597.

72. Battile J, Langbein WE, Weaver F, Maloney C, Jost MB, Effect of exercise on perceived quality of life of individuals with Parkinson's disease. *J Rehabil Res Dev* 2000; **37**(5):529–534.

73. Higginson CI, Fields JA, Troster AI, Which symptoms of anxiety diminish after surgical interventions for Parkinson disease? *Neuropsych Neuropsychol Behav Neurol* 2001; **14**:117–121.

74. Martinez-Martin P, Valldeoriola F, Tolosa E et al, Bilateral subthalamic nucleus stimulation and quality of life in advanced Parkinson's disease. *Mov Disord* 2002; **17**(2):372–377.

chapter 10

Psychosis

Laura Marsh

Introduction

Psychotic symptoms occur in up to one-half of patients with Parkinson's disease (PD). Treating psychosis is often challenging since antiparkinsonian medications contribute to psychopathology, antipsychotic medications can aggravate motor and cognitive impairments, and the patients tend to have advanced-stage PD with its attendant motor complications, dementia, medical and other psychiatric co-morbidities, and increased caregiver strain.[1,2] Even though prognosis has improved with use of atypical anti-psychotics, psychosis is the most important risk factor for nursing home placement in PD[3] and is associated with increased mortality.[4] This chapter reviews the phenomenology, pathophysiology, and treatments of psychosis in PD. It emphasizes awareness of the various presentations of psychosis, attention to modifiable risk factors, and application of a variety of treatment strategies with knowledge of how these impact motor function and drug interactions.

Epidemiology

Psychotic symptoms in PD include hallucinations, delusions, and their associated behavioral changes.[2,5] Depending on the study sample and the definitions of psychosis, cognitive impairment, or PD, prevalence estimates for psychosis in PD range from 8% to 40%. Rates tend to be lower in community-based samples[1] and higher in patients with dementia (40% versus 15% in non-demented patients). If minor visual hallucinations (Table 10.1) are included, prevalence increases to 70% in patients with dementia.[1]

Table 10.1 Forms of hallucinations in Parkinson's disease

Type	Definition	Examples
Minor hallucinations[5]		
Presence	Vivid sensation or perception of another person or animal somewhere in the room, including behind the person, but when the patient turns "nothing is there"	An uncle, who is deceased, is perceived as lying next to the patient in bed
Passage	Brief visions of a person, animal, or shadow of something that passes sideways in the peripheral visual fields	A person walking; a shadowy form of a lady in a blue dress passing through the dark corner of a parking garage; a mouse running
Illusions	Sensory distortions or transformations of actual objects (and thus not technically hallucinations). On closer inspection, the actual object is identified	A stick looks like a snake; a bush looks like a lurking person; flowers appear in the toilet bowl
Other hallucinations		
Visual-unformed[22]	Light, patterns, shadowy facial images without clear details; less common in PD	A ball-like form looking perhaps like an insect; a flash of light; zig-zag patterns on a floral rug
Visual-complex[22]	Vivid, well-formed figures, usually in full-color and often of people (adults or children), animals, or objects, sometimes in groups and possibly moving about; may be normal in size or miniaturized; figures may be familiar or strangers. Usually silent and non-threatening, but not always; may have affiliated secondary delusions	Children standing at the foot of the bed; men chopping trees in the yard; a group of adults playing cards; elaborate spider webs on a house plant; a "Victorian gentleman" sitting in a chair; lobsters in the toilet

Table 10.1 continued

Type	Definition	Examples
Auditory[2,5,7]	Can involve voices talking, commands, hearing ones name called, music, or indistinct whispering; may or may not be related to visual hallucinations[2,75]	People talking somewhere in the house; indistinct voices; Religious chanting
Olfactory[75,76]	Sensations of smells that are otherwise not present; may be pleasant or unpleasant	An "electric or metallic" odor; a food odor in the car
Gustatory[20]	Tastes in the mouth when nothing is there; pleasant or unpleasant	The taste of baking soda in the mouth
Somatic/tactile/ cenesthetic[2,8,77]	Sensations of things occurring in or to the body. Cenesthetic hallucinations are visceral in origin. Tactile hallucinations often involve sensations of animals or bugs and may be associated with somatic or paranoid delusions	A bug on the skin; a burning sensation

Visual hallucinations are the most common psychotic symptom, experienced by 15–40% of patients cross-sectionally and by nearly 50% of patients over the course of PD.[5] Other types of hallucinations and delusions usually occur in patients with visual hallucinations.[2,5] Auditory hallucinations are reported in 8–13%.[2,5-7] Olfactory, tactile, and somatic hallucinations are less common.[2,8] Prevalence of delusions varies from 3% to 30%.[2,9]

Clinical characteristics

There are three main categories of PD-related psychosis.[10] The term "benign" psychosis generally refers to hallucinations of any modality with retained insight into the "non-real" nature of the perception. The hallucination itself has no behavioral impact, but patients may express concerns about having hallucinations. Furthermore, the term "benign" is probably a misnomer in

this setting given the prognostic significance of the presence of hallucinations.[3,11] A second category includes hallucinations or delusions in a clear
sensorium, but with diminished insight. Some patients are indifferent to the
content of their hallucinations or delusions while others are preoccupied or
distressed. Delusions may lead to behavioral problems, including aggression.
A third group includes hallucinations and delusions in the context of
delirium, which can be superimposed on chronic PD-related psychosis.
Demarcations between these categories are not always clear. Some patients
become certain that their hallucinations are abnormal perceptions only after
they pause for a "reality check."

Hallucinations

Hallucinations are abnormal perceptions that occur in the absence of a
stimulus. In PD, hallucinations can involve any sensory modality (Table 10.1).
Minor visual hallucinations and illusions are most common (26%).[5] These are
usually fleeting and rarely cause behavioral disturbances; patients may not
reveal their occurrence unless specifically asked. However, for some patients,
the abnormal visual perceptions are distracting and affect safety while driving
or walking at night, even with retained insight. Visual hallucinations frequently present in dim light, but they can occur any time of day, inside or
outside, and often in the same visual field. Patients with compromised insight
may react to visual hallucinations, showing consideration or aggression,
depending on whether or not the hallucination is regarded as threatening.
Some patients prepare food for their night-time "visitors." Others may become
seriously injured, for example, when they lunge at a hallucination of a stranger
in the bedroom and instead fall into a nightstand. The content of hallucinations can vary, but many describe recurrent phenomena.

Delusions

Delusions are fixed, false idiosyncratic beliefs that are maintained despite
incontrovertible evidence. In PD, most delusions are paranoid in content
and focus on a single subject. Common themes include spousal infidelity,
fears of being poisoned, injured, or filmed, and elaborate conspiracies.[12] Less
commonly, patients describe somatic or grandiose delusions or bizarre delusions of control or passivity experiences, similar to phenomena described by
patients with schizophrenia. One patient maintained that the cycles of the
washing machine caused a back and forward motion within his body and
that others committed actions that aggravated his motor symptoms.

Delusional misidentification (e.g., Capgras phenomena) has also been reported.[13] Mood congruent delusions can occur as a component of a depressive disorder, but delusional ideation in PD patients is usually independent of a co-morbid mood disorder.[2,14] Similarly, delusions often occur with visual hallucinations, but the content may be unrelated or associated with other psychopathology, such as hypersexual or manic phenomena. Patients with non-motor fluctuations may have persecutory delusions when "off" and grandiose delusions when "on."

Longitudinal course

Longitudinal studies in new-onset idiopathic PD are needed to clarify when psychosis is most likely to develop. Early onset of psychosis before onset of dopaminergic replacement therapy (DRT) or shortly afterwards, i.e., within the first 3 months, is atypical for PD and suggests alternative diagnoses. In most patients, psychosis persists after initial onset and can fluctuate over time.[11] Severe psychosis usually requires chronic antipsychotic therapy for symptom control.[15] The need for antipsychotic therapy is also associated with development and progression of dementia and greater likelihood of nursing home placement and mortality.[3,4,16] However, long-term prognosis with respect to these issues has improved with use of atypical antipsychotic treatments such as clozapine.[17]

Neuropsychiatric co-morbidities

Presence of one non-motor psychiatric symptom in PD increases the likelihood of additional psychiatric disturbances[18] and this, along with the tendency to have advanced PD, is perhaps what makes management of psychosis most challenging. For clinicians, the major tasks are to characterize the psychotic phenomena, determine their relationship to other psychiatric, cognitive, and motor disturbances, and develop a treatment plan that accounts for these relationships and targets specific symptoms, in part with respect to their acuity. While some patients benefit most when each disturbance is addressed independently, a comprehensive but focused approach from the outset often simplifies treatment and yields multiple desirable outcomes. For example, treatment with an antipsychotic might also ameliorate insomnia, thereby enhancing daytime function and cognition and reducing caregiver burden. Alternatively, antidepressant treatment may improve mood and insomnia, with subsequent reduction in psychosis.[19]

Affective disorders

As described in Chapter 8, a number of studies show that depressive symptoms frequently co-occur with psychosis and add to functional impairment.[1,2,5,14,20–22] Furthermore, at least half of patients with psychosis (hallucinations and/or delusions) have an additional syndromic affective disturbance, including depression (71%), anxiety (21%), or apathy (14%).[2] This additional psycho-pathology is associated with greater cognitive impairment and caregiver distress. Psychotic affective syndromes, i.e., mania or depression with mood-congruent delusions, are relatively infrequent,[1,2,14] but patients can have both mood-congruent and an unrelated psychotic symptom. For example, an 80-year-old woman with recurrent depressive episodes throughout her 20-year course of PD described paranoia about possible torture by Japanese intelligence officers in the context of a severe depressive episode, but she also experienced chronic visual hallucinations of birds in her house.

Disruptive behaviors

Chapter 12 reviews the range of behavioral disturbances that occur in PD such as hypersexuality, pathological gambling and shopping, perseverative behaviors, and levodopa abuse, or in association with mania. Like psychosis, these are related to DRT and, most likely, underlying disease progression.[23] However, the psychotic phenomena and behavioral alterations are not always related and each may respond differently to DRT adjustments and antipsychotic medications. For example, a patient with increased libido and excessive masturbation experienced paranoid delusions and auditory hallucinations of neighbors commenting that they thought he was a homosexual. The psychotic symptoms improved with clozapine, but he continued to have excessive masturbation that he attributed to boredom. Another patient had pathological gambling, sexual promiscuity involving contacts through the internet, and paranoid delusions that he was being followed by police officers and that bugging devices were implanted in kitchen appliances. His behavioral symptoms diminished when his dose of dopamine agonist was reduced, but his psychotic symptoms were controlled only by quetiapine, except when he used additional doses of levodopa to combat akinesia.

Cognitive impairment and dementia

Chapters 7, 8, and 9 review cognitive impairment in PD. Cognitive impairment is one of the most consistently reported correlates of psy-chosis.[1,5,14,20,21] The average prevalence of dementia ranges from 15% to 30%, but more severe and widespread deficits consistent with dementia develop in up to 75%.[24] It is therefore of prognostic and perhaps diagnostic interest whether certain cognitive deficits predict onset of psychosis. For example, greater executive dysfunction is associated with transition to dementia,[25] but it is unclear whether such selective impairments represent a risk factor or marker for development of psychosis and might be a therapeutic target. Cross-sectionally, hallucinators show greater deficits on letter fluency as well as global cognitive performance.[21] Another study showed impaired object perception, recognition memory, and non-verbal recall in visual hallucinators compared to non-hallucinators and non-PD age-matched controls.[26] In a separate series, global and frontal lobe functions were more impaired in hallucinating and/or delusional patients compared to patients without psychiatric disturbances.[2]

Etiology and risk factors

The pathophysiology of psychosis in PD is unknown, but appears to at least involve a variety of brain regions and structures and related neuro-chemical systems (Table 10.2).[27] In addition, a primary role for DRT is supported by the infrequent occurrence of psychosis in idiopathic PD before the advent of levodopa therapy.[28] While dopamine agonists carry a higher risk, all forms of DRT, including dopamine agonists, amantadine, and lev-odopa, can induce psychosis that will improve with dose reductions. Selegiline and catecho-O-methyl-transferase inhibitors, which affect dopamine catabolism, can also be associated with the onset of psychotic symptoms. The most popular explanation attributes psychosis to sec-ondary dopamine receptor hypersensitivity and overstimulation by dopaminergic medications in mesocortical and mesolimbic regions.[21] Con-sistent with evidence for greater frontal dysfunction in association with psychosis, a recent positron emission tomography (PET) functional imaging study showed relative frontal hypermetabolism in PD patients with visual hallucinations compared to non-hallucinators.[29] Similarly, using functional magnetic resonance imaging, hallucinators with PD showed greater frontal and subcortical activation and non-hallucinators showed greater visual cortical activation in response to visual stimuli, sug-gesting disruption of attentional processes in visual circuitry.[30] Since DRT reduces serotonin levels, other theories invoke an imbalance between dopaminergic and serotonergic systems[31] or overstimulation of seroton-ergic receptors by DRT.[32]

Table 10.2 Risk factors for psychosis in Parkinson's disease

Primary factors
Dopaminergic therapies
Dopamine agonists (pergolide, bromocriptine, ropinirole, pramipexole), levodopa
Catecho-O-methyl-transferase inhibitors (entacapone)

Additional factors
Psychoactive medications
Antiparkinsonian agents: anticholinergics, selegeline, amantadine
Other agents: benzodiazepines, other anticholinergics, antihistamines, various hypnotics, steroids, narcotics, and other pain medications

Medical illnesses
Systemic conditions, dehydration, pain, undetected intracranial injury or fractures, acute or subacute infections, especially urinary tract infections, pneumonias, constipation, cellulitus

Other co-morbid neuropsychiatric conditions
Depressive symptoms, depressive syndromes, dementia, mania, levodopa abuse

Sleep disturbances
Sleep fragmentation, periodic leg movements, restless leg phenomena, REM-related behavioral disturbances

Non-dopaminergic neurotransmitter systems are also relevant to the pathophysiology of psychosis. Most notably, this is suggested by the lack of a direct relationship between psychosis and the dose of dopaminomimetic medications[1] or levodopa plasma level.[33] Cognitive impairment, particularly dementia, older age, longer disease duration, more severe PD, sleep/wake disturbances, and depression are also consistently cited as well as relevant patient-related factors.[1,5,14,20,34,35] Concurrent medical conditions can also lead to psychosis, including in the context of delirium, as can medications, including anticholinergic agents and psychoactive medications, e.g., benzodiazepines, opiates, and certain antidepressants, that may be prescribed for a variety of reasons besides PD or psychiatric conditions. Presence of rapid eye movement sleep behavior disorder[36] and sleep disturbances in general[37] are also associated with visual hallucinations in PD, suggesting a link with sleep pathophysiology. Visual dysfunction is another risk factor.[5,20] Genetic factors are not established, but are under investigation.[38]

Since cognitive deficits in PD are associated with cholinergic deficits[39] and the most consistent clinical correlate of psychosis is cognitive impairment, cholinergic deficits are thought to play a role in development of psychosis. Anticholinergic medications are associated with delirium as well as psychotic symptoms in a clear sensorium. Cortical Lewy body pathology may be related to development of psychosis in later stages of PD, including delirium-like states of fluctuating consciousness that are present in DLB.

Overlap of psychosis in PD with dementia (PDD) and dementia with Lewy bodies (DLB)

There is controversy as to whether PDD and DLB represent separate disorders or occur on a spectrum of a single disease entity related to synuclein pathology.[40,41] Clinically, both DLB and advanced-stage PD can present cross-sectionally with parkinsonism, dementia, and psychosis. Pathologically, Lewy bodies characterize both conditions, and some PDD patients have sufficient numbers of cortical Lewy bodies to meet neuropathological criteria for DLB. However, on clinical grounds, distinguishing DLB from PD-related psychosis is important because of differences in prognosis and treatment planning. These issues are discussed in detail in Chapter 7.

Clinical management

Table 10.3 provides guidelines for the treatment of psychosis. Given the implications of psychosis for long-term prognosis in PD, psychotic

---

Table 10.3 General steps in treatment of psychosis in Parkinson's disease[78]

1. Primary prevention – screen for and address risk factors that predispose to psychosis on an ongoing basis, especially when there are complaints of cognitive impairment
2. Recognition and treatment of additional medical conditions
3. Re-evaluation of the patient's entire medication regimen
4. Early recognition and treatment of mood and other co-morbid psychiatric illnesses
5. Address disrupted sleep
6. Non-pharmacologic strategies
7. Cholinesterase inhibitors
8. Trial of antipsychotic (neuroleptic) agents

symptoms should be assessed at every clinical visit, along with assessment of motor symptoms. As patients may have multiple clinicians who prescribe medications, the current regimen and patient adherence should also be evaluated. Coordination of care between clinicians is critical.

When psychosis is present, the severity of symptoms and the potential triggers in that individual guide the sequence of interventions. Treatment strategies will vary according to the different stages of the disease and according to the presence of other co-morbidities. Pharmacotherapy is complicated as antiparkinsonian medications contribute to psychosis and antipsychotic agents can aggravate motor and cognitive impairments. Psychosis with agitation may require emergent hospitalization to treat concurrent medical conditions, maintain safety of the patient and others, and control behavior, yet enable adequate motor function while adjusting medications or adding antipsychotics. Given the complexity of management and frailty of patients, inability of the patient (or caregiver) to adhere to the prescribed treatment is also justification for hospitalization.

"Benign" symptoms may only need education and reassurance, but it is always best to consider remediable factors that affect overall function even when the psychotic symptoms are not particularly disruptive. For example, a patient with major depression and panic disorder experienced occasional visual hallucinations of her deceased mother standing in the yard. The hallucinations were less frequent after cataract removal. A relapse of her depressive syndrome and problems with impaired concentration prompted a change in her antidepressant from paroxetine, which has anticholinergic properties, to escitalopram. Her mood and cognitive functioning improved and she no longer experienced any hallucinations. The hallucinations along with confusion recurred several months later when her urologist prescribed oxybutynin, an anticholinergic agent, for problems with urinary frequency. In this context, the patient was unable to follow her medication regimen correctly, and forgetfulness led her to take additional doses of her DRT and develop increased dyskinesias and gait instability, even though her hallucinations remained "benign."

Non-pharmacological treatments

Education is a critical component of management. Before starting DRT, patients and family members should be informed about the potential for psychotic symptoms and to report them if they do occur. When psychosis is already present, patients and caregivers often need reassurance that they are not "going crazy." It may help to know that certain tactics can diminish the effects of hallucinations, such as looking away, focusing on the hallucinated object, reassuring oneself, or distracting oneself by interacting with others.[42] Family members need instructions on management, including how to react when patients lack insight and respond to hallucinations or delusions, assess for environmental triggers of confusion, psychosis, or agitation, and when to seek additional help. Since presence of hallucinations is suggestive of increased cognitive impairment that affects daily functioning, we find it helpful to arrange home visits by nurses or occupational therapists who can assess home safety, the patient's ability to comply with the prescribed medication regimen, and identify factors that might increase the likelihood of hallucinations (e.g., dim lighting). When the patient's function is more compromised, assistance with referrals for respite care, adult day programs, or institutionalized placement is also incorporated into treatment. When patients have dementia, we routinely recommend that family and other informal caregivers read *The 36 Hour Day*.[43] It is an excellent resource for caregivers on caring for the loved one with dementia and addressing related behavioral issues.

Medication adjustments

After evaluating their utility and redundancy, DRT and other medications should be either eliminated or reduced to the lowest effective dose. "Drug holidays" from DRT are no longer recommended as patients experience extreme discomfort and there are medical risks, including neuroleptic malignant syndrome.[44] Among the antiparkinsonian agents, levodopa is best tolerated and provides optimal motor symptom control. Before reducing levodopa, other agents are usually eliminated or reduced in the following order, based on their likelihood of contributing to psychosis: anticholinergics, selegiline, amantadine, and catechol-*O*-methyltransferase inhibitors.[45] As medications are reduced, motor symptoms may increase, and relative effects on psychiatric status, mobility, and caregiver burden need to be considered. As discussed in Chapter 3, motor response tends to be more predictable with standard levodopa formulations than with sustained-release preparations.

Treatment of other neuropsychiatric conditions

Affective disorders

All patients with psychosis should be screened for mood disorders, namely depressive disturbances. Conversely, patients with mood disorders should be screened for psychosis.[2] Anxiety disturbances are also overlooked.[46] These affective disturbances are generally treated with antidepressants, though non-pharmacologic therapies may be effective for milder cases. Importantly, mood disorders should be treated aggressively with the goal of remission. As discussed in Chapter 8, selection of antidepressant medications is based on their side-effect profile and controlled studies of antidepressants for treatment of depression are underway. Benzodiazepine use is generally discouraged for treatment of anxiety or insomnia associated with depression. While tempting to prescribe in the short-term to reduce anxiety, benzodiazepines, in this population, generally result in adverse cognitive effects and aggravate psychosis. While there are exceptions in which patients with anxiety actually benefit from chronic benzodiazepine treatment, trazodone or an antipsychotic often serve as effective first-line alternatives for treatment of anxiety or insomnia.

Electroconvulsive therapy

The main indication for electroconvulsive therapy (ECT) is severe depression, especially with mood-congruent delusions. ECT, including maintenance ECT, has been used to treat psychosis in PD,[47,48] but parkinsonism and on-off fluctuations also improve.[49] Thus, ECT is an option when psychosis is resistant to medications or antipsychotic medications are not tolerated.

Sleep disturbances

Resolution of psychosis often improves sleep patterns. However, psychosis with disrupted sleep creates a cycle of nocturnal agitation and daytime somnolence that may improve with direct treatment of insomnia. Treatment of sleep disturbances is discussed in detail in Chapter 11. DRT may need adjusting to avoid nocturnal "wearing off" and improve sleep consolidation. Trazodone, beginning at 25–50 mg and repeating if needed up to 200 mg is often effective. Low doses of sedating antidepressants, e.g., nortiptyline (10–25 mg), mirtazipine (7.5–15 mg), and trazodone (25–200 mg), can be effective hypnotics. Low-dose quetiapine (6.25–50 mg) is a common hypnotic and antipsychotic in this population. Trazodone (25 mg q 6 hours prn) can be effective for daytime agitation and avoids increased sedation from benzodiazepines or antipsychotics. Benzodiazepine hypnotics, antihistamines, and new-generation non-benzodiazepine hypnotics (e.g., zolpidem) tend to increase confusion, while they may be initially effective. Nocturia and sleep apnea should be addressed. Daily exercise and activity facilitate nocturnal sleep. Modafanil or amfetamines may promote daytime wakefulness, although they also carry the risk of psychosis.

Cognitive impairment

The initial use of acetylcholinesterase inhibitors (AChEIs) for treatment of psychosis in PD was based on the established evidence for a cholinergic deficit in PD and studies using AChEIs in patients with Alzheimer's disease and DLB that showed improved cognitive and neuropsychiatric symptoms without aggravation of parkinsonism.[50] Several small open-label studies in patients with PD and dementia showed improved psychosis and cognition with tacrine,[51] rivastigmine,[52] donepezil,[53] and galantamine,[54] but some patients had poor tolerance and worse hallucinations. Recent small controlled trials showed improved cognitive test performance in donepezil-treated patients compared to placebo, including selective improvements in memory.[55,56] The effects of AChEIs on psychosis in these studies cannot be evaluated because samples were small and not all subjects had psychosis. While AChEIs aggravated parkinsonism, especially tremor, in some patients, others had improved motor function.[56] Importantly, abrupt withdrawal of AChEIs can have adverse cognitive and behavioral consequences and is ill-advised.[53] Other classes of cognitive-enhancing agents, e.g., memantine, in PD-related psychosis or dementia have not been studied, but some patients benefit cognitively from memantine in anecdotal experience.

Neuroleptic medications

Antipsychotic medications are indicated when other efforts to treat psychosis or agitation have failed or if antiparkinsonian medications cannot be reduced without sacrificing motor function. Importantly, antipsychotic medications enable increases in antiparkinsonian medications. Since "typical" antipsychotics block D2 receptors and lead to increased parkinsonism, only "atypical" antipsychotics with a low potential for inducing parkinsonism (rigidity, bradykinesia, and tremor) are used. Among those currently available (clozapine, risperidone, olanzapine, quetiapine, ziprasidone, and aripiprazole), only quetiapine and clozapine are consistently recommended.

Clozapine is regarded as the gold standard of antipsychotic agents in PD given its demonstrated safety and efficacy in controlled trials without worsening parkinsonian symptoms.[57-59] The starting dose is usually 6.25–12.5 mg at night. Sedation or confusion occurs at low doses in this fragile population and most patients respond to less than 50 mg/day, though some require higher doses or an additional low dose in the mornings. The most common side-effects are sedation, orthostasis, confusion, and drooling. Seizures can be a dose-related side-effect. Motor fluctuations worsen in some patients, but dystonia, dyskinesias, and tremor can improve.[60,61] As hematologic monitoring for potential agranulocytosis is required for the first 6 months and then biweekly thereafter, clozapine use is usually restricted to patients who are otherwise refractory to treatment. However, the inconvenience of monitoring white blood cell counts is often offset by therapeutic benefits.

Quetiapine resembles clozapine pharmacologically and is a common first choice in PD because it does not require white blood cell monitoring. While quetiapine has not been subject to large-scale controlled trials, a number of open-label studies show that it has a favorable safety and efficacy profile, although some patients experience inadequate symptom control or increased parkinsonism or motor fluctuations.[62] Thus, a general consensus is that quetiapine is slightly less effective than clozapine, but often provides adequate symptom control to warrant its continued use relative to the risks and burdens associated with clozapine. Initial doses range from 6.25 mg to 25 mg, usually at night, but the effective dose range in PD is up to 400 mg.[63] Lower doses are recommended initially because patients with hypotension or orthostasis may not tolerate higher amounts. Sedation and confusion are common side-effects, but a recent open-label study showed improved cognitive functioning on quetiapine.[63]

The ongoing search for novel antipsychotics without motor side-effects has resulted in development of additional agents that have been tried in PD, but without the same tolerability and effectiveness as clozapine or quetiapine. Aripiprazole, the most recently available atypical antipsychotic, is a D2 and 5-HT1a receptor partial agonist and a 5-HT2a antagonist. Its pharmacological properties may confer a lower risk of inducing parkinsonism as well as the weight gain or glucose dysregulation observed with other atypical antipsychotics. Clinical experience on its use in PD patients with psychosis and published reports provide mixed results. While tolerated and effective at doses ranging from 5 mg to 40 mg daily,[64] we and others have observed worse motor function,[65,66] including after a single dose. Therefore, a recommended starting dose for PD patients is 5 mg. Results of controlled trials to evaluate the safety, tolerability, and effectiveness of aripiprazole in PD with psychosis are pending.

The remaining atypical antipsychotic agents are generally less well-tolerated in PD. Initial open-label studies of olanzapine were favorable in terms of effectiveness and safety,[67] but this was not shown in controlled trials.[68,69] Risperidone is an effective antipsychotic, but is poorly tolerated in PD, even at doses less than 1.0 mg/day.[70] Ziprasidone, another more recently available atypical antipsychotic, has not been used widely in PD patients. Cautious use of ziprasidone is recommended as its pharmacological profile suggests it is more likely to worsen parkinsonism than clozapine or quetiapine.[71] As the smallest oral dose of ziprasidone is available in a 20 mg capsule, it is difficult to initiate ziprasidone at the lower doses usually used in PD patients. While ziprasidone at 20–40 mg daily was well-tolerated and effective in a clinical series of PD patients with psychosis,[72] another report described precipitation of neuroleptic malignant syndrome with ziprasidone in a PD patient.[6] However, we are also aware of anecdotal use of intramuscular ziprasidone at lower doses to treat acute agitation effectively and safely in PD patients.

Acute management

Acute agitation can occur in PD patients and is extremely challenging to manage for several reasons: (1) the mental and motor state is even more unstable compared to the usual baseline, (2) there are often active medical issues, and (3) the medication regimen is often complicated.[73] Such patients often present to emergency rooms or psychiatric units where clinicians may have less experience with PD symptoms and their management, including the need for regular dosing of DRT, is often under-appreciated. Comanagement with a movement disorder specialist is strongly encouraged. When a local specialist is not available, it is appropriate to contact one of the Parkinson's disease foundations or a regional movement disorder center to identify clinicians who can provide advice and perhaps assist in follow-up care. A list of PD Foundations is provided in Appendix B.

In acute settings, the general steps in Table 10.3 should be followed, but some more urgently than others. Benzodiazepines (intramuscular or oral) are recommended for severe acute agitation that presents a danger to the patient or others; neuroleptics may not be as readily effective, although quetiapine has been used satisfactorily.[73] Typical neuroleptics, namely haloperidol, that are used to treat agitation or delirium in non-PD patients are not recommended as they induce severe parkinsonism. This can result in medical complications such as deep venous thrombosis, aspiration pneumonia, decubiti, and fractures. Odansentron, a 5HT-3 blocker, can be given intravenously, intramuscularly, or orally and can be useful in emergency situations without causing parkinsonism.[32] The high cost of odansentron and similar agents prohibits its long-term use. As above, we are also aware of use of low-dose intramuscular ziprasidone in acute settings with favorable results.

Since many PD patients with severe agitation are managed on psychiatric or long-term care units, it is important for staff and clinicians to be aware of the potential for a neuroleptic malignant syndrome (NMS)-like condition. This can occur with neuroleptic exposure, after withdrawal of antiparkinsonian medications, or spontaneously.[74] The usual signs of NMS – rigidity, altered consciousness, elevated creatine kinase, hyperpyrexia, and autonomic instability – can be difficult to identify in PD patients with psychosis and acute agitation, who have some of these symptoms anyway, especially if there is a concurrent infection.[6,44]

Conclusion

Patients with advanced PD, who are already challenging to manage, often develop psychosis, which can be accompanied by multiple other co-morbidities, including dementia, mood disorders, behavioral disturbances, medical illnesses, and adverse medication effects. Assessment and treatment of psychosis in PD patients requires careful attention to the multiple factors that contribute to its development and overall morbidity. Early recognition of psychosis, patient and caregiver education, elimination or modification of risk factors, and thoughtful use of antiparkinsonian and other psychoactive medications are integral to treatment. Since treatment of psychiatric co-morbidities reduces burdens of the disease, clinicians should screen patients regularly for psychotic and other neuropsychiatric symptoms. Whether potential advances in the treatment of PD that focus on modification of the underlying disease processes, such as the use of neuroprotective agents, will modify the incidence and impact of psychosis in PD remains to be seen. In the meantime, ongoing development of new antipsychotic agents that do not cause parkinsonism or carry the adverse side-effect profile of clozapine offer the hope of improved clinical management.

References

1. Aarsland D, Larsen JP, Cummings JL, Laake K, Prevalence and clinical correlates of psychotic symptoms in Parkinson disease. A community-based study. *Arch Neurol* 1999; **56**:595–601.

2. Marsh L, Williams JR, Rocco M, Grill S, Munro C, Dawson TM, Psychiatric comorbidities associated with psychosis in patients with Parkinson's disease. *Neurology* 2004; **63**(2):293–300.

3. Goetz CG, Stebbins GT, Risk factors for nursing home placement in advanced Parkinson's disease. *Neurology* 1993; **43**:2227–2229.

4. Factor S, Feustel PJ, Friedman J et al, Longitudinal outcome of Parkinson's disease patients with psychosis. *Neurology* 2003; **60**:1756–1761.

5. Fénelon G, Mahieux F, Huon R, Ziégler M, Hallucinations in Parkinson's disease. Prevalence, phenomenology, and risk factors. *Brain* 2000; **123**:733–745.

6. Gray NS, Ziprasidone-related neuroleptic malignant syndrome in a patient with Parkinson's disease: a diagnostic challenge. *Hum Psychopharmacol* 2004; **19**(3):205–207.

7. Inzelberg R, Kipervasser S, Korczyn AD, Auditory hallucinations in Parkinson's disease. *J Neurol Neurosurg Psychiatry* 1998; **64**:533–535.

8. Fénelon G, Thobois S, Bonnet AM, Broussolle E, Tison F, Tactile hallucinations in Parkinson's disease. *J Neurol* 2002; **249**:1699–1703.

9. Cummings JL, Neuropsychiatric complications of drug treatment in Parkinson's disease. In: Huber SJ, Cummings JL (eds) *Parkinson's Disease: Neurobehavioral Aspects*. Oxford University Press: New York, 1992; 314–327.

10. Peyser CE, Naimark D, Zuniga R, Jeste DV, Psychoses in Parkinson's disease. *Semin Clin Neuropsychiat* 1998; **3**(1):41–50.

11. Goetz CG, Leurgans S, Pappert EJ, Raman R, Stemer AB, Prospective longitudinal assessment of hallucinations in Parkinson's disease. *Neurology* 2001; **57**:2078–2082.

12. Factor SA, Molho ES, Podskalny GD, Brown D, Parkinson's disease: drug-induced psychiatric states. *Adv Neurol* 1995; **65**:115–138.

13. Roane DM, Rogers JD, Robinson JH, Feinberg TE, Delusional misidentification in association with parkinsonism. *J Neuropsychiat Clin Neurosci* 1998; **10**(2):194–198.

14. Giladi N, Treves TA, Paleacu D et al, Risk factors for dementia, depression, and psychosis in long-standing Parkinson's disease. *J Neural Transm* 2000; **107**:59–71.

15. Fernandez HH, Trieschmann ME, Okun MS, Rebound psychosis: Effect of discontinuation of antipsychotics in Parkinson's disease. *Mov Disord* 2005; **20**(1):104–105.

16. Goetz CG, Stebbins GT, Mortality and hallucinations in nursing home patients with advanced Parkinson's disease. *Neurology* 1995; **45**:669–671.

17. Fernandez HH, Donnelly EM, Friedman JH, Long-term outcome of clozapine use for psychosis in parkinsonian patients. *Mov Disord* 2004; **19**(7):831–833.

18. Shulman LM, Taback RL, Bean J, Weiner WJ, Comorbidity of the nonmotor symptoms of Parkinson's disease. *Mov Disord* 2001; **16**(3):507–510.

19. Voon V, Lang AE, Antidepressants in the treatment of psychosis with comorbid depression in Parkinson disease. *Clin Neuropharmacol* 2004; **27**(2):90–92.

20. Holroyd S, Currie L, Wooten GF, Prospective study of hallucinations and delusions in Parkinson's disease. *J Neurol Neurosurg Psychiat* 2001; **70**:734–738.

21. Graham JM, Grunewald RA, Sagar HJ, Hallucinations in idiopathic Parkinson's disease. *J Neurol Neurosurg Psychiat* 1997; **63**:434–440.

22. Barnes J, David AS, Visual hallucinations in Parkinson's disease: a review and phenomenological survey. *J Neurol Neurosurg Psychiat* 2001; **70**:727–733.

23. Kurlan R, Disabling repetitive behaviors in Parkinson's disease. *Mov Disord* 2003; **19**(4):433–469.

24. Aarsland D, Andersen K, Larsen JP, Lolk A, Nielsen H, Kragh-Sørensen P, Risk of dementia in Parkinson's disease. A community-based prospective study. *Neurology* 2001; **56**:730–736.

25. Woods SP, Tröster AI, Prodromal frontal/executive dysfunction predicts incident dementia in Parkinson's disease. *J Int Neuropsychol Soc* 2003; 9(1):17–24.
26. Barnes J, Boubert L, Harris J, Lee A, David AS, Reality monitoring and visual hallucinations in Parkinson's disease. *Neuropsychologia* 2003; 41:565–574.
27. Diederich NJ, Goetz CG, Stebbins GT, Repeated visual hallucinations in Parkinson's disease as disturbed external/internal perceptions: Focused review and a new integrative model. *Mov Disord* 2005; 20(2):130–140.
28. Young BK, Camicioli R, Ganzini L, Neuropsychiatric adverse effects of antiparkinsonian drugs. Characteristics, evaluation and treatment. *Drugs Aging* 1997; 10(5):367–383.
29. Nagano-Saito A, Washimi Y, Arahata Y et al, Visual hallucination in Parkinson's disease with FDG PET. *Mov Disord* 2004; 19(7):801–806.
30. Stebbins GT, Goetz CG, Carrillo MC et al, Altered cortical visual processing in PD with hallucinations. An fMRI study. *Neurology* 2004; 63:1409–1416.
31. Birkmayer W, Riederer P, Responsibility of extrastriatal areas for the appearance of psychotic symptoms. *J Neural Transm* 1975; 37:175–182.
32. Zoldan J, Friedberg G, Weizman A, Melamed E, Ondansetron, a 5-HT3 antagonist for visual hallucinations and paranoid delusional disorder associated with chronic L-DOPA therapy in advanced Parkinson's disease. *Adv Neurol* 1996; 69:541–544.
33. Goetz CG, Pappert EJ, Blasucci LM, Intravenous levodopa in chronically-treated hallucinating Parkinson's patients: high dose pharmacological challenge does not precipitate visual hallucinations. *Neurology* 1998; 50:515–517.
34. Naimark D, Jackson E, Rockwell E, Jeste DV, Psychotic symptoms in Parkinson's disease patients with dementia. *J Am Ger Soc* 1996; 44(3):296–299.
35. Sanchez-Ramos JR, Ortoll R, Paulson GW, Visual hallucinations associated with Parkinson disease. *Arch Neurol* 1996; 53(12):1265–1268.
36. Manni R, Pacchetti C, Terzaghi M, Sartori FM, Nappi G, Hallucinations and sleep–wake cycle in PD: A 24-hour continuous polysomnographic study. *Neurology* 2002; 59:1979–1981.
37. Pappert EJ, Goetz CG, Niederman FG et al, Hallucinations, sleep fragmentation, and altered dream phenomena in Parkinson's disease. *Mov Disord* 1999; 14:117–121.
38. Goldman JG, Goetz CG, Berry-Kravis E, Leurgans S, Zhou L, Genetic polymorphisms in Parkinson disease subjects with and without hallucinations: an analysis of the cholecystokinin system. *Arch Neurol* 2004; 61(8):1280–1284.
39. Nakano I, Hirano A, Parkinson's disease: neuron loss in the nucleus basalis without concomitant Alzheimer's disease. *Ann Neurol* 1984; 15:415–418.
40. Richard IH, Papka M, Rubio A, Kurlan R, Parkinson's disease and dementia with Lewy bodies: One disease or two? *Mov Disord* 2002; 17(6):1161–1165.
41. McKeith IG, Spectrum of Parkinson's disease, Parkinson's dementia, and Lewy body dementia. *Neurol Clin* 2000; 18(4):865–902.
42. Diederich NJ, Pieri V, Goetz CG, Coping strategies for visual hallucinations in Parkinson's disease. *Mov Disord* 2003; 18(7):831–832.
43. Mace NL, Rabins PV, *The 36-Hour Day*, 3rd edn. Warner Books: New York, 1999.
44. Gordon PH, Frucht SJ, Neuroleptic malignant syndrome in advanced Parkinson's disease. *Mov Disord* 2001; 16(5):960–962.
45. Henderson MJ, Mellers JDC, Psychosis in Parkinson's disease: "between a rock and a hard place." *Int Rev Psychiat* 2000; 12:319–334.
46. Marsh L, Anxiety disorders in Parkinson's disease. *Int Rev Psychiat* 2000; 12(4):307–318.
47. Factor SA, Molho ES, Brown DL, Combined clozapine and electroconvulsive therapy for the treatment of drug-induced psychosis in Parkinson's disease. *J Neuropsychiat Clin Neurosci* 1995; 7(3):304–307.

48. Shulman RB, Maintenance ECT in the treatment of PD. Therapy improves psychotic symptoms, physical function. *Geriatrics* 2003; **58**(11):43–45.

49. Andersen K, Balldin J, Gottfries CG et al, A double-blind evaluation of electroconvulsive therapy in Parkinson's disease with "on-off" phenomena. *Acta Neurol Scand* 1987; **76**(3):191–199.

50. Cummings JL, Cholinesterase inhibitors: a new class of psychotropic compounds. *Am J Psychiat* 2000; **157**(1):4–15.

51. Hutchinson M, Fazzini E, Cholinesterase inhibition in Parkinson's disease (letter). *J Neurol Neurosurg Psychiat* 1996; **61**:324–325.

52. Reading PJ, Luce AK, McKeith IG, Rivastigmine in the treatment of parkinsonian psychosis and cognitive impairment: preliminary findings from an open trial. *Mov Disord* 2001; **16**(6):1171–1195.

53. Minett TS, Thomas A, Wilkinson LM et al, What happens when donepezil is suddenly withdrawn? An open label trial in dementia with Lewy bodies and Parkinson's disease with dementia. *Int J Geriatr Psychiat* 2003; **18**(11):988–993.

54. Aarsland D, Hutchinson M, Larsen JP, Cognitive, psychiatric and motor response to galantamine in Parkinson's disease with dementia. *Int J Geriatr Psychiat* 2003; **18**:937–941.

55. Aarsland D, Laake K, Larsen JP, Janvin C, Donepezil for cognitive impairment in Parkinson's disease: a randomized controlled study. *J Neurol Neurosurg Psychiat* 2002; **72**:708–712.

56. Leroi I, Brandt J, Reich SG et al, Randomized placebo controlled trial of donepezil in cognitive impairment in Parkinson's disease. *Int J Geriatr Psychiat* 2004; **19**(1):1–8.

57. Pollak P, Tison F, Rascol O et al, Clozapine in drug induced psychosis in Parkinson's disease: a randomised, placebo controlled study with open follow up. *J Neurol Neurosurg Psychiat* 2004; **75**(5):689–695.

58. The French Clozapine Parkinson Study Group, Clozapine in drug-induced psychosis in Parkinson's disease. *Lancet* 1999; **353**:2041.

59. Parkinson Study Group, Low-dose clozapine for the treatment of drug-induced psychosis in Parkinson's disease. *New Engl J Med* 1999; **340**(10):757–763.

60. Durif F, Vidailhet M, Assal F, Roche C, Bonnet AM, Agid Y, Low-dose clozapine improves dyskinesias in Parkinson's disease. *Neurology* 1997; **48**(3):658–662.

61. Friedman JH, Koller WC, Lannon MC, Busenbark K, Swanson-Hyland E, Smith D, Benztropine versus clozapine for the treatment of tremor in Parkinson's disease. *Neurology* 1997; **48**(4):1077–1081.

62. Fernandez HH, Trieschmann ME, Burke MA, Jacques C, Friedman JH, Long-term outcome of quetiapine use for psychosis among Parkinsonian patients. *Mov Disord* 2003; **18**(5):510–514.

63. Juncos JL, Roberts VJ, Evatt ML et al, Quetiapine improves psychotic symptoms and cognition in Parkinson's disease. *Mov Disord* 2004; **19**(1):29–35.

64. Gupta S, Chohan M, Madhusoodanan S, Treatment of acute mania with aripiprazole in an older adult with noted improvement in coexisting Parkinson's disease. *Prim Care Companion J Clin Psychiat* 2004; **6**(1):50–51.

65. Fernandez HH, Trieschman ME, Friedman JH, Aripiprazole for drug-induced psychosis in Parkinson's disease: preliminary experience. *Clin Neuropharmacol* 2004; **27**(1):4–5.

66. Schonfeldt-Lecuona C, Connemann BJ, Aripiprazole and Parkinson's disease psychosis. *Am J Psychiat* 2004; **161**(2):373–374.

67. Wolters EC, Jansen EN, Tuynman-Qua HG, Bergmans PL, Olanzapine in the treatment of dopaminomimetic psychosis in patients with Parkinson's disease. *Neurology* 1996; **47**(4):1085–1087.

68. Goetz CG, Blasucci LM, Leurgans S, Pappert EJ, Olanzapine and clozapine. Comparative effects on motor function in hallucinating PD patients. *Neurology* 2000; **55**:789–794.

69. Breier A, Sutton VK, Feldman PD et al, Olanzapine in the treatment of dopamimetic-induced psychosis in patients with Parkinson's disease. *Biol Psychiat* 2002; **52**:438–445.

70. Friedman JH, Fernandez HH, Atypical antipsychotics in Parkinson-sensitive populations. *J Geriatr Psychiat Neurol* 2002; **15**:156–170.

71. Tarsy D, Baldessarini RJ, Tarazi FI, Effects of newer antipsychotics on extrapyramidal function. *CNS Drugs* 2002; **16**(1):23–45.

72. Lopez DV, Santos S, Quetiapine and ziprasidone in the treatment of the psychotic disorders in Parkinson's disease. *Rev Neurol* 2004; **39**(7):661–667.

73. Factor SA, Molho ES, Emergency department presentations of patients with Parkinson's disease. *Am J Emer Med* 2000; **18**(2):209–215.

74. Ueda M, Hamamoto M, Nagayama H et al, Susceptibility to neuroleptic malignant syndrome in Parkinson's disease. *Neurology* 1999; **52**:777–781.

75. Tousi B, Frankel M, Olfactory and visual hallucinations in Parkinson's disease. *Parkinsonism Relat Disord* 2004; **10**(4):253–254.

76. Sandyk R, Olfactory hallucinations in Parkinson's disease. *South Afr Med J* 1981; **60**(25):950.

77. Jimenez-Jimenez FJ, Orti-Pareja M, Gasalla T, Tallon-Barranco A, Cabrera-Valdivia F, Fernandez-Lliria A, Cenesthetic hallucinations in a patient with Parkinson's disease. *J Neurol Neurosurg Psychiat* 1997; **63**(1):120.

78. Marsh L, Psychosis in Parkinson's disease. *Curr Treat Options Neurol* 2004; **6**(3):181–189.

chapter 11

Sleep

Matthew Menza, Humberto Marin and Roseanne DeFronzo Dobkin

Introduction

Disturbances of sleep are one of the most common problems experienced by people with Parkinson's disease (PD). This is not surprising as sleep disorders are very prevalent in the elderly and in the medically ill.[1] However, a variety of surveys now suggest that sleep is even more of a problem for patients with PD than it is for the general population, or medical controls, of a similar age.[2,3]

Until recently, the pattern of sleep in people with Parkinson's disease (PD) received relatively little attention from the research community.[4] Nonetheless, it is a common and very disabling complication with which patients, caregivers, and clinicians struggle. In fact, sleep problems are a significant factor in the quality of life for both patients and their caregivers. In this chapter, we review clinical issues relevant to the practicing physician and the patient suffering from disrupted sleep. These issues include the type of sleep disturbances seen in PD, the prevalence of these problems, the relationships between sleep and other clinical characteristics of PD, and lastly, recommendations on treatment.

Insomnia

Insomnia, the inability to sleep, is generally divided into difficulty falling asleep (sleep initiation), staying asleep (sleep fragmentation), and awakening too early in the morning. While all three may be found in patients with

PD, typically the most difficulty is with sleep fragmentation.[5] For instance, Nausieda et al.[2] found that 74% of a group of patients with PD whom he surveyed had sleep fragmentation complaints. If one includes difficulties such as an inability to turn over in bed and frequent nocturnal urination, the rate may be as high as 98%.[6] It is important to remember that aging is associated with worsening sleep, with approximately 40% of the elderly experiencing sleep problems, especially in the presence of physical and psychological illness.[7] However, community-based surveys consistently report a greater prevalence of sleep problems in patients with PD compared to healthy controls, matched for age and gender. Furthermore, these studies also show an increased prevalence of sleep disorders compared to patients with other medical disorders like diabetes. For instance, Tandberg et al.[3] found that 60% of people with PD report sleeping problems, compared to 46% of patients with diabetes mellitus and 33% of healthy controls, matched for age and gender. Sleep fragmentation was found in 39% of patients with PD and only 12% of controls. Sleep initiation problems were equally prevalent in patients and controls. These findings on insomnia have been consistently reported over the past 20 years.[5,8–11]

Parasomnias

The parasomnias, a group of disorders characterized by abnormal behavior during sleep, are also common in patients with PD. They may include rapid eye movement (REM) behavior disorder, vivid dreams, nightmares, sleepwalking, and night terrors.

REM behavior disorder (RBD)

RBD deserves special attention as it can result in significant injury. RBD is a syndrome of abnormal behavior during rapid eye movement (REM) sleep. Under normal circumstances, voluntary muscles are atonic (not moving) when one enters REM sleep, resulting in limb paralysis. However, the absence of this normal atonia in patients with RBD leads to the acting out of dreams. Thus, an individual who experiences being chased in a dream may flee the bed or attempt to punch his pursuer. The response may range from relatively mild restlessness to more severe, wild punching and thrashing in which patients may leap out of bed or strike their bed partner. We have seen one patient who broke his femur in three places after leaping out of bed into his dresser. Thus, RBD is potentially dangerous for the patient and his or her bed partner and prompt identification and treatment is warranted.

RBD occurs in 15–50% of patients with PD.[12,13] RBD is uncommon in individuals without neurological disease; patients with PD account for a significant percentage of the cases that a sleep center sees. Among 93 consecutive patients with RBD from the Mayo Sleep Disorder Center, 49 also had PD, dementia, or multiple system atrophy. Furthermore, half of the patients with PD and RBD had developed RBD prior to the onset of their movement disorder.[14] RBD is likely the result of degenerative changes in the brain, possibly representing an underlying common pathology across neurological illness.[15]

Sleep attacks

Sleep attacks are abrupt and unavoidable transitions from wakefulness to sleep. These "attacks" are of particular concern as the patient may have little warning that they are about to fall asleep. Obviously, if these attacks occur during potentially dangerous activities, such as driving or walking down stairs, harm may result.

There has been debate over this issue since the first reports by Frucht et al.[16] of sleep attacks in patients with PD taking dopaminergic agonists. The prevalence of sleep attacks in patients with PD varies across studies, from 0–30%.[17,18] The debate has involved the issue of whether or not sleep attacks are largely the result of tiredness or if they are specifically related to dopaminergic agonists. In the end, while many reports specifically implicate pramipexole and ropinirole, it is probably a class effect of all dopamine agonists and probably all dopamine replacement therapies.[18] Given the potential for harm, an inquiry into the presence of sleep attacks should be a routine in all patients with PD.

Sleep-disordered breathing

Sleep-disordered breathing occurs when the individual has episodes of not breathing (apnea) during deep sleep. The problem may be a lack of breathing drive in the brain (central sleep apnea) or a problem with the passage of air through the breathing passages (obstructive sleep apnea – OSA). In OSA, the breathing passages are blocked by relaxed muscles and tissues of the throat and neck. If the passage of air is severely obstructed, breathing may stop, leading to a decrease in blood oxygen level that eventually results in sufficient awakening to restore breathing. As the patient remains in light sleep, they may be unaware of these awakenings, which may happen hundreds of times a night. Consequently, the patient experiences little deep restorative sleep at night and extreme daytime sleepiness. Since the patient may be unaware of the problem, one needs to query a bed partner who will be aware of loud snoring, gasping, and periods of no breathing.

Apnea has been found in as many as 50% of patients with PD.[19] A significant incidence of obstructive and central apnea has been found in PD, generally developing later in the illness.[20] Snoring and apneic episodes may be up to three times more common in PD (12%) than in the general population.[12]

Restless legs syndrome and periodic leg movements of sleep

Persistent motor symptoms that occur during sleep include periodic limb movement of sleep (PLMS) and restless legs syndrome (RLS). RLS tends to occur at the beginning of sleep or as one is trying to fall asleep and is a disagreeable restless feeling that is often only relieved by moving one's legs. PLMS are rhythmic moving or jerking of the limbs during sleep. Both of these disorders may interfere with the quantity and quality of sleep. RLS and PLMS are common in patients with PD, occurring in up to 30% of patients and can lead to disrupted sleep and excessive daytime sleepiness.[11,21]

Vivid dreaming

An increase in dreaming is common in patients on dopaminergic therapy.[4] Survey data suggest that about 30% of patients develop vivid dreams on dopaminergic therapies[22] and our clinical experience suggests that the majority of patients with PD experience them. Because vivid dreams are often a prodrome of daytime hallucinations[23] one should query patients concerning increases in vivid dreaming.

Excessive daytime sleepiness and fatigue

Tiredness during the day is one of the more common difficulties experienced by people with PD. EDS (the tendency to fall asleep during the day) should be differentiated from fatigue (difficulty in initiating and sustaining mental and physical tasks), though in clinical practice it is often difficult to separate the two. Fatigue is characterized by excessive tiredness, lack of energy and motivation, but without sleepiness, or the likelihood of falling asleep if one lies down. Both EDS and fatigue are common and troubling to patients with PD.[9] Estimates of the occurrence of EDS range from 15–50%[3,24,25] and fatigue is found in up to 59% of patients.[26,27] The presence of both EDS and fatigue are significantly correlated with more severe disease, more disability, cognitive decline, and depression.[27,28]

There are a variety of possible explanations for this degree of EDS and fatigue. Included in these possibilities are insomnia, the effects of aging, sedating effects of medications, an effect of the central illness on sleep and wake centers in the brain, intrinsic sleep disorders such as apnea, and the presence of co-morbid illness such as depression.

The impact of sleep disorders in PD: Quality of life

Parkinson's disease clearly has a deleterious impact on quality of life[29,30] with patients reporting significant difficulties with physical mobility and social functioning.[31] In a large national survey of American veterans, patients with PD reported more impairment in quality of life than those with other chronic medical or neurological conditions such as heart disease, arthritis, chronic pain, diabetes, and stroke.[32]

Sleep difficulties are a critical factor in the poor quality of life in PD.[33–35] These sleep difficulties have not only been associated with the PD patients' reduced enthusiasm for daily events but have also been found to negatively impact the quality of life of their spousal caregivers.[36] Although sleep disturbance strongly correlates with patient distress, the interaction between sleep difficulties, depression, and impairment in activities of daily living may be the most important predictor of low quality of life for PD patients.[34] There are, therefore, a variety of reasons for us to address sleep problems in patients with PD.

Relationship between depression and sleep in Parkinson's disease

Sleep disturbances have an intimate and complex relationship with depression.[37] Depression is one of the two most common causes of insomnia[38] and sleep disturbance is one of the most common presenting symptoms of depression. Mendelson et al.[39] reported that more than 90% of depressed patients complain about impairments of sleep quality. Typically, depressed patients suffer from difficulties in falling asleep, frequent nocturnal awakenings, and early morning awakening, with the most common complaint involving difficulties with maintaining sleep throughout the night.

Depression and anxiety are very common in PD.[40,41] The effects of depression and anxiety on sleep in PD patients has not been carefully studied but clinically the impact is clear. Surveys have, however, confirmed what is clinically apparent, that patients with PD and depression have more difficulty with sleep.[42] In a questionnaire study from our group, anxiety and depression were associated with sleep quality though disease severity and age had larger effects.[43] In a separate study, Pal et al.[36] found that PD patients with more severe sleep dysfunction had greater depression and anxiety but observed no significant association between sleep disturbance and age, severity, or duration of PD. While the relationship between these variables warrants further investigation, it is nonetheless prudent to assume that depression and anxiety will adversely affect sleep; one needs therefore, to address these issues.

The etiology of sleep disorders in Parkinson's disease

The interactions between PD and sleep are complicated. Many of the degenerative changes that are occurring in the brain may directly affect sleep/wake mechanisms and lead to sleep disruption.[44] In particular, brain neurotransmitters that mediate sleep functions (norepinephrine (noradrenaline), serotonin, dopamine, and GABA) are damaged in PD, although to different degrees.[45,46] Furthermore, motor difficulties, such as inability to move in bed, dystonic movements, and pain from leg cramps may all interfere with sleep maintenance. While dopaminergic replacement therapy (DRT) may improve sleep in patients experiencing night-time motor dysfunction, DRT can also disrupt normal sleep architecture and may be stimulating to some patients. Lastly, many other primary sleep disorders, such as sleep apnea, restless legs, etc., occur commonly in individuals with PD, as previously discussed.

Superimposed on these complex interactions are age-related sleep and circadian changes. Approximately 40% of the elderly experience sleep difficulties and these problems tend to be more common in those elderly with physical and psychological problems.[47] These problems tend to be difficulties falling asleep, staying asleep and taking more daytime naps.

Treatment of sleep disorders in Parkinson's disease

Accurate diagnosis is the first principle in the treatment of sleep disturbances in patients with PD. For most patients, this can be accomplished with a thorough clinical history, but it will sometimes require a polysomnogram at a sleep center. The most common disorders of sleep are listed in Table 11.1. Once a diagnosis is established, the following stepwise approach should be taken (Table 11.2). The first of these steps is to assure that the night-time control of the PD is maximized. Difficulty sleeping is sometimes related to increasing rigidity during sleep and this may be managed with a long-acting dopaminergic agent. Some patients find the effect of the dopaminergic stimulating and the dose, in these situations, may be reduced at night.

The second step is to insure that other common medical conditions, such as depression, anxiety, nocturia, or incontinence, are treated – if these are not adequately treated the sleep will likely remain disturbed.

Table 11.1 Sleep disorders commonly found with PD

Insomnia
REM behavior disorder (RBD)
Sleep attacks
Sleep disordered breathing
Periodic limb movements in sleep (PLMS)
Restless legs syndrome
Vivid dreaming
Excessive daytime sleepiness and fatigue

Table 11.2 Principles of the treatment of sleep disorders in PD

Diagnosis
Maximize night-time control of PD
Treat co-morbid conditions, depression, anxiety, nocturia, etc.
Treat specific sleep disorder, such as RLS, REM behavior disorder, OSA, etc.
Treat non-specific insomnia with CBT, and/or sleep medication
Address environmental issues
    Early bedtime
    Bedtime out of phase with caretaker (nursing home, caretaker)
    Boring daytime environment

After all contributing medical and psychiatric disorders have been evaluated and treated, efforts should be directed at the specific sleep disorder. Unfortunately, there are few research data, specific to PD, from which to derive treatment recommendations. To our knowledge, there have been few controlled trials examining the treatment of sleep disruption in PD. Nonetheless, one can, based on clinical experience and controlled data in the non-PD geriatric population, develop some general principles and make some recommendations on treating sleep disorders in PD. Each of the disorders previously discussed will be addressed in turn below.

Insomnia

While no specific trials have examined the treatment of insomnia in patients with PD, both non-pharmacologic and pharmacologic measures have been shown to be beneficial in the treatment of insomnia in the general population and in the elderly.

Psychologically based treatments for insomnia are widely recommended and have potential advantages in at least three areas. First, psychological treatments are generally benign and free of adverse side-effects. Second, psychological interventions appear to engender more lasting changes following treatment cessation.[48] Additionally, psychological treatments are designed to target key maintaining, if not precipitating or causal, factors underlying the patient's sleep difficulties. Other potential benefits include positive changes in self-efficacy and generalizability to other areas of self-management. Patients also report a preference for psychological therapy overall compared to pharmacotherapy for insomnia.[49] Potential limitations for psychologically based treatments include a shortage of trained therapists, costs associated with treatment and variable insurance reimbursement, and the widespread assumption that medications are more efficacious.

Despite these limitations, significant evidence exists in support of psychologically based treatments for insomnia. Two meta-analyses of a large number of treatment trials support the efficacy of psychological interventions for primary insomnia.[50,51] These studies suggest that approximately 80% of patients with persistent insomnia show improvements in sleep with psychologically based treatments, with sleep latency (the delay in sleep onset) and sleep efficiency returning to normal values in most instances.

Cognitive-behavioral therapy (CBT) for insomnia consists of several components, including stimulus control (associating the bedroom environment with sleep), sleep restriction (limiting the amount of time in bed), cognitive therapy (modifying self-defeating cognitions related to sleep), relaxation therapy (somatic and cognitive relaxation techniques) and sleep hygiene education. Sleep hygiene measures that are useful for nearly all patients with insomnia are listed in Table 11.3.

Pharmacotherapy is the most widely used treatment for insomnia in clinical practice.[52,53] In patients with PD living in the community, 40% were found to be using sleeping pills, compared to 23% of the controls.[3]

A variety of medications are available for use in patients with insomnia, including benzodiazepines, the non-benzodiazepine hypnotics, antihistamines, and the sedating antidepressants.[54] Table 11.4 lists the common medications and doses used for these patients.

Numerous large studies have found the benzodiazepines (such as temazepam, flurazepam, and lorazepam) to be superior in short-term use to placebo for sleep latency and for total sleep time.[55,56] While these medications are widely used and clearly effective, one should use them with caution in the elderly as they increase risk for fall and fractures by 50% or more.[57] In addition, benzodiazepines are associated with tolerance and are associated with a risk of cognitive impairment in this age group.[58] Nonetheless, when used carefully with appropriate caution they may be helpful, especially for short-term use.

A newer class of medications is the non-benzodiazepine hypnotics (zolpidem and zaleplon) that also work via the benzodiazepine receptor but have an improved side-effect profile. As with the benzodiazepines, these

Table 11.3 Sleep hygiene measures

Establish a sleep-conducive environment
   Familiar space, right temperature, no bright light, low noise
Regular exercise
Reduce evening fluid intake to limit nocturia (use bedpan, bedside commode or condom catheter if necessary)
Use bed only for sleep
Warm bath before bedtime
If necessary, instrumental aids for getting in and out of bed
Allow reading or watching TV at night to reduce initial insomnia, but out of bed
Maintain a fixed wake-up time regardless of the quality or quantity of sleep
Avoid daytime naps over half an hour
Avoid evening large meals, caffeine, and alcohol

Table 11.4 Sleep medications for insomnia

Antihistamines	Diphenhydramine or hydroxyzine, 25–50 mg
Non-benzodiazepine hypnotics	Zolpidem 5–10 mg, zaleplon 5–10 mg
Benzodiazepines	Lorazepam 0.25–1 mg
	Clonazepam 0.25–1 mg
	Temazepam 15–30 mg
Sedating antidepressants	Nortriptyline 10–50 mg
	Amitriptyline 10–50 mg
	Trazodone 25–100 mg
	Mirtazapine 15 mg
Atypical antipsychotics	Quetiapine 25–100 mg

medications are effective for the short term treatment of both difficulty falling asleep and difficulty staying asleep in non-Parkinson's groups.[59] While one small study suggested that zolpidem may have a beneficial effect on the motor components of PD,[60] no studies have specifically examined the effect of these drugs for insomnia in individuals with PD. The non-benzodiazepines generally cause less confusion and morning sedation than the benzodiazepines, but caution is still advised in using these agents, as they have been associated with an increase in hip fractures from falls.[61]

Sedating antidepressants, especially trazodone, are now widely used for insomnia.[62] There is no specific information available as to its use in PD, though it is sometimes helpful in other elderly populations. Over-the-counter medications such as the antihistamines (diphenhydramine (Benadril™)) are also widely used and may be useful in some patients.[63] A significant issue with both the sedating antidepressants and the antihistamines in PD is their anticholinergic effects, which may increase both constipation and cognitive impairment. Other over-the-counter aids, including herbal supplements have not been studied and we generally do not recommend their use in individuals with PD.

In patients with significant cognitive impairment, psychosis, or very vivid dreaming (often heralding daytime psychosis) the atypical antipsychotics quetiapine or clozapine may be of use. These medications have not been studied for insomnia in any patient group but, as discussed in Chapters 10 and 12, have been studied in PD for psychosis and used to treat a variety of disinhibited behaviors.[64] In general, PD patients tolerate these medications, but in very low doses. One must also be cautious about sedation and a worsening of the motor components of the illness. Of special note is that clozapine may only be used with frequent white blood cell monitoring (every week for the first 6 months) because of the risk of agranulocytosis.

Other new treatments that target the movements of PD may also have positive effects on sleep. For instance, deep brain stimulation (DBS), an effective therapeutic option for the treatment of advanced Parkinson's disease, has been shown to improve sleep in PD. It is likely that the treatment is effective because it improves the night-time control of the motor movements of PD, rather than having a specific effect on sleep.[65]

In summary, when using medications for insomnia in individuals with PD, we generally begin with a non-benzodiazepine hypnotic such as zaleplon or zolpidem. Alternatives include trazodone (25–50 mg with a repeat dose if needed) and the benzodiazepine, if used cautiously. In any case, patients or caregivers should be asked about any adverse effects that might be evident the next day or after several nights of use. Both of the non-benzodiazepine and benzodiazepine classes of medications are best if used intermittently, from three to five times a week, which may decrease tolerance. In situations in which there is significant cognitive impairment, or psychosis, one should probably switch to quetiapine.

REM behavior disorder

There are relatively little data on treating RBD in patients with PD. In one widely cited study using clonazepam, a long-acting benzodiazepine, Schenck et al.[66] reported that 90% of the 57 treated patients improved on moderate doses. Another small case series describes melatonin as useful.[67] Because of the study by Schenck et al., and clinical experience, clonazepam is currently the standard treatment for RBD in patients with PD. One does, however, need to remember the caution concerning benzodiazepines, sedation and confusion.

RLS and PLMS

If tolerated, an increase in dopaminergic treatment at night is helpful with RLS and PMLS, as they decrease periodic limb movements during sleep and significantly improve early-morning motor function.[68] Gabapentin is sometimes used for the treatment of RLS.[69] Other treatments that have received some support include benzodiazepines and the opiates.[4]

Sleep attacks

Treatment of sleep attacks involves a number of approaches. The first is to identify the problem by systematic patient inquiry and then to educate patients about the risks associated with the problem. One should also consider reducing or eliminating the direct dopamine agonists if sleep attacks are occurring with little warning or are significantly affecting functioning. As sleep attacks generally occur in the context of EDS, one should also address this problem. This approach is dealt with in the next section.

Excessive daytime sleepiness and fatigue

As discussed above, the main causes of EDS and fatigue that should be considered in treatment planning are insufficient or unsatisfactory sleep, co-morbid medical and psychiatric disorders and the effects of drug therapy. Therefore, the first approach is to re-evaluate the patient's sleep. A review of medical and psychiatric disorders, such as depression and anxiety should also be a priority. Among medications, consider a "hangover" from hypnotics and other psychotropics such as antidepressants and antipsychotics. Many other medications that patients take may also induce EDS and fatigue so one needs to review the entire medication list. Special attention should be directed to the direct dopamine agonists as discussed in the previous section.

Besides elimination of aggravating medications, treatment includes a variety of environmental and behavioral approaches that, while not studied in PD, have been found to be helpful in other populations. Regular mild exercise is a mainstay of the treatment of fatigue and should usually be recommended. A stimulating daytime environment and exposure to intense light in early morning may be of use. Stimulant medications should be considered in refractory situations. Two small controlled trials of modafinil (marketed for the treatment of excessive daytime sleepiness associated with narcolepsy or sleep apnea) have found a modest effect on EDS in PD patients.[70,71] Other stimulants, such as methylphenidate, may improve EDS and fatigue, though there are no controlled studies addressing this issue.

Obstructive sleep apnea

The treatment of sleep apnea involves, first, the identification of the problem through clinical vigilance, and then confirmation with a polysomnogram. Some patients are resistant to the idea of a polysomnogram because it generally involves sleeping at a sleep center, hooked to a variety of sensors.

Nonetheless, patients should be reassured that the vast majority of people find the experience non-aversive. Patients with OSA then have a variety of treatment options, generally administered through a sleep center. These may involve night-time appliances, like CPAP (continuous positive airway pressure) machines, among others.

Vivid dreaming

Many patients do not find vivid dreaming to be a significant problem and may not want to expend effort in treatment. Remembering that vivid dreams may be a prodrome to daytime hallucinations, even if treatment is not required, the issue should be followed clinically. As the problem is generally related to dopaminergic therapy, the first approach may be to reduce the night-time dopaminergic dose. If this is not tolerated or not helpful, the addition of the atypical antipsychotic quetiapine is generally helpful. Because it does not require hematological monitoring (as with clozapine), quetiapine is the best tolerated of the atypical antipsychotics in patients with PD. While it has not been formally studied, a consensus exists about its usefulness and tolerability in this setting.

Conclusions

Sleep problems are very common in individuals with PD, affecting about three-quarters of individuals. The problem most commonly involves difficulty staying asleep through the night, but may involve virtually any aspect of sleep. Other co-occurring sleep disorders, such as sleep apnea, REM behavior disorder, and restless legs syndrome are also very common. These sleep problems are associated with poor quality of life, for both the patient and the caregiver. Anyone who has had a sleepless night knows the discomfort of the problem, and these individuals have many sleepless nights. In addition, sleep disorders are associated with excessive daytime tiredness and poor control of the motor symptoms of the illness. Accordingly, clinicians need to attend to diagnosis and treatment of sleep problems.

The treatment of sleep disturbances in PD is largely unstudied but recommendations based on clinical experience in PD and research studies in other geriatric populations can be made. The first step is proper diagnosis. The next step is to treat the specific sleep disorder or the co-occurring disorder that is interfering with sleep, as many conditions, such as RBD, RLS, etc., have specific treatments. Special attention should be paid to depression and anxiety, which frequently travel with PD and nearly always interfere with sleep. The control of the motor aspects of PD must also be paramount, as night-time movements will interfere with sleep. In the case of insomnia, symptomatic treatments, both pharmacologic and non-pharmacologic are generally helpful.

While these disorders are not well studied in PD, there has been significant progress recently. Researchers and clinicians have begun to recognize that these non-motor aspects of PD often are as important to the patient's quality of life as is control of the motor symptoms of the illness. Hopefully, research on the treatment of sleep problems in PD will continue apace and help to improve quality of life while we wait for the eventual cure of this illness.

Acknowledgment

This work was supported by R01NS43144-01A1 and 3R01NS043144-01A1S1 from NINDS.

References

1. Ancoli-Israel S, Insomnia in the elderly: a review for the primary care practitioner. *Sleep* 2000; **23**(Suppl 1):S23–S30.
2. Nausieda PA, Weiner WJ, Kaplan LR, Weber S, Klawans HL, Sleep disruption in the course of chronic levodopa therapy: an early feature of the levodopa psychosis. *Clin Neuropharmacol* 1982; **5**(2):183–194.
3. Tandberg E, Larsen JP, Karlsen K, A community-based study of sleep disorders in patients with Parkinson's disease. *Mov Disord* 1998; **13**(6):895–899.
4. Garcia-Borreguero D, Larrosa O, Bravo M, Parkinson's disease and sleep. *Sleep Med Rev* 2003; **7**:115–129.
5. Factor SA, McAlarney T, Sanchez-Ramos JR, Weiner WJ, Sleep disorders and sleep effect in Parkinson's disease. *Mov Disord* 1990; **5**:280–285.
6. Lees AJ, Blackburn NA, Campbell VL, The nighttime problems of Parkinson's disease. *Clin Neuropharmacol* 1988; **6**:512–519.
7. Ganguli M, Reynolds CF, Gilby JE, Prevalence and persistence of sleep complaints in a rural older community sample: The MoVIES project. *J Am Geriatr Soc* 1996; **44**:778–784.
8. Shulman LM, Taback RL, Bean J, Weiner WJ, Comorbidity of the nonmotor symptoms of Parkinson's disease. *Mov Disord* 2001; **16**:507–510.
9. Van Hilton JJ, Weggerman M, VanderVelde EA, Korkhof GA, VanDijk JG, Roos RAC, Sleep, excessive sleepiness and fatigue in Parkinson's disease. *J Neural Transm* 1993; **5**:235–244.
10. Goetz CG, Wilson RS, Tanner CM, Garron DC, Relationships among pain depression and sleep alterations in Parkinson's disease. In: Yahr MD, Bergmann KD (eds) *Advances in Neurology*. Raven Press: New York, 1986; **45**:345–347.
11. Wetter TH, Collado-Seidel V, Pollmacher T, Yassouridis A, Trenkwalder C, Sleep

and periodic leg movement patterns in drug-free patients with Parkinson's disease and multiple system atrophy. *Sleep* 2000; **23**(3):361–367.

12. Oerlemans WG, de Weerd AW, The prevalence of sleep disorders in patients with Parkinson's disease: A self-reported, community-based survey. *Sleep Med* 2002; **3**:147–149.

13. Gagnon JF, Bedard MA, Fantini ML et al, REM sleep behavior disorder and REM sleep without atonia in Parkinson's disease. *Neurology* 2002; **59**:585–589.

14. Olson EJ, Boeve BF, Silber MH, Rapid eye movement sleep behavior disorder: demographic, clinical and laboratory findings in 93 cases. *Brain* 2000; **123**:331–339.

15. Boeve BF, Silber MH, Parisi JE et al, Synucleinopathy pathology and REM sleep behavior disorder plus dementia or parkinsonism. *Neurology* 2003; **61**(1):40–45.

16. Frucht S, Rogers JD, Geen PE et al, Falling asleep at the wheel: motor vehicle mishaps in persons taking pramipexole and ropinirole. *Neurology* 1999; **52**:1908–1910.

17. Montastruc JL, Brefel-Courbon D, Senard JM et al, Sleep attacks and antiparkinsonian drugs: a pilot prospective pharmacoepidemiologic study. *Clin Neuropharmacol* 2001; **24**:A181–A183.

18. Homann CH, Wnzel K, Suppan K, Ivanic G, Crevenna R, Ott E, Sleep attacks – facts and fiction: A critical review. Parkinson's disease. *Ad Neurol* 2003; **91**:335–341.

19. Greulich W, Shafer D, Georg WM, Schlafke ME, Sleep behaviour in patients with PD. *Somnology* 1998; **2**:163–171.

20. Hardie RJ, Efthimiou J, Stern GM, Respiration and sleep in Parkinson's disease. *J Neurol Neurosurg Psychiat* 1986; **50**:1326.

21. Trenkwalder C, Garcia-Borreguero D, Montagna P et al, Ropinirole in the treatment of restless legs syndrome: Results from the TREAT RLS 1 study, a 12 week randomized placebo controlled study in 10 European countries. *J Neurol Neurosurg Psychiatr* 2004; **75**:92–97.

22. Sharf B, Moskovitz C, Lupton MD et al, Dream phenomena induced by chronic levodopa therapy. *J Neural Transm* 1978; **43**:143–151.

23. Moskovitz C, Moses K, Klawans HL, Levodopa-induced psychosis: a kindling phenomenon. *Am J Psychiat* 1978; **135**:669–675.

24. Kumar S, Bhatia M, Behari M, Sleep disorders in Parkinson's disease. *Mov Disord* 2002; **17**:775–781.

25. Ondo WG, Dat Vuong K, Buong K et al, Daytime sleepiness and other sleep disorders in Parkinson's disease. *Neurology* 2001; **57**(8):1392–1396.

26. Schenkman M, Wei Zhu C, Cutson TM, Whetten-Goldstein K, Longitudinal evaluation of economic and physical impact of Parkinson's disease. *Parkinsonism Relat Disord* 2001; **8**(1):41–50.

27. Friedman JH, Chou KL, Sleep and fatigue in Parkinson's disease. *Parkinsonism Rel Disord* 2004; **10**:S27–S35.

28. Tandberg E, Larsen JP, Karlsen K, Excessive daytime sleepiness and sleep benefit in Parkinson's disease: a community-based study. *Mov Disord* 1999; **14**(6):922–927.

29. Katsarou Z, Bastantjopoulou S, Peto V et al, Assessing quality of life in Parkinson's disease: Can a short-form questionnaire be useful? *Mov Disord* 2004r; **19**(3):308–312.

30. Kuopio AM, Marttila RJ, Helenius H et al, The quality of life in Parkinson's disease. *Mov Disord* 2000; **15**(2):216–223.

31. Schrag A, Jahanshahi M, Quinn N, How does Parkinson's disease affect quality of life? A comparison with quality of life in the general population. *Mov Disord* 2000; **15**(6):1112–1118.

32. Gage H, Hendricks A, Zhang S, Kazis L, The relative health related quality of life of veterans with Parkinson's disease. *J Neurol Neurosurg Psychiat* 2003; **74**(2):163–169.

33. Scaravilli T, Gasparoli E, Rinaldi F et al, Health related quality of life and sleep disorders in Parkinson's disease. *Neurol Sci* 2003; **24**(3):209–210.

34. Karlsen KH, Tanberg E, Arsland D, Larsen JP, Health related quality of life in Parkinson's disease: A prospective longitudinal study. *J Neurol Neurosurg Psychiat* 2000; **69**:584–589.

35. Caap-Ahlgren M, Lannerheim L, Dehlin O, Older Swedish women's experiences of living with symptoms related to Parkinson's disease. *J Adv Nurs* 2002; **39**(1):87–95.

36. Pal PK, Thennarasu K, Fleming J et al, Nocturnal sleep disturbances and daytime dysfunction in patients with Parkinson's disease and in their caregivers. *Parkinsonism Relat Disord* 2004; **10**(3):157–168.

37. Benca RM, Obermeyer WH, Thisted RA, Gillin JC, Sleep and psychiatric disorders: A meta-analysis. *Arch Gen Psychiatr* 1992; **49**:651–668.

38. Ware JC, Morewitz J, Diagnosis and treatment of insomnia and depression. *J Clin Psychiat* 1991; **52**:55–61.

39. Mendelson JC, Wyatt RD, *Human Sleep and its Disorders*. New York: Plenum Press, 1977.

40. Menza MA, Robertson-Hoffmann DE, Bonapace AS, Parkinson's disease and anxiety: comorbidity with depression. *Biol Psychiat* 1993; **34**:465–470.

42. Starkstein SE, Preziosi TJ, Robinson RG, Sleep disorders, pain and depression in Parkinson's disease. *Eur Neurol* 1991; **31**:352–355.

43. Menza MA, Rosen R, Sleep in Parkinson's disease: The role of depression and anxiety. *Psychosomatics* 1995; **36**:262–266.

44. Hogl BE, Gomez-Arevalo G, Garcia S et al, A clinical pharmacologic and polysomnographic study of sleep benefit in Parkinson's disease. *Neurology* 1998; **50**(5):1332–1339.

45. Agid Y. Cervera P, Hirsch E et al, Biochemistry of Parkinson's disease 28 years later: a critical review. *Mov Disord* 1989; **4**(Suppl 1):S126–S144.

46. Hornykiewicz O, Kish SJ, Biochemical pathophysiology of Parkinson's disease. *Adv Neurol* 1986; **45**:19–34.

47. Ganguli M, Reynolds CF, Gilby JE, Prevalence and persistence of sleep complaints in a rural older community sample: The MoVIES project. *J Am Geriatr Soc* 1996; **44**:778–784.

48. Morin CM, Colecchi C, Stone J, Sood R, Brink D, Behavioral and pharmacological therapies for late-life insomnia: A randomized controlled trial. *JAMA* 1999; **281**(11):991–999.

49. Morin CM, Gaulier B, Barry T, Kowatch RA, Patients' acceptance of psychological and pharmacological therapies for insomnia. *Sleep* 1992; **15**(4):302–305.

50. Morin CM, Culbert JP, Schwarz SM, Nonpharmacological interventions for insomnia: a meta-analysis of treatment efficacy. *Am J Psychiat* 1994; **151**:1172–1180.

51. Murtagh DR, Greenwood KM, Identifying effective psychological treatments for insomnia: a meta-analysis. *J Consult Clin Psychol* 1995; **63**:79–89.

52. Hohagen F, Kappler C, Schramm E et al, Prevalence of insomnia in elderly general practice attenders and the current treatment modalities. *Acta Psychiat Scand* 1994; **90**:102–108.

53. Kupfer DJ, Reynolds CF, Management of insomnia. *New Engl J Med* 1997; **336**:341–346.

54. Sateia MJ, Pigeon WR, Identification and management of insomnia. *Med Clin North Am* 2004; **88**(3):567–596.

55. Nowell PD, Mazumdar S, Buysse DJ, Dew MA, Reynolds CF, Kupfer DJ, Benzodi-

azepines and zolpidem for chronic insomnia: a meta-analysis of treatment efficacy. *JAMA* 1997; **278**:2170–2177.

56. Holbrook AM, Crowther R, Lotter A, Chang C, King D, Meta-analysis of benzo-diazepine use in the treatment of insomnia. *Can Med Assoc J* 2000; **162**:225–233.

57. Wang PS, Bohn RL, Glynn RJ et al, Hazardous benzodiazepine regimens in the elderly: effects of half-life, dosage, and duration on risk of hip fracture. *Am J Psychiat* 2001; **158**:892–898.

58. Hanlon JT, Horner RD, Schmader KE et al, Benzodiazepine use and cognitive function among community-dwelling elderly. *Clin Pharmacol Ther* 1998; **64**:684–692.

59. Hajak G, Bandelow B, Safety and tolerance of zolpidem in treatment of disturbed sleep: A post-marketing surveillance of 16,944 cases. *Int Clin Psychopharmacol* 1998; **13**:157–167.

60. Daniele A, Albanese A, Gainotti G et al, Zolpidem in Parkinson's disease. *Lancet* 1997; **349**:1222–1223.

61. Wang PS, Bohn RL, Glynn RJ et al, Zolpidem use and hip fractures in older people. *J Am Geriatr Soc* 2001; **49**:1685–1690.

62. Walsh JK, Schweitzer PK, Ten-year trends in the pharmacological treatment of insomnia. *Sleep* 1999; **22**:371–375.

63. Rickels K, Morris RJ, Newman H, Rosenfeld H, Schiller H, Weinstock R, Diphenhy-dramine in insomniac family practice patients: a double-blind study. *J Clin Pharmacol* 1983; **23**:234–242.

64. Morgante L, Epifanio A, Spina E et al, Quetiapine and clozapine in parkinsonian patients with dopaminergic psychosis. *Clin Neuropharmacol* 2004; **27**(4):153–156.

65. Cicolin A, Lopiano L, Zibetti M et al, Effects of deep brain stimulation of the sub-thalamic nucleus on sleep architecture in parkinsonian patients. *Sleep Med* 2004; **5**(2):207–210.

66. Schenck CH, Mahowald MW, Polysomnographic, neurologic, psychiatric, and clinical outcome report of 70 consecutive cases with the REM sleep behavior disorder (RBD): Sustained clonazepam efficacy in 89.5% of 57 treated patients. *Clev Clin J Med* 1990; **57**:10–24.

67. Boeve BF, Silber MH, Ferman TJ, Melatonin for treatment of REM sleep behavior disorder in neurologic disorder: Results in 14 patients. *Sleep Med* 2003; **4**:281–284.

68. Trenkwalder C, Garcia-Borreguero D, Montagna P et al, Ropinirole in the treatment of restless legs syndrome: Results from the TREAT RLS 1 study, a 12 week randomized placebo controlled study in 10 European countries. *J Neurol Neurosurg Psychiat* 2004; **75**:92–97.

69. Garcia-Borregureo D, Larrosa O, de la Llave Y et al, Treatment of restless legs syndrome with gabapentin: A double-blind, cross-over study. *Neurology* 2002; **59**:1573–1579.

70. Adler CH, Caviness JN, Hentz JG, Lind M, Tiede J, Randomized trial of modafinil for treating subjective daytime sleepiness in patients with Parkinson's disease. *Mov Disord* 2003; **18**(3):287–293.

71. Adler CH, Caviness JN, Hentz JG, Lind M, Tiede J, Randomized trial of modafinil for treating subjective daytime sleepiness in patients with Parkinson's disease. Mov Disord 2003; **18**(3):287–293.

chapter 12

Behavioral disturbances

Laura Marsh

Introduction

Parkinson's disease (PD) and its dopaminergic treatments are associated with several types of behavioral disturbances. These behavioral alterations are less common than affective disturbances or psychosis, but they can be quite dramatic with serious social consequences. Included are hyperactive and disruptive behaviors as well as hypoactive but still disabling behavioral changes such as apathy. In general, behavioral disturbances in PD have received less attention and their relevance to PD is not always recognized. Furthermore, the behaviors may be embarrassing or covert and patients or families may therefore not reveal their presence without specific inquiry. This chapter focuses on the distinguishing features, pathophysiology, and potential interventions for the range of behavioral disturbances that occur in PD. We also describe neuropsychiatric disturbances associated with neurosurgical interventions.

There are several ways to categorize the spectrum of behavioral disturbances in PD. As several behaviors resemble one another superficially, we have subdivided them according to whether their primary characteristics involve a deficit state, impulsivity, or repetitive, ritualistic activities (Table 12.1). For example, both impulsive and compulsive behaviors involve repetitive behaviors and inability to inhibit or delay acting on the behaviors. However, the prospect of pleasure or gratification drives impulsive behaviors whereas compulsive behaviors are conducted to reduce anxiety and avoid harm. These differences may also underlie pharmacological responsiveness. Table 12.2 lists instruments used in research studies that may be used for screening in clinical settings.

Table 12.1 Types of behavioral disturbances in PD

Deficit	Impulse control	Repetitive
Apathy	Disinhibition	Non-motor behavioral fluctuations
Confusion with hypoactive delirium	Hypomania/mania	Obsessive-compulsive disorder
Hyposexuality	Hypersexuality	Punding
	Pathological gambling	
	Pathological shopping	
	Abuse of dopaminergic medications	
	Hedonistic homeostatic dysregulation	
	Aggression	

Suggested interventions in this chapter are based on case reports, clinical experience with PD patients, and treatment of similar disturbances in non-PD patients.[1] Until there are definitive treatments, optimal management includes judicious use of antiparkinsonian and psychiatric medications and non-pharmacological strategies (Table 12.3). Treatment is challenging because dopaminergic replacement therapy (DRT) influences behavioral disturbances and many patients have a narrow therapeutic margin between the ability of DRT to control motor deficits versus cause motor or psychiatric complications. Poor insight, additional psychiatric co-morbidities, cognitive impairment, caregiver strain, and motor and neuropsychiatric side-effects of psychiatric medications also add to treatment complexity.

Deficit behaviors

Apathy
Prevalence and impact
Apathy, a state of diminished goal-directed speech, motor activity, and emotions, is common in PD.[2] Apathy may be a symptom of other neuropsychiatric conditions such as depression, delirium, or dementia or a syndrome when it is the primary manifestation of the behavioral disturbance. Prevalence of apathetic symptoms in PD ranges from 16.5% to nearly 50%.[2–4] Rates of syndromic apathy are not known, but apathetic symptoms coexisted

Table 12.2 Rating scales for behavioral disturbances

Scale	Comments
Apathy Evaluation Scale (AES)[80]	Has clinician-rated, informant-rated, and patient-rated versions. 18 items
Modified Apathy Scale[3]	Modification of AES. Clinician-administered patient and informant versions. 14 items. Validated in PD samples
Disinhibition Scale[81]	Self-administered by patient or informant. 26 items. Validated in Alzheimer's disease. Yields 4 factors: abnormal motor behavior, hypomania, loss of insight and geocentricism, and poor self-care
Frontal Behavioral Inventory[82]	Clinician-administered to informant. 24 items. Developed for diagnosis of frontotemporal dementia syndromes. Inquires about specific temperamental changes, deficit behaviors, and disinhibited behaviors
Frontal Systems Behavior Scale[83]	Self-administered with versions for patient and informant (Family Rating Form). 46 items. Provides total score and 3 subscores: disinhibition, apathy, and executive dysfunction
Neuropsychiatric Inventory[84]	Clinician-administered to informant. Assesses ten psychiatric disturbances common to neurodegenerative disorders: delusions, hallucinations, agitation, depression/dysphoria, anxiety, euphoria/elation, apathy/indifference, disinhibition, irritability/lability, and aberrant motor behavior. Used extensively to assess range of psychopathology in PD and other CNS disorders

Note: Patients with behavioral disturbances tend to lack insight into the presence or severity of their condition, so clinical assessments and inventories require input from informants. The sensitivity and specificity of these instruments as screening measures has not been evaluated in PD samples. For example, without specific inquiry, problems with gambling, shopping, hypersexuality, or medication abuse may not be endorsed when using the above inventories.

Table 12.3 General strategies for treating behavioral disturbances

Characterization of the primary behavior and its co-morbidities
Identify target behaviors for treatment
Identify co-morbid psychiatric disorders and their treatment options

Review of all medications for effectiveness and interactions
Evaluate all PD, psychiatric, non-PD, and over the counter medications
As feasible, eliminate psychoactive and redundant medications
Use lowest effective dosages, especially for psychoactive medications
Adjust antiparkinsonian regimen, balancing effects on motor and behavioral
symptoms

Non-pharmacological strategies
Educate patient and caregiver about the problem behavior and the role of PD and
its medications
Limit patient's responsibility for medication administration
Neuropsychological assessment to quantify cognitive deficits that impact behaviors
and devise compensatory strategies, e.g., simplify tasks in patients with executive
dysfunction
Occupational therapy to address deficits and maximize functioning
Structured environments, day programs, supervision, caregiver respite

Add psychiatric medications judiciously
Target specific behaviors and monitor for specific therapeutic effects, e.g.,
quetiapine may reduce the drive for pathological gambling
Monitor for other potential beneficial effects, e.g., quetiapine may also reduce
insomnia and anxiety
Monitor for potential adverse somatic, cognitive, and psychiatric effects, e.g.,
quetiapine may aggravate parkinsonism and cause orthostasis, daytime sedation, or
delirium; benzodiazepines may reduce anxiety but aggravate cognitive deficits and
disinhibited behavior
Continue treatment based on ongoing risk/benefit assessment

Consider admission to medical day programs or in-patient psychiatric units
Enables longitudinal observation and characterization of behaviors and their
relationship to antiparkinsonian medications and other motor, cognitive, and
psychiatric disturbances
Structured environment may facilitate control over behaviors and provide control
over medication administration
May be needed to maintain safety of patient or others
Provides caregiver respite

with depression in 30% of patients and were independent in 12% of patients.[3] Apathy profoundly impacts self-management of a chronic disease such as PD; patients are less motivated to comply with treatment or self-care, socialize, or exercise.[5] Inactivity, deconditioning, and fatigue promote disability and dependency.

Mechanisms

Goal-directed behavior is associated with intact dopaminergic and cortical-subcortical circuits involving the thalamus, basal ganglia, and frontal cortex. Presence of apathy is associated with dysfunction of forebrain dopaminergic systems in PD.[6] Dorsolateral prefrontal dysfunction is associated with executive dysfunction,[7] which is evident at higher rates in apathetic patients[3,4,6] and affects planning and monitoring of goal-directed behaviors. Orbitofrontal damage is associated with disinhibited behaviors that accompany apathy. Noradrenergic dysfunction is suggested by a relationship between bradyphrenia and neuronal loss in the locus coeruleus in PD.[8]

Several medical causes of apathy are amenable to treatment. Suboptimal motor control with DRT or reduced dosing of DRT after effective deep brain stimulation (DBS) treatment can aggravate anergy and apathy that is reversible with higher-dose DRT. Hypotestosteronemia (<325 ng/dl total serum testosterone) was found in nearly 50% of non-demented men with PD and free testosterone levels correlated significantly with apathy scores.[9] Selective serotonin uptake inhibitors (SSRIs), the most frequently prescribed antidepressants in PD,[10] can cause apathy.[11] Other causes to consider include delirium, strokes, endocrinologic dysfunction, and other medication effects.

Clinical presentation

A central feature is a reduction in goal-directed activity as a result of diminished motivation.[12] Table 12.4 describes several types of apathy. Patients tend to sit idly, but generally go along with planned activities, often enjoying them and showing greater animation. Apathy can accompany depressive or disinhibited conditions.[13] Some patients describe "mental emptiness," but most have no concerns. Family members report that the patient "sits around doing nothing" and rarely initiates conversations or activities. This indifference and lack of initiative often strains caregivers who may attribute symptoms to fatigue, depression, dementia, or general effects of PD. Parkinsonian symptoms such as akinesia, bradyphrenia, hypomimia, and hypophonia can mimic or mask the presence of apathy.

Table 12.4 Common types of apathy

Type	Feature
Motoric	Lack of initiative
Motivational	Absence of motivation to start activities or persevere once a task is started
Emotional	Indifference with decreased curiosity or concern for oneself or others
Cognitive	Lack of spontaneous ideas or conversation

It is important to distinguish primary apathy from: (1) apathy that is a feature of a depressive syndrome or delirium and (2) decreased interest resulting from motor and cognitive deficits in PD. Apathy and depression can involve a loss of interest as well as anhedonia, the inability to experience pleasure. Dysphoria, loss of interest, and anhedonia are prominent in PD-related depression.[14] Yet, while PD patients with high apathy levels show reduced "hedonic tone," they are not more likely to be depressed than patients with low apathy levels.[6] Finally, in the absence of depression or apathy, patients who lose interest in activities because of physical or intellectual effects of PD will redirect their activities and interests to other pleasurable pursuits.

Treatment

After addressing other causes and ensuring optimal treatment of motor symptoms with DRT, treatment includes behavioral and pharmacological interventions. Educating caregivers about apathy reduces misinterpretations of the patient's behavior as deliberate or insensitive and is a critical first-step. Families benefit from ongoing supportive therapy and help with problem-solving. Because of executive dysfunction, patients often benefit from structured environments, cueing, and simplification of tasks into fewer steps. Day programs can provide structured and enriched environments for patients and respite for caregivers.

There are no formal studies on pharmacologic treatment of apathy in PD. Presumed impairments of mesocortical and mesolimbic dopaminergic pathways in apathy suggest a role for stimulant and dopamine agonist drugs. In patients with neurological disorders, dopamine receptor agonists are regarded as the most effective treatment for apathy.[15] Reported mean (range) doses are bromocriptine 10 (2.6–60) mg/day and pergolide 3 (1–5) mg/day. Dosing of ropinirole or pramipexole for treatment of apathy is not reported. Other dopaminergic agents (levodopa, selegeline, amantadine, and bupro-prion) have shown benefits in some cases. In non-PD patients, amfetamines have been used for amotivation and fatigue with variable results. A single case report of an 82-year-old man with PD described beneficial effects of methylphenidate 5 mg twice daily for apathy.[16] Further study is needed on the role of cognitive enhancing agents, but benefits were seen for treatment of apathy in Alzheimer's disease.[17] Study of testosterone as a treatment for apathy is also indicated.[9]

Hyposexuality

Prevalence and impact

Decreased rates of sexual activity are common in PD. About 60% of patients report sexual problems,[18] including diminished desire, decreased satisfaction, or sexual dysfunction. Gender differences affect prevalence, with more women reporting arousal or orgasmic difficulties and men reporting erectile dysfunction. Since patients remain interested in sex as an aspect of their function, assessment and intervention are warranted.[19]

Mechanisms

Causes of sexual dysfunction include PD itself, other medical conditions, psychiatric disturbances, medications, age-related changes, and various psychological and social factors. Erectile dysfunction is associated with other medical conditions, depression, prostatectomy, dopamine agonists, anti-depressants, and more advanced PD. Whereas dopamine depletion results in reduced desire and erectile dysfunction, DRT also has negative effects on sexual function. Less commonly, DRT will cause increased sexual desire and penile erections.[20] Acquired sexual dysfunction along with pre-morbid low sexual desire, intimacy, and sexual satisfaction can contribute to cessation of sexual activity.[21]

Clinical presentation

Fatigue, immobility, rigidity, bradykinesia, tremor, and difficulty with fine finger movements affect performance of intimate activities needed for sexual arousal and pleasure. Changes in appearance and relationship roles, drooling, excessive sweating, and gait problems can negatively affect self-esteem, body image, and attractiveness. Among younger patients, depression and employment status influenced perception of sexual functioning even when actual function was no different from a control population.[22] Sexual dysfunction may also be evident in partners.[23]

Treatment

Assessment and intervention early in the course of PD may help avoid deterioration of sexual function. After investigating medical causes, sexual counseling can help. There are several treatments for erectile and orgasmic dysfunction, including sildefanil.[24] DRT may facilitate sexual relationships when it increases sexual function.[20] The role of treatment of testosterone deficiency in PD needs investigation.[9,25]

Impulse control disorders

Pathophysiology

The core feature of an impulse control disorder is the inability to resist an impulse, drive, or temptation that is harmful to the individual or others. A number of brain systems and neurotransmitters are implicated in the development of impulse control disorders.[26] The mesolimbic dopaminergic system is associated with cognitive and reward-related processing. The serotonergic system has a role in harm-avoidance and impulsivity is associated with serotonergic dysfunction. The noradrenergic system also has a role in arousal and novelty-seeking behaviors. While reduced novelty seeking and increased harm avoidance is more common among PD patients, treatment-induced stimulation of mesolimbic dopamine receptors may influence novelty- and reward-seeking behaviors, including impulsivity.[27] In experimental studies, DRT improves or impairs neuropsychological functioning, depending on the nature of the task and the basal level of dopamine function in cortico-striatal circuitry[28] and may underlie fluctuating effects of DRT on cognitive and behavioral functions. Other brain regions in the limbic cortico-striatal-thalamic circuit that interact with the mesolimbic dopamine pathway are also involved in impulse control disorders.[29] For example, the orbitofrontal cortex is implicated in decision-making and emotional-related learning and is involved in the representation of abstract rewards and punishments, such as winning and losing money.

Several factors influence the phenotypic variability of impulse control disturbances in PD. One factor may be asymmetric patterns of dopamine activity in PD and differential effects on novelty seeking and harm avoidance.[30] Functional polymorphisms of genes that regulate central dopaminergic transmission could also affect phenotypic variation, including the development of cognitive and behavioral disturbances in response to DRT. For example, catechol-*O*-methyl transferase (COMT) genotypes in PD affect performance on the Tower of London task, a test of planning that requires working memory.[31] Genetic variation in the dopamine receptor D1 gene and interactions between genetic variants of dopamine receptor genes may also play a role in addictive behaviors.[32] Dysfunction of serotonergic and dopaminergic neurotransmitter systems, particularly in the ventral striatal-orbitofrontal circuits, is also linked to impulsivity.

Disinhibition

Prevalence and impact

Disinhibition refers to inappropriate social and interpersonal behaviors or a loss of social cognition. While aware of social norms and manners, patients have limited insight into their indiscreet or impulsive behaviors or the feelings of others. In PD, prevalence of disinhibitory symptoms, based on the Neuropsychiatric Inventory (NPI), ranges from 6.5%[2] to 18%.[33]

Clinical presentation

Like apathy, disinhibition can be a characteristic of another condition or an independent syndrome. The disinhibitory syndrome in PD is not well-characterized. In our experience, patients are distractible and impulsive and act on a range of ideas or emotions without regard for potential consequences. The impulsive behaviors can be dangerous or merely socially awkward and tactless, often involving executive dysfunction with poor planning and problem-solving. One patient brought a large saucepan into the formal living room where she joined her family and proceeded to eat directly from the pan. Another patient phoned remote acquaintances to re-establish contact. The same patient made overfamiliar comments, sometimes with sexual connotations, to staff and other patients in a day program. While there was no evidence for enhanced libido, the behaviors compromised his ability to remain in that program. Another patient with poor vision and postural instability would slip away to use power tools in the basement, cook on the stove, or walk in the neighborhood. Such unpredictable and risky impulsive behaviors pose safety hazards and management difficulties. There may be overactivity, irritability, and excitement, but usually not a sustained hypomanic syndrome with grandiosity, as described below. Impulse control disorders, such as pathological gambling or hypersexuality, may also be present.

Differential diagnosis

Profound alterations in social cognition suggest alternative diagnoses. Frontotemporal dementia (FTD) is associated with more severe and global behavioral declines than PD. FTD with parkinsonism linked to chromosome 17 (FTDP-17) involves an autosomal dominant mutation in the tau gene, but this syndrome is distinct from idiopathic PD. One study showed higher rates of apathetic and disinhibitory symptoms, based on the NPI, in PSP compared to PD.[34]

Treatment

There are no reports on the treatment of disinhibitory behaviors in PD. In addition to the general principles in Table 12.3, patients generally need structured environments and 24-hour supervision to minimize risks to self or others. Unpredictable behaviors can limit options for long-term care. SSRIs, beta-blockers, trazodone, and mood stabilizers have been used.[1] In two of the cases described above, caregivers reported substantial reductions in impulsivity after treatment with low-dose atomoxetine (10–20 mg/day). There is a need for further study of atomoxetine, a norepinephrine (noradrenaline) reuptake inhibitor indicated for attention deficit hyperactivity disorder, which is also associated with hyperactivity and impulsivity.

Hypersexuality

Prevalence and impact

Hypersexuality is estimated to occur in 0.9% to 3% of PD patients.[35] There is not a clear relationship with premorbid sexual behaviors or stage of disease.[36] It is more common in men with PD. Hypersexuality occurs with all dopaminergic medications and selegiline or after neurosurgical treatments, including pallidotomy and DBS. In many cases, the onset of paraphilias and aberrant desires has catastrophic consequences. Patients may become preoccupied by their sexual impulses, at the expense of other personal and social activities and despite legal ramifications or distress to others. Spontaneous penile erections are a potential side-effect of DRT, including agonists, and may or may not be associated with an increased sexual drive.[20]

Clinical presentation

Hypersexuality is characterized by an excessive sexual drive or the development of deviant sexual behaviors. In many cases, the behaviors occur within a few months after an increase in DRT or after neurosurgery, but many patients will have had longstanding PD.[37] Commonly, there are intrusive sexual thoughts and urges, frequent masturbation, and increased demands for sexual intercourse, sometimes despite erectile dysfunction. Use of pornographic materials, phone lines, and internet sites may be covert until discovered by a family member, often via credit card records. Other reports describe onset of sexually inappropriate remarks, indiscriminate sexual encounters or use of prostitutes, sado-masochism, cross-dressing, voyeurism, exhibitionism, pedophilia, and zoophilia.[38–40] In the context of the hypersexuality, there may be anxiety, mood lability, disturbed sleep, restlessness, and irritability and anger, especially at the spouse who may be perceived as sexually unavailable or intolerant. Co-morbid disorders can include gambling, DRT abuse, psychosis or mania. A range of sexually inappropriate behaviors may occur in patients with more cognitive impairment, especially in nursing home settings.[41] These include cuddling, touching the genitals, sexual remarks, propositioning, grabbing and groping, use of obscene language, and masturbation without shame. Associated behaviors can include aggression, agitation, and irritability.

Treatment

In most cases, reduction or withdrawal of antiparkinsonian medications eliminates hypersexuality.[38] This may result in significantly increased parkinsonism. Interestingly, one dopamine agonist may be associated with development of hypersexuality and another will be tolerated without causing hypersexuality. If downward adjustments in DRT have no effect on behavior or are not tolerated from the standpoint of motor symptoms, certain atypical antipsychotics (clozapine and quetiapine) can reduce hypersexual behaviors and allow adequate dosing with DRT for control of motor symptoms. One report described patient benefit with addition of sodium valproate, a mood stabilizer, to clozapine.[37] There are a few favorable reports on use of gabapentin in patients with non-PD dementia and inappropriate sexual behaviors.[41] Antiandrogens, estrogens, and SSRIs have also been used.[41] Patient, family, and caregiver education and the importance of patient supervision are important non-pharmacological interventions. Informing patients and families about the potential for hypersexuality as a side-effect when antiparkinsonian medications are prescribed may facilitate earlier detection.

Mania and hypomania

Prevalence and impact

Mania and hypomania are affective syndromes that involve prominent behavioral features. In PD, mania and hypomania present in two main circumstances. First, patients with earlier histories of bipolar disorder may experience an exacerbation of symptoms in response to DRT. Secondly, patients without a history of bipolar disorder can develop mania following treatment with levodopa, dopamine agonists, selegiline, adrenal medullary transplant, pallidotomy, or DBS. A 1.5% incidence rate of hypomania was reported in a large clinical series soon after levodopa became available.[35] It is not established whether antidepressant medications induce hypomania or mania in the setting of DRT in patients without a history of bipolar disorder, and the respective contributions of an antidepressant versus DRT would be difficult to delineate. "On-off" fluctuations can be associated with transient mood changes, but other features of a mood syndrome are not necessarily present. In one series, about 25% of patients reported slight elation and 12% of patients experienced moderate elation during "on" states.[42]

Clinical presentation

Mania is a mood disorder characterized by a persistent change in mood and self-attitude. In hypomania, the symptoms are less severe. Both are manifest by an elevated, expansive, or irritable mood and an inflated sense of self-confidence or self-esteem or grandiosity. Other features include racing thoughts, flight of ideas, pressured speech, hypertalkativeness, increased goal-directed activity, and a decreased need for sleep. Manic and hypomanic patients are more likely to act impulsively and become excessively involved in pleasurable behaviors that may have untoward consequences, such as gambling or sexual activity. However, pathological gambling or hypersexuality are not necessarily present. The behavioral changes in hypomanic states may be relatively harmless. One frail patient with hypomania post-pallidotomy wanted to redecorate the clinic and start a support group for patients considering a second pallidotomy. Another reported an elevated mood, despite significant progression of her motor symptoms, along with a tendency to speak with strangers about personal matters, something she had never done before. Manic syndromes involve more extreme, hyperactive, grandiose, and irresponsible behaviors, including initiation of extravagant business plans, reckless driving, excessive and indiscriminate spending or sexual activities, agitation, pressured speech, racing thoughts, sleeplessness, and psychosis.

Treatment
In most reports and in our experience, treatment requires reductions in the total dose of antiparkinsonian medications. Atypical antipsychotics may be needed to control symptoms. There is a need for further study of treatment with mood-stabilizing drugs and the role of antidepressants in inducing manic states in PD patients.

Pathological gambling
Prevalence and impact
Pathological gambling (PG) refers to the presence of recurrent and mal-adaptive gambling behaviors. The progressive inability to resist the impulse to gamble becomes severely disruptive, causing financial hardship, bank-ruptcy, divorce, arrest, unemployment, incarceration, and suicide attempts.[26] In the United States, prevalence of PG is 1–3.4% among adults. A recent review[43] cited 29 reported cases of PG in PD; there may be underdetection since it is not always reported spontaneously. Incidence was 0.05% over one year in a United States sample.[44] Prevalence was 4.8% in a Spanish PD sample, compared to a <2% prevalence in the general Spanish population.[45] In a longitudinal study on social disability in 101 PD patients under 65 years of age (Bassett SS, unpublished data), 3% had PG that developed in the absence of prior previous psychiatric history and after the onset of DRT.

Clinical presentation
All forms of gambling have been observed in PD patients, including playing at casinos as well as internet and television-based gambling sites, slot machines, and lottery games with scratch cards or arcade-like games. Like non-PD pathological gamblers, patients may gamble to try to pay back their losses, sell belongings to enable further gambling, and borrow or steal money from family. There can be mood lability, with irritability and tension relieved by gambling, and sleeplessness. In our experience, losses range from several thousand dollars to over $500 000. At least initially, patients deny the extent of their problem, even when their families are severely affected, with depletion of savings and considerable debt.

In PD,[44,45] men are more often affected than women and a number of patients have young onset PD, but only a minority report impulse control problems before PD. Duration of PD ranges from 1 to 22 years, with a tendency towards more advanced stages with motor fluctuations. Onset of PG often corresponds to a period after a decline in motor symptoms and associated increases in the dose of DRT, especially with dopamine agonists.[44,45] Patients with mania or hypomania may gamble impulsively or gamble exclusively during the "on" period,[45] but patients with PG do not manifest a sustained hypomanic or manic syndrome. Concurrent impulse control disorders may include DRT abuse,[43,46] hypersexuality, or alcohol or other substance abuse[45] as well as psychosis or depressive or anxiety disorders.[45]

Treatment

Initial treatment includes reductions in the dose of DRT, especially dopamine agonists. In many cases, PG will resolve with this change alone. Switching from one agonist to another may be sufficient, or there may be a need to initiate or increase levodopa therapy to treat motor symptoms. We recommend using regular release levodopa when there are behavioral changes since motor and mood effects can be less predictable with controlled-release levodopa preparations. DBS is associated with occasional emergence of PG,[45] but successful surgery can also enable significant reductions in DRT with remission of PG. Inpatient treatment may be needed to manage the patient's behavior and control administration of DRT. Families may need to gain complete control over the patient's ability to conduct financial transactions.

There are no controlled trials on treatment of gambling in PD. Medications used to treat gambling in non-PD patients can be tried, but benefits may be limited;[26] in non-PD patients, SSRIs tend to show high placebo response rates for treatment of PG and short-lived anti-impulsive effects (in contrast to the anti-compulsive effects of SSRIs). A cautionary note is that SSRIs can induce hypomania, causing further impulsivity. Atypical antipsychotics, using guidelines discussed in Chapter 10, can help control gambling behaviors; DRT may need to be adjusted upward for the worsened parkinsonism.[47] When there are co-morbid psychiatric symptoms, initial treatment may target those conditions, such as antidepressants for co-morbid depression. In non-PD samples, mood stabilizers such as lithium and valproate and naltrexone (an opioid antagonist) improved PG.

Patients and families benefit from education about DRT and PG, including when first prescribing DRT. Suicidal risk should be monitored and treated aggressively. Patients may enter specific behavioral treatment programs for gambling or become involved with Gamblers Anonymous. In our experience, such programs do not uniformly appreciate the role of PD and DRT in gambling, and therefore co-management with a movement disorder specialist should be encouraged.

Pathological shopping

Pathological shopping refers to excessive or poorly controlled preoccupations, urges, or behaviors regarding shopping and spending, which lead to adverse consequences. We have observed pathological shopping clinically and there are isolated reports of pathological shopping in PD, usually in association with other impulse control behaviors.[45] Prevalence in the United States ranges from 2% to 8%, with women affected nearly ten times more often than men.[48] Co-morbid mood disorders and other impulse-control disorders are common. As with PG, the role of DRT should be evaluated with dose reductions to try to reduce the behaviors. Antidepressants can be used to treat co-morbid mood disorders. The role of substance abuse and eating disorders should be considered. There are high placebo response rates in studies on non-PD patients, but one controlled study showed benefits with citalopram.[49]

Abuse of dopaminergic replacement therapy (DRT)

Prevalence

Some patients develop a pattern of excessive use of DRT accompanied by drug-seeking behaviors, a phenomenon first described in 1985.[50] A number of terms are used to describe this behavior: levodopa abuse, compulsive DRT use, DRT addiction, dopamine dysregulation,[51] and hedonistic homeostatic dysregulation.[52] While occurrence is rare, DRT abuse is extremely difficult to manage and there may be a heavier concentration in tertiary care centers where prevalence estimates are 3–4%.[52,53] Occurrence of DRT abuse is more common in patients with young-onset PD and in men.[51] The behavior results in extreme psychosocial disability.

Clinical presentation

Whereas motor symptoms ordinarily drive adjustments in antiparkinsonian therapy, patients with DRT abuse describe a powerful psychological affective response to levodopa and other forms of DRT that fuels its abuse. The phenomenon also occurs with stimulator settings after DBS. Soon after initiation of DRT, patients complain of "unbearable" motor and affective symptoms, and insist upon dose increases to address what appears to be a tolerance to the psychological response to DRT along with dependence. In this regard, the phenomena are similar to those of a drug addiction, although there is a fundamental requirement for dopamine in PD. Doses of DRT soon exceed what is needed to control motor symptoms. Consequently, despite minimal motor symptoms, patients develop unpredictable motor fluctuations with severe dyskinesias and use of inordinately high doses of DRT with short dosing intervals given their duration of PD. Corresponding to the DRT dosing schedule, which becomes erratic, mood lability is intense. In response to DRT, patients experience a "rush" or "high" and may have paranoid and/or hypomanic symptoms with euphoria, increased energy and libido, reduced sleep, and pressured speech with a mild thought disorder. Depression, dysphoria, irritability, and anxiety occur when "off," although perceptions of "on-off" states are markedly distorted in such patients.

Despite their maladaptive behaviors, patients have poor insight and resist reduction or withdrawal of levodopa. Patients will contact other physicians to obtain additional medications and may hoard stashes. Covert drug use, drug craving, and other psychiatric symptoms, usually depression, develop when DRT is limited. Suicidal behavior can occur when medications are withdrawn. Other disturbances have accompanied DRT abuse including psychosis, agitation, aggression, punding, akathisia, abuse of alcohol or other substances, and pathological gambling, shopping, or sexual behaviors.

Treatment

Awareness of the possibility for DRT abuse should encourage preventive measures early in PD management, including referral to a movement disorder specialist. A questionnaire is available for screening purposes.[54] Treatment requires institution of a medication regimen that targets appropriate control of motor symptoms along with withdrawal and reduction of antiparkinsonian medications. Poor insight, covert use of DRT, and affective lability make management difficult. Patients should be encouraged to keep "on-off" diaries to track motor and mood symptoms, as reducing DRT to levels that control motor symptoms improves mood lability. Hospitalization may be needed initially to gain control over medication administration since patients thwart efforts by others to restrict medications and can become aggressive. Afterwards, medications still need to be rationed, including any booster doses of levodopa. Atypical antipsychotics can help psychosis, sleep, and hypomanic symptoms, but they can be followed by worse depression.[52] Antidepressants reportedly help with the ensuing depression, but the long-term course of the mood disturbance may be protracted and suicidality can occur.[52] The long-term course and prognosis of the mood disorder has not been characterized. Treatment with mood stabilizers has not been described.

Repetitive behaviors

Non-motor behavioral fluctuations

As discussed in Chapter 3, fluctuating non-motor symptoms can develop with long-term DRT and may be more disabling than motor symptoms. There are three subtypes of non-motor fluctuations: autonomic, psychiatric, and sensory.[55] In addition to clinically significant mood fluctuations, which occur in about 7% of PD patients,[56] behavioral symptoms also occur. The stereotyped and predictable nature of these fluctuating behaviors places them in the category of "repetitive behaviors." Akathisia, irritability, abulia, mutism, and aggressive behaviors occur mostly during the "off" state.[57] As described above, euphoria, manic symptoms, sexual and other impulse control disorders as well as screaming or hyperactivity are more likely to occur in the "on" state. Psychiatric fluctuations tend to be associated with higher doses of levodopa.[57,58] Changes in DRT that decrease "off" time and improve motor function usually help non-motor fluctuations. It can be more difficult to control problematic behaviors that occur in the "on" state since reducing medicines increases motor symptoms.

Obsessive-compulsive behaviors

Prevalence and impact

Obsessive-compulsive disorder (OCD), in which there are recurrent and disabling obsessions or compulsions, occurs in about 2% of the general population. Some PD patients have OCD, but there is no evidence for increased rates of OCD in PD.[59] However, since frontal-striatal circuits play a role in obsessive-compulsive phenomena, a few studies have examined obsessive-compulsive symptoms (OCS) in PD;[60–63] some patients develop OCS in the context of a depressive disorder and others have isolated OCS with a limited clinical impact.

Mechanisms

OCD is commonly co-morbid with tic disorders, which also involve basal ganglia pathology. An association between a predominance of left-sided PD symptoms and OCS is reported, suggesting a role for right hemisphere dysfunction.[59,63] OCD and OCS can co-occur with other psychiatric conditions, including depression and other anxiety disorders. As discussed in Chapter 15, obsessive personality traits may be common in patients who eventually develop PD, but it is not known if these are related to development of ritualistic behaviors.

Clinical presentation

As there can be other repetitive abnormal behaviors in PD, it is important to distinguish OCS from other psychiatric phenomena. Obsessions are recurrent, persistent, and unwanted stereotyped images, impulses, or thoughts that are intrusive and distressing. Patients regard their obsessions as inappropriate and often try to suppress them or neutralize their distress by other thoughts or actions. Compulsions are repetitive but senseless behaviors that are performed ritualistically and in a driven manner to combat the anxiety brought on by obsessions. Examples of obsessions include concerns with order or symmetry, fears of dirt or contamination, or unwanted sexual or religious thoughts. Examples of compulsions include excessive handwashing, checking locks and doors, and arranging items in a precise order.

Differential diagnosis

Obsessions should be distinguished from excessive worries, ruminations, or preoccupations about real-life issues, interests, or addictions. Despite their similar names, OCD is not the same as obsessive-compulsive personality (OCP) disorder. The latter involves a personality pattern characterized by rigidity, inflexibility, an excessive devotion to work, and a preoccupation with rules, schedules, and lists. Some studies suggest that OCP phenomena may be a premorbid characteristic related to dopamine depletion and associated with later development of PD.[64] While repetitive behaviors are their common feature, compulsive behaviors are not the same as impulsive behaviors, in which thoughts do *not* precede actions, addictive behaviors, which are not stereotyped and are driven by the need to gratify a craving rather than a true obsession, or punding behaviors (see below).

Treatment

Education, psychotherapy (cognitive-behavioral therapy) and medications that inhibit serotonin reuptake are the cornerstones of therapy. Subthalamic deep brain stimulation (DBS) improved both motor and psychiatric symptoms in three patients with PD and severe OCD,[65,66] suggesting an alternative application of DBS.

Punding

Prevalence

Punding refers to a form of stereotyped behavior in which there is repetitive performance of useless tasks. It is most often associated with amfetamine and cocaine abuse and its prevalence in PD is not established. Punding tends to occur in patients with advanced PD on high-dose DRT or who use excessive doses of apomorphine or "rescue" doses of levodopa.[67–69] There may be higher rates than are clinically recognized or reported spontaneously; in a movement disorders clinic, 14% of patients on high-dose DRT endorsed punding behaviors on a specially developed questionnaire.[69]

Mechanisms

Occurrence of punding with high-dose DRT suggests a relationship to hyper-dopaminergic states. However, the behaviors often persist even when the dose of DRT is reduced, implicating underlying neurodegeneration.[70] The relationship of punding to cognitive dysfunction has not been examined.

Clinical presentation

Punding can be manifest by a variety of severe and disabling behaviors. There may be intense fascination with assembling and disassembling equipment, often in a prolonged or bizarre manner, or repetitive handling, examination, or sorting and arranging of objects, such as buttons, paperwork, or items in one's pocketbook.[69,70] Past work-related behaviors or hobbies may shape the type of behavior. Patients tend to find the repetitive behaviors calming and become irritable or dysphoric when forced to stop, even though they recognize them as pointless and disruptive. Unlike OCD, however, obsessive or compulsive phenomena are absent. In more severe cases, patients forego social obligations and may stay awake all night, neglecting their need to sleep, eat, or take medications. Consequently, motor symptoms are worse and, if punding is undetected, patients are at risk for receiving higher doses of DRT.

Evaluation requires identification of co-morbid psychiatric conditions as well as discrimination from disturbances with overlapping features. Hyper-sexuality, gambling, or DRT abuse may co-occur, but not hypomanic mood changes or goal-directed hyperactivity. The relationship of punding to goal-directed and purposeful behaviors, such as artistic or other projects that some PD patients pursue well into the night, has not been examined. With the latter, patients find it calming to work undisturbed, but they may neglect their sleep, which aggravates parkinsonism and cognitive complaints.

Treatment

Like DRT abuse, treatment of punding can be challenging because of the dis-organization in the daily lives of patients and their non-adherence to pre-scribed therapy. Patients and caregivers require education about the role of DRT in treating motor symptoms and the importance of restorative sleep and a daily schedule of balanced activities. Medications, especially rescue medications, have to be limited, and doses may have to be rationed, espe-cially during the night. The sleep disturbance can be treated with hypnotics such as trazodone or antipsychotics such as quetiapine, but this can be met with resistance by the patient. SSRIs were ineffective in reported cases. There are no reports on the use of anti-seizure medicines used for mood-stabilization or impulse-control. In-patient psychiatric hospitalization may be necessary to control behaviors and medication administration, especially when a dedicated caregiver is lacking.

Effects of neurosurgical treatments on behavior

Neurosurgical procedures such as ablative lesions of the globus pallidus interna (GPi, pallidotomy) and deep brain stimulation (DBS) of the sub-thalamic nucleus (STN) or ventral intermediate thalamus (VIM) are effective treatments for advanced PD with medically uncontrolled motor fluctuations and levodopa-induced involuntary movements. Ideal candidates are physi-cally healthy and psychiatrically stable, younger patients without significant cognitive impairment. With carefully selected patients, there are clinically trivial, if any, immediate or longer-term postoperative effects on cognitive function. On average, there are mild changes in mood, including relative increases in apathy and decreased depression ratings.[71,72] As mentioned above, STN DBS can improve OCD and is potentially a therapy for refractory OCD without PD.[73] A small study showed mild but significantly improved sexual functioning after bilateral STN DBS in men with PD under 60 years of age, but not in women or older men.[74] Effects of STN-DBS on mood fluctuations have not been well-studied, but some cases showed improvements.

Behavioral and cognitive complications after surgical treatments for PD are less common. However, dramatic changes occur and underscore the importance of pre- and postoperative psychiatric assessments and careful management of pharmacological and stimulation treatments.[75] There are several reports of hypomania or mania in the immediate postoperative period.[76] This may be accompanied by psychosis and can last several months. Abulia, aggression, disinhibition, hypersexuality, pathological gambling, and lowered mood, including suicidality, also occur.[77-79] Cognitive losses affect attention, working memory, declarative memory, associative learning, and verbal fluency.

Mechanisms
Potential mechanisms for psychiatric complications[75] include the influence of lesions or DBS on non-motor associative and limbic cortico-subcortical loops, in addition to effects on motor circuits. Stimulation may also result in acute neurotransmitter effects that have psychoactive effects. Hyperactive behaviors or elevated mood may be related to additive effects of DRT and STN stimulation, including effects of stimulation on nearby neural circuits that affect emotional and affective behavior. Electrode misplacement into adjacent areas could also stimulate cells that project to anterior cingulate, ventral striatal, and frontal regions and have psychotropic effects.

Treatment
Psychiatric assessments before neurosurgical procedures should help identify pre-existing disturbances and provide a baseline for tracking postoperative status. Patients and families should be counseled about the potential for behavioral or mood changes after DBS and to report them immediately. Clinicians should be aware of the potential for psychiatric effects resulting from combined effects of stimulation and medications and vigilant about behavioral changes and the need for prompt interventions.

Conclusions

An array of behavioral disturbances occur in PD and these often have serious consequences. As part of routine care, patients and families should be educated about the potential for these disturbances, as the status of DRT is often an important factor. Since patients or families may not be forthcoming about symptoms, clinicians should screen for the development of behavioral complications and adjust therapy accordingly. Few studies have addressed specific treatment of these disturbances. Future studies should include controlled trials that target the various behavioral disturbances in PD.

Acknowledgment

Support for Dr Marsh provided by grants from the NIH (P50-NS-58366 and NIH RO1-MH069666).

References

1. Campbell JJ, Duffy JD, Salloway SP, Treatment strategies for patients with dysexecutive syndromes. In: Salloway SP, Malloy PF, Duffy JD (eds) *The Frontal Lobes and Neuropsychiatric Illness.* American Psychiatric Publishing. Inc.: Washington, DC, 2002; 153–163.
2. Aarsland D, Larsen JP, Lim NG et al, Range of neuropsychiatric disturbances in patients with Parkinson's disease. *J Neurol Neurosurg Psychiat* 1999; **67**:492–496.
3. Starkstein SE, Mayberg HS, Preziosi TJ, Andrezejewski P, Leiguarda R, Robinson RG, Reliability, validity, and clinical correlates of apathy in Parkinson's disease. *J Neuropsychiat Clin Neurosci* 1992; **4**(2):134–139.
4. Isella V, Melzi P, Grimaldi M et al, Clinical, neuropsychological, and morphometric correlates of apathy in Parkinson's disease. *Mov Disord* 2002; **17**(2): 366–371.
5. Shulman LM, Apathy in patients with Parkinson's disease. *Intern Rev Psychiat* 2000; **12**(4):298–306.
6. Pluck GC, Brown RG, Apathy in Parkinson's disease. *J Neurol Neurosurg Psychiat* 2002; **73**:636–642.
7. Rogers D, Lees AJ, Smith E, Bradyphrenia in Parkinson's disease and psychomotor retardation in depressive illness: an experimental study. *Brain* 1987; **110**:761–776.
8. Mayeux R, Stern Y, Sano M, Clinical and biochemical correlates of bradyphrenia in Parkinson's disease. *Neurology* 1987; **37**:1130–1134.
9. Ready RE, Friedman J, Grace J, Fernandez H, Testosterone deficiency and apathy in Parkinson's disease: a pilot study. *J Neurol Neurosurg Psychiat* 2004; **75**(9): 1323–1326.
10. Richard IH, Kurlan R, Parkinson Study Group, A survey of antidepressant usage in Parkinson's disease. *Neurology* 1997; **49**:1168–1170.
11. Gelenberg AJ, Apathy and new antidepressants. *Biol Ther Psychiat Newsletter* 1991; **14**:925.
12. Marin RS, Differential diagnosis and classification of apathy. *Am J Psychiat* 1990; **147**(1):22–30.
13. Levy ML, Cummings JL, Fairbanks LA et al, Apathy is not depression. *J Neuropsychiat Clin Neurosci* 1998; **10**(3):314–319.
14. Leentjens AFG, Marinus J, Van Hilten JJ, Lousberg R, Verhey FRJ, The contribution of somatic symptoms to the diagnosis of depressive disorder in Parkinson's disease: a discriminant analytic approach. *J Neuropsychiat Clin Neurosci* 2003; 15:74–77.

15. Campbell J, Duffy JD, Treatment strategies in amotivated patients. *Psychiatr Ann* 1997; **27**(1):44–49.
16. Chatterjee A, Fahn S, Methylphenidate treats apathy in Parkinson's disease (letter). *J Neuropsychiat Clin Neurosci* 2002; **14**(4):461–462.
17. Wynn ZJ, Cummings JL, Cholinesterase inhibitor therapies and neuropsychiatric manifestations of Alzheimer's disease. *Dement Geriatr Cogn Disord* 2004; **17**(1–2): 100–108.
18. Singer C, Weiner WJ, Sanchez-Ramos J, Ackerman M, Sexual function in patients with Parkinson's disease. *J Neurol Neurosurg Psychiat* 1991; **54**(10):942.
19. Yu M, Roane DM, Miner CR, Fleming M, Rogers JD, Dimensions of sexual dysfunction in Parkinson disease. *Am J Geriatr Psychiat* 2004; **12**(2):221–226.
20. Fine J, Lang AE, Dose-induced penile erections in response to repinirole therapy for Parkinson's disease. *Mov Disord* 1999; **14**(4):701.
21. Bronner G, Royter V, Korczyn AD, Giladi N, Sexual dysfunction in Parkinson's disease. *J Sex Marital Ther* 2004; **30**(2):95–105.
22. Jacobs H, Vieregge A, Vieregge P, Sexuality in young patients with Parkinson's disease: a population based comparison with healthy controls. *J Neurol Neurosurg Psychiat* 2000; **69**(4):550–552.
23. Brown RG, Jahanshahi M, Quinn N, Marsden CD, Sexual function in patients with Parkinson's disease and their partners. *J Neurol Neurosurg Psychiat* 1990; **53**(6):480–486.
24. Frohman EM, Sexual dysfunction in neurologic disease. *Clin Neuropharmacol* 2002; **25**(3):126–132.
25. Okun MS, Walter BL, McDonald WM et al, Beneficial effects of testosterone replacement for the nonmotor symptoms of Parkinson's disease. *Arch Neurol* 2002; **59**:1750–1753.
26. Sood ED, Pallanti S, Hollander E, Diagnosis and treatment of pathologic gambling. *Curr Psychiat Rep* 2003; **5**(1):9–15.
27. Czernecki V, Pillon B, Houeto JL, Pochon JB, Levy R, Dubois B, Motivation, reward, and Parkinson's disease: influence of dopatherapy. *Neuropsychologia* 2002; **40**(13):2257–2267.
28. Cools R, Barker RA, Sahakian BJ, Robbins TW, L-dopa medication remediates cognitive inflexibility, but increases impulsivity in patients with Parkinson's disease. *Neuropsychologia* 2003; **41**(11):1431–1441.
29. Chau DT, Roth RM, Green AI, The neural circuitry of reward and its relevance to psychiatric disorders. *Curr Psychiat Rep* 2004; **6**(5):391–399.
30. Tomer R, Aharon-Peretz J, Novelty seeking and harm avoidance in Parkinson's disease: effects of asymmetric dopamine deficiency. *J Neurol Neurosurg Psychiat* 2004; **75**(7):972–975.
31. Foltynie T, Goldberg TE, Lewis SG et al, Planning ability in Parkinson's disease is influenced by the COMT val158met polymorphism. *Mov Disord* 2004; **19**(8):885–891.
32. Comings DE, Gade R, Wu S et al, Studies of the potential role of the dopamine D1 receptor gene in addictive behaviors. *Mol Psychiat* 1997; **2**(1):44–56.
33. Ringman JM, Diaz-Olavarrieta C, Rodriguez Y, Fairbanks L, Cummings JL, The prevalence and correlates of neuropsychiatric symptoms in a population with Parkinson's disease in Mexico. *Neuropsychiat Neuropsychol Behav Neurol* 2002; **15**(2):99–105.
34. Aarsland D, Litvan I, Larsen JP, Neuropsychiatric symptoms of patients with progressive supranuclear palsy and Parkinson's disease. *J Neuropsychiat Clin Neurosci* 2001; **13**(1):42–49.
35. Goodwin FK, Psychiatric side effects of levodopa in man. *JAMA* 1971; **218**:1915–1920.

36. Uitti RJ, Tanner CM, Rajput AH, Goetz CG, Klawans HL, Thiessen B, Hypersexuality with antiparkinsonian therapy. *Clin Neuropharmacol* 1989; **12**(5):375–383.
37. Roane DM, Yu M, Feinberg TE, Rogers JD, Hypersexuality after pallidal surgery for Parkinson's disease. *Neuropsychiat Neuropsychol Behav Neurol* 2002; **15**(4):247–251.
38. Quinn NP, Toone B, Lang AE, Marsden CD, Parkes JD, Dopa dose-dependent sexual deviation. *Br J Psychiat* 1983; **142**:296–298.
39. Riley D, Reversible transvestic fetishism in a man with Parkinson's disease treated with selegiline. *Clin Neuropharmacol* 2002; **25**(4):234–237.
40. Mendez MF, O'Connor SM, Lim GT, Hypersexuality after right pallidotomy for Parkinson's disease. *J Neuropsychiat Clin Neurosci* 2004; **16**(1):37–40.
41. Alkhalil C, Tanvir F, Alkhalil B, Lowenthal DT, Treatment of sexual disinhibition in dementia: case reports and review of the literature. *Am J Ther* 2004; **11**(3):231–235.
42. Nissenbaum H, Quinn NP, Brown RG, Toone B, Gotham AM, Marsden CD, Mood swings associated with the "on-off" phenomenon in Parkinson's disease. *Psychol Med* 1987; **17**(4):899–904.
43. Avanzi M, Uber E, Bonfa F, Pathological gambling in two patients on dopamine replacement therapy for Parkinson's disease. *Neurol Sci* 2004; **25**(2):98–101.
44. Driver-Dunckley E, Samanta J, Stacy M, Pathological gambling associated with dopamine agonist therapy in Parkinson's disease. *Neurology* 2003; **61**(3):422–423.
45. Molina JA, Sainz-Artiga MJ, Fraile A et al, Pathological gambling in Parkinson's disease: a behavioral manifestation of pharmacologic treatment? *Mov Disord* 2000; **15**(5):869–872.
46. Gschwandtner U, Aston J, Renaud S, Fuhr P, Pathologic gambling in patients with Parkinson's disease. *Clin Neuropharmacol* 2001; **24**(3):170–172.
47. Seedat S, Kesler S, Niehaus DJH, Stein DJ, Pathological gambling behavior: emergence secondary to treatment of Parkinson's disease with dopaminergic agents. *Depression Anxiety* 2000; **11**(4):185–186.
48. Black DW, Compulsive buying disorder: definition, assessment, epidemiology and clinical management. *CNS Drugs* 2001; **15**(1):17–27.
49. Koran LM, Chuong HW, Bullock KD, Smith SC, Citalopram for compulsive shopping disorder: an open-label study followed by double-blind discontinuation. *J Clin Psychiat* 2003; **64**(7):793–798.
50. Nausieda PA, Sinemet "abusers." *Clin Neuropharmacol* 1985; **8**:318–327.
51. Lawrence AD, Evans AH, Lees AJ, Compulsive use of dopamine replacement therapy in Parkinson's disease: reward systems gone awry? *Lancet Neurology* 2003; **2**:595–604.
52. Giovannoni G, O'Sullivan JD, Turner K, Manson AJ, Lees AJ, Hedonistic homeostatic dysregulation in patients with Parkinson's disease on dopamine replacement therapies. *J Neurol Neurosurg Psychiat* 2000; **68**(4):423–428.
53. Pezzella FR, Colosimo C, Vanacore N et al, Prevalence and clinical features of hedonistic homeostatic dysregulation in Parkinson's disease. *Mov Disord* 2005; **20**(1):77–81.
54. Pezzella FR, Di Rezze S, Chianese M et al, Hedonistic homeostatic dysregulation in Parkinson's disease: a short screening questionnaire. *Neurol Sci* 2003; **24**(3):205–206.
55. Riley DE, Lang AE, The spectrum of levodopa-related fluctuations in Parkinson's disease. *Neurology* 1993; **43**(8):1459–1464.
56. Racette BA, Hartlein JM, Hershey T, Mink JW, Perlmutter JS, Black KJ, Clinical features and comorbidity of mood fluctuations in Parkinson's disease. *J Neuropsychiat Clin Neurosci* 2002; **14**(4):438–442.

57. Witjas T, Kaphan E, Azulay JP et al, Nonmotor fluctuations in Parkinson's disease: frequent and disabling. *Neurology* 2002; **59**(3):408–413.
58. Gunal DI, Nurichalichi K, Tuncer N, Bekiroglu N, Aktan S, The clinical profile of nonmotor fluctuations in Parkinson's disease patients. *Can J Neurol Sci* 2002; **29**(1):61–64.
59. Maia AF, Pinto AS, Barbosa ER, Menezes PR, Miguel EC, Obsessive-compulsive symptoms, obsessive-compulsive disorder related disorders in Parkinson's disease. *J Neuropsychiat Clin Neurosci* 2003; **15**(3):371–374.
60. Alegret M, Junqué C, Valldeoriola F, Vendrell P, Martí MJ, Tolosa E, Obsessive-compulsive symptoms in Parkinson's disease. *J Neurol Neurosurg Psychiat* 2001; **70**:394–396.
61. Muller N, Putz A, Kathmann N, Lehle R, Gunther W, Straube A, Characteristics of obsessive-compulsive symptoms in Tourette's syndrome, obsessive-compulsive disorder, and Parkinson's disease. *Psychiat Res* 1997; **70**(2):105–114.
62. Hollander E, Cohen L, Richards M, Mullen L, DeCaria C, Stern Y, A pilot study of the neuropsychology of obsessive-compulsive disorder and Parkinson's disease: basal ganglia disorders. *J Neuropsychiat Clin Neurosci* 1993; **5**(1):104–107.
63. Tomer R, Levin BE, Weiner WJ, Obsessive-compulsive symptoms and motor asymmetries in Parkinson's disease. *Neuropsychiat Neuropsychol Behav Neurol* 1993; **6**:26–30.
64. Menza MA, Forman NE, Goldstein HS, Golbe LI, Parkinson's disease, personality, and dopamine. *J Neuropsychiat Clin Neurosci* 1990; **2**:282–287.
65. Fontaine D, Mattei V, Borg M et al, Effect of subthalamic nucleus stimulation on obsessive-compulsive disorder in a patient with Parkinson disease. Case report. *J Neurosurg* 2004; **100**(6):1084–1086.
66. Mallet L, Mesnage V, Houeto JL et al, Compulsions, Parkinson's disease, and stimulation. *Lancet* 2002; **360**(9342):1302–1304.
67. Fernandez HH, Friedman J, Punding on L-dopa. *Mov Disord* 1999; **14**:836–838.
68. Friedman J, Punding on L-dopa. *Biol Psychiat* 1994; **36**:350–351.
69. Evans AH, Katzenshlager R, Paviour D et al, Punding in Parkinson's disease: its relation to the dopamine dysregulation syndrome. *Mov Disord* 2004; **19**(4):397–405.
70. Kurlan R, Disabling repetitive behaviors in Parkinson's disease. *Mov Disord* 2003; **19**(4):433–469.
71. Perozzo P, Rizzone M, Bergamasco B et al, Deep brain stimulation of the sub-thalamic nucleus in Parkinson's disease: comparison of pre- and postoperative neuropsychological evaluation. *J Neurol Sci* 2001; **192**(1–2):9–15.
72. Funkiewiez A, Ardouin C, Caputo E et al, Long term effects of bilateral sub-thalamic nucleus stimulation on cognitive function, mood, and behaviour in Parkinson's disease. *J Neurol Neurosurg Psychiat* 2004; **75**(6):834–839.
73. Nuttin BJ, Gabriels L, van Kuyck K, Cosyns P, Electrical stimulation of the anterior limbs of the internal capsules in patients with severe obsessive-compulsive disorder: anecdotal reports. *Neurosurg Clin N Am* 2003; **14**(2):267–274.
74. Castelli L, Perozzo P, Genesia ML et al, Sexual well being in parkinsonian patients after deep brain stimulation of the subthalamic nucleus. *J Neurol Neurosurg Psychiat* 2004; **75**(9):1260–1264.
75. Piasecki SD, Jefferson JW, Psychiatric complications of deep brain stimulation for Parkinson's disease. *J Clin Psychiat* 2004; **65**(6):845–849.
76. Kulisevsky J, Berthier ML, Gironell A, Pascual-Sedano B, Molet J, Pares P, Mania following deep brain stimulation for Parkinson's disease. *Neurology* 2002; **59**(9):1421–1424.
77. Houeto JL, Mesnage V, Mallet L et al, Behavioural disorders, Parkinson's disease and subthalamic stimulation. *J Neurol Neurosurg Psychiat* 2002; **72**:701–707.

78. Sensi M, Eleopra R, Cavallo MA et al, Explosive-aggressive behavior related to bilateral subthalamic stimulation. *Parkinsonism Relat Disord* 2004; **10**(4):247–251.
79. Berney A, Vingerhoets F, Perrin A et al, Effect on mood of subthalamic DBS for Parkinson's disease: a consecutive series of 24 patients. *Neurology* 2002; **59**(9):1427–1429.
80. Marin RS, Biedrzycki RC, Firinciogullari S, Reliability and validity of the Apathy Evaluation Scale. *Psychiat Res* 1991; **38**:143–162.
81. Starkstein SE, Garau ML, Cao A, Prevalence and clinical correlates of disinhibition in dementia. *Cog Behav Neurol* 2004; **17**(3):139–147.
82. Kertesz A, Nadkarni N, Davidson W, Thomas AW, The Frontal Behavioral Inventory in the differential diagnosis of frontotemporal dementia. *J Int Neuropsychol Soc* 2000; **6**(4):460–468.
83. Grace J, Malloy P, Frontal Systems Behavior Scale (FrSBe). Psychological Assessment Resources, Inc.: Lutz, PL, 2001.
84. Cummings JL, The Neuropsychiatric Inventory: assessing psychopathology in dementia patients. *Neurology* 1997; **48**(5(Suppl 6)):10–16.

chapter 13

Disability

Susan Spear Bassett

Introduction

Parkinson's disease (PD), a chronic, progressive neurodegenerative disorder of unknown etiology, affects approximately 1% of the population over age 50 and up to 2.5% of the population over age 70. United States government figures from 1994 estimate annual societal costs related to PD at $20 billion dollars,[1] and much of this appears related to higher hospitalization rates and longer length of stay[2] with accompanying disability driving much of the healthcare utilization among these patients.[3] Community studies have found that PD patients have greater physical, social, and emotional disability than that experienced by individuals with other chronic conditions such as diabetes mellitus.[4] While the societal burden is measured in dollars, the impact on patients and by extension their families, requires additional metrics. This chapter will present information on the disabilities that often accompany Parkinson's disease, including definitions of key concepts in the disability field, examples of the major areas of disability, means of assessment, a discussion of factors that influence both the presentation and extent of these disabilities and finally suggestions for intervention and management.

Definitions

Impairments

Parkinson's disease (PD), a neurodegenerative disorder, is characterized by significant changes in the functioning of multiple body systems. These abnormalities of function are termed impairments. In PD the primary impairments are of the motor system and include a slowing of movements (bradykinesia), rigidity of the muscles, a resting tremor, poor posture, and an expressionless face. In addition to these defining motor impairments, PD patients also experience psychiatric impairments of mood and drive, which can manifest as depression and apathy for a great many patients, and include a reduction in spontaneity and initiation. Finally, there are impairments of the intellect, which, for the majority of patients are not global, but rather specific and include impairments of attention, concentration, problem solving, and memory. Other body systems are also affected, producing impairments of fatigue, sleep disturbance, and temperature sensitivity, to name a few. Impairments are generally documented by clinical assessment and objective testing, rather then patient report.

Disability

The impairments discussed above, as well as others, plus co-morbid conditions, individually and in concert, produce significant disability for most patients. Disability here refers to the inability to perform normal activities or roles in the manner considered normal.[5] These changes in activity level and role performance span all aspects of patients' lives from home-life to the workplace. Normal physical, social, and occupational activities can become disrupted and produce significant distress. It is, in fact, the disabilities, rather than the impairments, that form the basis for much of the dialogue between patients and their physicians, as patients attempt to describe the impact of the disease for them personally as well as for their family. Disability therefore is a self-report subjective measure in contrast to the objective measurement of impairments. Table 13.1 presents a summary of body systems that are affected in PD, the impairments that result and examples of disabilities that can arise. Table 13.2 provides a summary of disability rating scales, focused on specific areas of disability, which can be useful for clinicians in understanding and monitoring the impact of PD on patients' daily lives.

Physical disability

In general, physical disability is focused on tasks necessary for independent living, and is the area of functioning most often assessed by clinicians. Included here are tasks related to self-care, such as bathing, dressing,

Table 13.1 Common impairments and disabilities in PD

Body systems	Impairments	Disabilities
Intellectual	Memory, planning	Completing tasks at work and home
Sensory	Seeing, hearing, pain	Social isolation
Emotion	Mood regulation, volition	Interacting with family members
Language	Voice, speech	Problems communicating at work
Motor	Muscle, joint movement	Putting on clothes, eating
Digestive	Weight maintenance	Lose of strength for tasks
Metabolic	Thermoregulation	Embarrassment due to sweating
Sleep regulation	Fatigue, disrupted sleep	Poor driving

Table 13.2 Instruments for the assessment of disability

Functional area	Instruments	Reference
Physical functioning	Schwab & England ADL Scale	11
	Northwestern University Disability Scale	12
	Unified PD Rating Scale, Section II	13
	Lawton IADL Scale	15
Social functioning	PsychoSocial Questionnaire	48
	Social Adjustment Scale	49
	Groningen Social Disabilities Schedule	51
Occupational functioning	Self-Assessment of Occupational Functioning	71
	Social Adjustment Scale	49
Quality of life	Extensive Disability Scale	54
	Parkinson's Disease Questionnaire-39	55
	Parkinson's Disease Quality of Life Questionnaire	56
	Parkinson's Disease Quality of Life Scale	57
General health	Nottingham Health Profile	43
	Sickness Impact Profile	44
	Short Form Health Survey	45

grooming and toileting, as well as tasks related to the maintenance of independent living, including such things as maintaining household cleanliness, managing medications, and maintaining mobility in the home and community. Successful completion of these tasks generally requires both fine and gross motor skills. Increasing disability on these tasks is associated with the duration of disease, and improvement in these tasks is found with both pharmocologic and surgical treatment.[6–11]

Assessment

Assessment of basic skills which enable an individual to remain independent focus on what are referred to as activities of daily living (ADL) and utilize scales developed specifically for PD. These include the Schwab and England Scale,[12] the Northwestern University Disability Scale (NWDS)[13] and the ADL subscale of the Unified Parkinson's Disease Rating Scale (UPDRS).[14] The Schwab & England Scale rates the patient's overall capacity to complete basic activities as a percentage of their normal abilities, ranging from 0% which reflects an individual who is bed-ridden and unable to complete any self-care to 100% for the individual whose daily tasks remain at pre-morbid levels. The NWDS asks the patient to rate their performance on six functions (walking, dressing, speech, hygiene, eating, and feeding), using a 10-point scale with the use of descriptors for each point on the scale. The UPDRS includes assessment of 12 activities, including such things as turning over in bed, writing, using eating utensils, graded on a 5-point scale with higher scores reflecting greater severity. A recent comparison of these scales reported that the UPDRS and NWDS have moderate to good reliability and validity.[15] Instrumental activities of daily life, which include household activities, driving, telephone use, and medication managements are part of the Lawton IADL Scale, where items are endorsed on an anchored scale of increasing difficulty.[16]

Interaction of impairments

While the impact of motor impairments on daily living task seems obvious, physical disability is also affected by impairments in other domains. The relationship of psychiatric impairments to physical disability in PD has received considerable attention. Most studies find that anxiety and ratings of physical disability are unrelated,[17–20] while the relationship between depression and physical disability is less clear. Several cross-sectional, as well as three longitudinal studies report a positive association between disability and depression.[21–27] These findings are interpreted as evidence of reactive depression in PD. However, as Brown notes from his follow-up of the original study cohort,[28] the relationship between depression and disability is not linear. Patients who were not depressed at the initial assessment, but were at follow-up showed an increase in ADL disability, but so did patients whose depression had remitted.[25] Interestingly, Cole found depression to be predictive of physical disability, as well as social disability, but only for males.[21] Other studies, however, find no relationship between the two,[29-34] supporting the view that depression reflects the underlying pathology of PD.[35] In addition, surgical outcome studies of pallidotomy in PD patients report reductions in depressive and anxiety symptoms independent of improvement in motor activity.[36-38]

Increasing physical disability has been reported to accompany intellectual decline in several studies.[30,32,39-41] Two of the studies[32,41] noted poorer cognitive performance associated with more severe bradykinesia. A longitudinal 12-month study documented decline in both cognition and ADL functioning in 92 PD patients and found this decline to accelerate in those patients with baseline depression, providing evidence for the synergistic effect of both cognitive and psychiatric impairments on physical functioning.[42] Finally, the contribution of multiple impairments to physical disability has been noted in a recent community study.[43]

Social disability

Social functioning focuses on the patient's interactions with others and their performance in family and social roles. The impairments that accompany PD can result in patients no longer sustaining their normal role function. Motor impairments, for example, may interfere with the normal household tasks, such as house cleaning, lawn maintenance, getting groceries, to name a few. This then necessitates a redistribution of tasks within the family, impacting all family members. It also may change role dynamics, that is, the individual who was responsible for the household now needs personal care from other family members. Restructuring roles within the family can often be difficult and requires forthright discussions among all members.

Maintaining social interaction outside the family unit also can be altered by the impairments that accompany PD. For example, when attending social gatherings, cognitive impairments, such as attention difficulties can make it difficult for patients to concentrate and attend to one conversation when there are others in the background. Cognitive problems with planning, organizing and sequencing can also have consequences for maintaining social contacts with friends and family members. Psychiatric and motor impairments can interact to induce social withdrawal in some patients and result in isolation.

Assessment

Assessment of social functioning has been included in several studies of treatment outcomes employing scales designed to assess the impact of illness, including the Nottingham Health Profile (NHP),[44] the Sickness Impact Profile (SIP)[45] and the Short Form Health Survey (SF-36).[46] These surveys contain items relating to social isolation, social functioning, or social support. Studies using these scales for the assessment of treatment outcomes following levodopa, pallidotomy and implants have all reported improvements in social functioning,[8-11] with a recent study suggesting that females show a greater improvement than males.[47] A recent report by Helofson and colleagues finds fatigue to have a significant impact on social functioning as measured by the SF-36.[48] These instruments include items related to social functioning but assess a variety of other areas. Two other self-report instruments provide a more focused assessment of social and role functioning. One, the PsychoSocial questionnaire asks patients to indicate on a 4-point scale the degree of difficulty or problems they have regarding 11 items.[49] The second, an instrument designed solely for social functioning, not normally used for PD assessment, which provides a more thorough examination is the Social Adjustment Scale, a self-report instrument that contains 42 questions that measure either instrumental or expressive role performance in six major areas of functioning.[50] These include work as a worker, housewife, or student; social and leisure activities; relationships with extended family; marital roles as a spouse, a parent, and a member of a family unit. The scale has been shown to be sensitive to improvement in patients with depression.[51] Finally, although more time consuming, the Groningen Social Disabilities Schedule, a semi-structured interview, provides for the opportunity to explore social functioning unconstrained by standardized questions. This schedule has been extensively used to examine social disability in psychiatric disorders.[52]

Global measures: quality of life

Concerns that the NHP, SIP, and SF-36 scales do not assess functions necessarily relevant to PD and may not be sensitive to subtle changes which might occur in PD[53,54] prompted development of several global measures of functioning targeted specifically to PD. These instruments are more comprehensive and have been designed to more fully document the effects of PD on the lives of patients. These include the Extensive Disability Scale (EDS),[55] the Parkinson's Disease Questionnaire-39 (PDQ-39),[56] the Parkinson's Disease

Quality of Life Questionnaire (PDQL),[57] and the Parkinson's Disease Quality of Life Scale (PDQUALIF).[58] All provide patients with a list, which includes both disease symptoms and life activities, and ask them to indicate how frequently they have these difficulties. The PDQL for example,[57] is self-administered and contains 37 items relating to parkinsonian symptoms, systemic symptoms, social functional, and emotional well-being. Patients indicate how often during the previous 3 months they had trouble with the item. Responses use a 5-point Leikert scale that ranges from "all of the time" to "never." Although these instruments contain items that are related to social functioning, with the PDQUALIF containing the most, they are really considered more global measures of "quality of life" and include assessment of both impairments and disabilities.

Interaction of impairments

A study by Hobson and colleagues[59] found greater difficulty on the PDQL was related to older age, greater depressive symptomatology, and poorer cognitive function. Thus a combination of impairments proved to be related to overall life quality. A similar pattern was reported using both the PDQ-39 and NHP, where among several predictors of poor QOL, depressive symptoms proved the most important.[60,61] A recent study also using the PDQ-39, found an increase in quality of life following unilateral pallidotomy, particularly in the areas of mobility, ADL, emotion, and pain. Interestingly, these improvements were unrelated to clinical evaluation of change.[62] Several studies have examined the relationship of motor impairments to physical disability looking at QOL or life satisfaction, finding motor impairments were related not only to physical disability but also to life satisfaction.[63,64] Finally, a comparison of young versus older-onset PD cases, found poorer QOL among the young-onset cases with more significant motor, and psychiatric impairments.[65]

Occupational disability

There has been little study of the impact of PD on other areas of normal activity, such as employment. Patient interviews indicate that the problems associated with PD go beyond activities that are related to motor impairments.[66–68] These problems affect all aspects of patients' lives, for example surveys of PD patients living in the community report up to 40% retire early and 71% give up driving because of their disease.[6,69] A recent survey of 148

PD patients who developed PD before the age of 65 found over 79% retired early, however no factors were identified that increased the risk of leaving work.[70] There are obviously many factors involved in the withdrawal from the workforce. For example, analysis of the Survey of Disability and Work, which included over 5000 men and women ages 35–64, found high self-esteem related to lower disability even among those with severe impairments, supporting the notion that non-medical factors are likely related to maintenance of work roles.[71]

Assessment of occupational disability does not easily lend itself to standardized questionnaires since job requirements vary greatly. However, there are certain areas that need to be examined and these include the quality and quantity of job performance as well as interactions with colleagues. The Self-Assessment of Occupational Functioning is a 23-item self-assessment of the patients' perceptions of their own strengths and weaknesses relative to occupational functioning.[72] Each item is rated on a 3-point ordinal scale indicating whether the individual perceives this item to be a personal strength, an adequate area of function, or an area that needs improvement. The test has been used with patients entering occupational rehabilitation. The Social Adjustment Scale[51] mentioned above, also contains items related to work roles.

It is not difficult to imagine the possible impact motor, psychiatric and cognitive impairments can have on staying in the workplace. Most jobs require organizing space and materials, completing work on time, developing plans for job completion, seeing tasks to completion, maintaining focus on tasks at hand, and interacting with co-workers. Disability can be reduced often with accommodations in the workplace. These usually have more to do with re-structuring the job demands than with altering the physical environment. These changes require a willing employer and a flexible workplace. For example, one patient, a 53-year-old engineer, was able to reduce his focus to one aspect of project management and then perform this for several projects, instead of handling all aspects of a single project. On the other hand, another patient, whose job involved traveling to see clients, was given poor performance ratings and ultimately fired because of the increased travel time required.

Personality and disability

There has been little study of individual patients' personal characteristics or attributes and how these might affect disability. One recent PD study examined 86 individuals between the ages of 51–87 to assess the effects of physical disability, stage of disease, depression, mastery and health locus of control on the patients' quality of life as rated on a 5-point scale. Their findings indicated that only the sense of mastery or control was related to the patient's rating of life quality.[73] Similar findings come from two recent epidemiological studies that report the relationship of psychological attributes to changes in disability status. A community-based longitudinal study of 575 elderly individuals found that feelings of perceived control or mastery were highly associated with the absence of disability.[74] The study by Schieman and Turner[75] found a synergistic relationship between age, disability and the sense of mastery. A more recent, smaller-scale study of 74 patients, also found that psychosocial adjustment was inversely related to perceptions of control.[76] Studies of personality in PD have focused on the search for premorbid traits which may represent latent disease[77–79] rather than examining personality traits as they may be related to disability in this disease.

Changes in disability in response to PD treatments

While, over the entire course of the disease, disability can be expected to increase,[80–82] current treatments for both motor and psychiatric impairments alter the trajectory of this disability. Standard treatments for PD reduce motor symptoms and thus in general reduce physical disability, as well as other areas of disability. For example, the reduction in tremor can reduce stigma and thus reduce social disability. However, treatment side-effects, such as the development of "on-off" motor states, for example, can add to the fluctuations in daily functioning and hence can increase disability.[83,84]

Pharmacologic treatments for the cognitive impairments in PD, primarily cholinesterase inhibitors, find some improvements in cognition,[85–87] however few studies examine accompanying changes in disability. One that has, a case series of patients receiving rivastigmine (Exelon), a drug that inhibits both acetylcholinesterase and butyrylcholinesterase, found improvement both in cognition and functional abilities.[88]

PD patients with severe motor impairments that can no longer be effectively treated with medications may undergo pallidotomy or deep brain stimulation (DBS). These procedures are very successful in reducing motor symptoms and subsequently generally improve physical disability, specifically activities of daily living, for most patients.[8,89–94]

Although almost all studies of surgical outcomes assess motor impairments and physical disability, there are several studies that have assessed other aspects of disability as well. A recent study by Lagrange and colleagues assessed quality of life in 60 patients prior to and 12 months following DBS, utilizing the PDQL.[95] In addition to improvements in ADLs, all patients showed improvement on the PDQL in all four domains, one of which is social functioning. Inspection of those data found improvement in motor impairments highly related to improvements in social functioning. This can be attributed to not only the improvement in mobility but also the reduction in stigma often attached to individuals with severe dyskinesias. Baron's study of 15 patients used the instrument from the Medial Outcomes Study to measure a number of areas of disability. Physical functioning, social functioning, and vitality all showed improvement at 3-month follow-up, with no further improvement at 12 months.[8] Emotional functioning did not show any change with the surgical procedure. Longer-term follow-up of surgical cases has reported sustained improved in quality of life for these patients.[96]

Finally, there have been several studies of comprehensive, multidisciplinary rehabilitation programs for individuals with PD, with diverging results. A study by Trend and colleagues[97] evaluated 118 patients, without cognitive impairment, enrolled in a 6-week program which included individual treatment from a specialist team and weekly group educational and relaxation activities. Assessment at the end of the program found a significant increase in quality of life, with those with more severe disease showing greater improvement. These improvements in global quality of life may be related to the improvement in mobility and gait and the reduction in depression noted in the study. In contrast, a similar study with longer follow-up did not find sustained improvement.[98] Wade and colleagues examined 144 patients, without serious cognitive impairments, at baseline and 6-month follow-up, 4 months after having received 6 weeks of group educational activities as well as individualized multidisciplinary rehabilitation services. This study examines patient status 4 months after services, rather then immediately following the intervention. In this case, while there was sustained improvement in selected motor abilities, patients showed significant decline in emotional health and overall quality of life. Thus, it may be that sustained or different services or interventions are required to reduce disability in PD where the nature of the disease is progressive.

Conclusions

In summary, PD patients suffer significant disability as a consequence of the motor, psychiatric, and cognitive impairments that occur with this disease. This disability affects all realms of the patient's life including the most obvious, self-care, as well as family roles, and occupational success. The level of impairments affects the subsequent disability but individual characteristics, such as personality traits, as well as environmental factors, such as an understanding boss, contribute to the variation seen in PD patients, and helps explain why patients with the same impairments can have a very different disability profile.

Improvement or stabilization of these disabilities requires a multi-focused approach. This can include physical therapy, individual psychological and family counseling, and employment counseling, which may need to be ongoing. Working provides a deep and sustaining sense of worth, contribution to one's family and the community, and general sense of satisfaction, and PD patients are no exception. Being creative in helping these patients retain all their roles, while perhaps adjusting their expectations, is critically important.

Acknowledgments

Dr Bassett's Parkinson's disease research is supported by a grant from the NIH, RO1 HD39822.

References

1. Cummings JL, Understanding Parkinson disease. *JAMA* 1999; **281**(4):376–378.
2. Guttman M, Slaughter PM, Theriault ME, DeBoer DP, Naylor CD, Burden of parkinsonism: a population-based study. *Mov Disord* 2003; **18**(3):313–319.
3. de Boer AG, Sprangers MA, Speelman HD, de Haes HC, Predictors of health care use in patients with Parkinson's disease: a longitudinal study. *Mov Disord* 1999; **14**(5):772–779.
4. Karlsen KH, Larsen JP, Tandberg E, Maland JG, Quality of life measurements in patients with Parkinson's disease: A community-based study. *Eur J Neurol* 1998; 5(5):443–450.
5. Jette AM, Concepts of health and methodological issues in functional assessment. In: Granger CV, Gresham GE (eds) *Functional Assessment in Rehabilitation Medicine*. Williams & Wilkins: Baltimore, 1984; 46–64.
6. Peterson GM, Nolan BW, Millingen KS, Survey of disability that is associated with Parkinson's disease. *Med J Aust* 1988; **18**:69–70.
7. Growdon JH, Kieburtz K, McDermott MP, Panisset M, Friedman JH, Levodopa

improves motor function without impairing cognition in mild non-demented Parkinson's disease patients. Parkinson Study Group. *Neurology* 1998; **50**(5): 1327–1331.

8. Baron MS, Vitek JL, Bakay RA et al, Treatment of advanced Parkinson's disease by posterior GPi pallidotomy: 1-year results of a pilot study [see comments]. *Ann Neurol* 1996; **40**(3):355–366.

9. Block G, Liss C, Reines S, Irr J, Nibbelink D, Comparison of immediate-release and controlled release carbidopa/levodopa in Parkinson's disease. A multicenter 5-year study. The CR First Study Group. *Eur Neurol* 1997; **37**(1):23–27.

10. McRae C, O'Brien C, Freed C, Quality of life among persons receiving neural implant surgery for Parkinson's disease. *Mov Disord* 1996; **11**:605–606.

11. Wilson RS, Goetz CG, Stebbins GT, Neurologic illness. In: Spilker B (ed.) *Quality of Life and Pharmacoeconomics in Clinical Trials.* Lippincott-Raven: Philadelphia, 1996; 903–908.

12. Schwab JF, England AC, Projection technique for evaluating surgery in Parkinson's disease. In: Gillingham FJ, Donaldson IM (eds) *Third Symposium On Parkinson's Disease.* Livingstone: Edinburgh, 1969; 152–157.

13. Canter GJ, de la Torre R, Mier M, A method for evaluating disability in patients with Parkinson's disease. *J Nervous Mental Dis* 1961; **133**:145–147.

14. Fahn S, Elton RL, Members of the UPDRS Development Committee, Unified Parkinson's disease rating scale. In: Fahn S, Marsden CD, Goldstein M (eds) *Recent Developments in Parkinson's Disease II.* Macmillan: New York, 1987; 153–163.

15. Ramaker C, Marinus J, Stiggelbout AM, Van Hilten BJ, Systematic evaluation of rating scales for impairment and disability in Parkinson's disease. *Mov Disord* 2002; **17**(5):867–876.

16. Lawton MP, Brody EM, Assessment of older people: self-maintaining and instrumental activities of daily living. *Gerontologist* 1969; **9**(3):179–186.

17. Menza MA, Robertson-Hoffman DE, Bonapace AS, Parkinson's disease and anxiety: comorbidity with depression. *Biol Psychiat* 1993; **34**:465–470.

18. Henderson R, Kurlan R, Kersun JM, Como P, Preliminary examination of the comorbidity of anxiety and depression in Parkinson's disease. *J Neuropsychiat Clin Neurosci* 1992; **4**(3):257–264.

19. Stein MB, Heuser IJ, Juncos JL, Uhde TW, Anxiety disorders in patients with Parkinson's disease. *Am J Psychiat* 1990; **147**:217–220.

20. Seimers ER, Shekhar A, Quaid K, Anxiety and motor performance in Parkinson's disease. *Mov Disord* 1993; **8**:501–506.

21. Cole SA, Woodard JL, Juncos JL, Kogos JL, Youngstrom EA, Watts RL, Depression and disability in Parkinson's disease. *J Neuropsychiat Clin Neurosci* 1996; **8**:20–25.

22. Kostic VS, Filipovic SR, Lecic D, Momcilovic D, Sokic D, Sternic N, Effect of age at onset on frequency of depression in Parkinson's disease. *J Neurol Neurosurg Psychiat* 1994; **57**:1265–1267.

23. Menza MA, Mark MH, Parkinson's disease and depression: the relationship to disability and personality. *J Neuropsychiat Clin Neurosci* 1994; **6**(2):165–169.

24. Tandberg E, Larsen JP, Aarsland D, Laake K, Cummings JL, Risk factors for depression in Parkinson disease. *Arch Neurol* 1997; **54**:625–630.

25. Brown RG, MacCarthy B, Gotham AM, Der GB, Marsden CD, Depression and disability in Parkinson's disease: a follow-up of 132 cases. *Psychol Med* 1988; **18**:49–55.

26. Mindham RH, Marsden CD, Parkes JD, Psychiatric symptoms during L-dopa therapy for Parkinson's disease and their relationship to physical disability. *Psychol Med* 1976; **6**(1):23–33.

27. Starkstein SE, Preziosi TJ, Bolduc PL, Robinson RG, Depression in Parkinson's disease. *J Nerv Ment Dis* 1990; **178**(1):27–31.

28. Gotham AM, Brown RG, Marsden CD, Depression in Parkinson's disease: a quantitative and qualitative analysis. *J Neurol Neurosurg Psychiat* 1986; **49**(4):381–389.

29. Ehmann TS, Beninger RJ, Gawel MJ, Riopelle RJ, Depressive symptoms in Parkinson's disease: a comparison with disabled control subjects. *J Geriatr Psychiat Neurol* 1990; **3**(1):3–9.

30. Huber SJ, Paulson GW, Shuttleworth EC, Relationship of motor symptoms, intellectual impairments and depression in Parkinson's disease. *J Neurol Neurosurg Psychiat* 1988; **51**:855–858.

31. Robins AH, Depression in patients with Parkinsonism. *Br J Psychiat* 1976; **128**:141–145.

32. Mayeux R, Stern Y, Rosen J, Leventhal J, Depression, intellectual impairment, and Parkinson disease. *Neurology* 1981; **31**(6):645–650.

33. Santanaria J, Tolosa E, Valles A, Parkinson's disease with depression: a possible subgroup of idiopathic parkinsonism. *Neurology* 1986; **36**:1130–1133.

34. Warburton JW, Depressive symptoms in Parkinson patients referred for thalamotomy. *J Neurol Neurosurg Psychiat* 1967; **30**(4):368–370.

35. Cummings JL, Depression and Parkinson's disease: a review. *Am J Psychiat* 1992; **149**(4):443–454.

36. Marsh L, Solvasson B, Cahn DA et al, Psychiatric outcome after pallidotomy for Parkinson's disease. *Biol Psychiat* 1997; 41:107S.

37. Masterman D, DeSalles A, Baloh RW et al, Motor, cognitive, and behavioral performance following unilateral ventroposterior pallidotomy for Parkinson disease. *Arch Neurol* 1998; **55**(9):1201–1208.

38. Riordan HJ, Flashman LA, Roberts DW, Neurocognitive and psychosocial correlates of ventroposterolateral pallidotomy surgery in Parkinson's disease. *Neurosurg Focus* 1997; **2**(3):e7.

39. Caparros-Lefebvre D, Pecheux N, Petit V, Duhamel A, Petit H, Which factors predict cognitive decline in Parkinson's disease? *J Neurol Neurosurg Psychiat* 1995; **58**(1):51–55.

40. Mortimer JA, Pirozzolo FJ, Hansch EC, Webster DD, Relationship of motor symptoms to intellectual deficits in Parkinson disease. *Neurology* 1982; **32**:133–137.

41. Marttila RJ, Rinne UK, Dementia in Parkinson's disease. *Acta Neurol Scand* 1976; **54**:431–441.

42. Starkstein SE, Mayberg HS, Leiguarda R, Preziosi TJ, Robinson RG, A prospective longitudinal study of depression, cognitive decline, and physical impairments in patients with Parkinson's disease. *J Neurol Neurosurg Psychiat* 1992; **55**:377–382.

43. Weintraub D, Moberg PJ, Duda JE, Katz IR, Stern MB, Effect of psychiatric and other nonmotor symptoms on disability in Parkinson's disease. *J Am Geriatr Soc* 2004; **52**(5):784–788.

44. Hunt SM, McEwen J, McKenna SP, *Measuring Health Status*. Croom Helm: London, 1986.

45. Bergner M, Bobbitt RA, Pollard WE, Martin DP, Gilson BS, The sickness impact profile: validation of a health status measure. *Med Care* 1976; **14**(1):57–67.

46. Ware JE Jr, Sherbourne CD, The MOS 36-item short-form health survey (SF-36). I. Conceptual framework and item selection. *Med Care* 1992; **30**(6):473–483.

47. Hariz GM, Lindberg M, Hariz MI, Bergenheim AT, Gender differences in disability and health-related quality of life in patients with Parkinson's disease treated with stereotactic surgery. *Acta Neurol Scand* 2003; **108**(1):28–37.

48. Herlofson K, Larsen JP, The influence of fatigue on health-related quality of life in patients with Parkinson's disease. *Acta Neurol Scand* 2003; **107**(1):1–6.

49. Marinus J, Visser M, Martinez-Martin P, van Hilten JJ, Stiggelbout AM, A short

psychosocial questionnaire for patients with Parkinson's disease: the SCOPA-PS. *J Clin Epidemiol* 2003; **56**(1):61–67.

50. Weissman MM, Bothwell S, Assessment of social adjustment by patient self-report. *Arch Gen Psychiat* 1976; **33**(9):1111–1115.

51. Weissman MM, Prusoff BA, Thompson WD, Harding PS, Myers JK, Social adjustment by self-report in a community sample and in psychiatric outpatients. *J Nerv Ment Dis* 1978; **166**(5):317–326.

52. Wiersma D, deJong A, Ormel J, The Groningen Social Disabilities Schedule: development, relationship with ICIDH and psychometric properties. *Int J Rehab Res* 1988; **11**:213–224.

53. Guyatt GH, Jaeschke R, Feeny DH, Patrick DL, Measurements in clinical trials: Choosing the right approach. In: Spilker B (ed.) *Quality of Life and the Pharmacoeconomics in Clinical Trials*. Lippincott-Raven: Philadelphia, 1996; 41–48.

54. Fitzpatrick R, Peto V, Jenkinson C, Greenhall R, Hyman N, Health-related quality of life in Parkinson's disease: a study of outpatient clinic attenders. *Mov Disord* 1997; **12**(6):916–922.

55. Ginanneschi A, Degl'Innocenti F, Maurello MT, Magnolfi S, Marini P, Amaducci L, Evaluation of Parkinson's disease: a new approach to disability. *Neuroepidemiology* 1991; **10**(5–6):282–287.

56. Peto V, Jenkinson C, Fitzpatrick R, PDQ-39: a review of the development, validation and application of a Parkinson's disease quality of life questionnaire and its associated measures. *J Neurol* 1998; **245**(Suppl 1):S10–S14.

57. de Boer AG, Wijker W, Speelman JD, de Haes JC, Quality of life in patients with Parkinson's disease: development of a questionnaire. *J Neurol Neurosurg Psychiat* 1996; **61**(1):70–74.

58. Welsh M, McDermott MP, Holloway RG, Plumb S, Pfeiffer R, Hubble J, Development and testing of the Parkinson's disease quality of life scale. *Mov Disord* 2003; **18**(6):637–645.

59. Hobson P, Holden A, Meara J. Measuring the impact of Parkinson's disease with the Parkinson's Disease Quality of Life Questionnaire. *Age Ageing* 1999; **28**:341–346.

60. The Global Parkinson's Disease Survey (GPDS) Steering Committee, Factors impacting on quality of life in Parkinson's disease: Results from an international survey. *Mov Disord* 2002; **17**(1):60–67.

61. Karlsen KH, Larsen JP, Tandberg E, Maeland JG, Influence of clinical and demographic variables on quality of life in patients with Parkinson's disease. *J Neurol Neurosurg Psychiat* 1999; **66**(4):431–435.

62. Martinez-Martin P, Valldeoriola F, Molinuevo JL, Nobbe FA, Rumia J, Tolosa E, Pallidotomy and quality of life in patients with Parkinson's disease: an early study. *Mov Disord* 2000; **15**:65–70.

63. Dural A, Atay MB, Akbostanci C, Kucukdeveci A, Impairment, disability, and life satisfaction in Parkinson's disease. *Disabil Rehabil* 2003; **25**(7):318–323.

64. Marras C, Lang A, Krahn M, Tomlinson G, Naglie G, Quality of life in early Parkinson's disease: impact of dyskinesias and motor fluctuations. *Mov Disord* 2004; **19**(1):22–28.

65. Schrag A, Hovris A, Morley D, Quinn N, Jahanshahi M, Young- versus older-onset Parkinson's disease: impact of disease and psychosocial consequences. *Mov Disord* 2003; **18**(11):1250–1256.

66. Abudi S, Bar-Tal Y, Ziv L, Fish M, Parkinson's disease symptoms – patients' perceptions. *J Adv Nurs* 1997; **25**:54–59.

67. Brod M, Mendelsohn GA, Roberts B, Patient's experiences of Parkinson's disease. *J Gerontol B Psychol Sci Soc Sci* 1998; **53**:P213–P222.

68. Lee KS, Merriman A, Owen A, Chew B, Tan TC, The medical, social and functional profile of Parkinson's disease patients. *Singapore Med J* 1994; **35**:265–268.
69. Mutch WJ, Strudwick A, Roy SK, Downie AW, Parkinson's disease: disability, review, and management. *Br Med J (Clin Res Ed)* 1986; **293**(6548):675–677.
70. Currie L, Bennett J, Harrison M, Trugman J, Wooten G, The effect of Parkinson's disease on employment. *Neurology* 2002; **58**(Suppl 3):A467–A468.
71. Mudrick NR, Predictors of disability among midlife men and women: differences by severity of impairment. *J Community Health* 1988; **13**:70–84.
72. Henry AD, Baron KB, Mouradian L, Curtin C, Reliability and validity of the self-assessment of occupational functioning. *Am J Occup Ther* 1999; **53**:482–488.
73. Koplas PA, Gans HB, Wisely MP et al, Quality of life and Parkinson's disease. *J Gerontol A Biol Sci Med Sci* 1999; **54**(4):M197–M202.
74. Kempen GI, van Sonderen E, Ormel J, The impact of psychological attributes on changes in disability among low-functioning older persons. *J Gerontol B Psychol Sci Soc Sci* 1999; **54**(1):23–29.
75. Schieman S, Turner HA, Age, disability, and the sense of mastery. *J Health Soc Behav* 1998; **39**(3):169–186.
76. McQuillen AD, Licht MH, Licht BG, Contributions of disease severity and perceptions of primary and secondary control to the prediction of psychosocial adjustment to Parkinson's disease. *Health Psychol* 2003; **22**(5):504–512.
77. Glosser G, Clark C, Freundlich B, Kliner-Krenzel L, Flaherty P, Stern M, A controlled investigation of current and premorbid personality: characteristics of Parkinson's disease patients. *Mov Disord* 1995; **10**(2):201–206.
78. Hubble JP, Venkatesh R, Hassanein RE, Gray C, Koller WC, Personality and depression in Parkinson's disease. *J Nerv Ment Dis* 1993; **181**(11):657–662.
79. Menza MA, The personality associated with Parkinson's disease. *Curr Psychiat Rep* 2000, **2**:421–426.
80. Webster DA, Critical analysis of the disability in Parkinson's disease. *Med Treat* 1968; **5**:257–282.
81. Hoehn MM, Yahr MD, Parkinsonism: onset, progression, and mortality. *Neurology* 1967; **17**(5):427–442.
82. Ilson J, Bressman S, Fahn S, Current concepts in Parkinson's disease. *Hosp Med* 1983; **19**:33.
83. Fitzsimmons B, Bunting LK, Parkinson's disease. Quality of life issues. *Nurs Clin North Am* 1993; **28**(4):807–818.
84. Factor SA, Molho ES, Podskalny GD, Brown D, Parkinson's disease: drug-induced psychiatric states. *Adv Neurol* 1995; **65**:115–138.
85. Pakrasi S, Mukaetova-Ladinska EB, McKeith IG, O'Brien JT, Clinical predictors of response to acetyl cholinesterase inhibitors: experience from routine clinical use in Newcastle. *Int J Geriatr Psychiat* 2003; **18**(10):879–886.
86. Aarsland D, Laake K, Larsen JP, Janvin C, Donepezil for cognitive impairment in Parkinson's disease: a randomised controlled study. *J Neurol Neurosurg Psychiat* 2002; **72**(6):708–712.
87. Leroi I, Brandt J, Reich SG et al, Randomized placebo-controlled trial of donepezil in cognitive impairment in Parkinson's disease. *Int J Geriatr Psychiat* 2004; **19**(1):1–8.
88. Bullock R, Cameron A, Rivastigmine for the treatment of dementia and visual hallucinations associated with Parkinson's disease: a case series. *Curr Med Res Opin* 2002; **18**(5):258–264.
89. Dogali M, Fazzini E, Kolodny E et al, Stereotactic ventral pallidotomy for Parkinson's disease. *Neurology* 1995; **45**(4):753–761.
90. Valldeoriola F, Martinez-Rodriguez J, Tolosa E et al, Four year follow-up study after

unilateral pallidotomy in advanced Parkinson's disease. *J Neurol* 2002; **249**(12):1671–1677.

91. Iacono RP, Shima F, Lonser RR, Kuniyoshi S, Maeda G, Yamada S, The results, indications, and physiology of posteroventral pallidotomy for patients with Parkinson's disease. *Neurosurgery* 1995; **36**(6):1118–1125.

92. Perrine K, Dogali M, Fazzini E et al, Cognitive functioning after pallidotomy for refractory Parkinson's disease. *J Neurol Neurosurg Psychiat* 1998; **65**(2):150–154.

93. Fine J, Duff J, Chen R et al, Long-term follow-up of unilateral pallidotomy in advanced Parkinson's disease. *New Engl J Med* 2000; **342**(23):1708–1714.

94. Lai EC, Jankovic J, Krauss JK, Ondo WG, Grossman RG, Long-term efficacy of posteroventral pallidotomy in the treatment of Parkinson's disease. *Neurology* 2000; **55**(8):1218–1222.

95. Lagrange E, Krack P, Moro E et al, Bilateral subthalamic nucleus stimulation improves health-related quality of life in PD. *Neurology* 2002; **59**(12):1976–1978.

96. Baron MS, Vitek JL, Bakay RA et al, Treatment of advanced Parkinson's disease by unilateral posterior GPi pallidotomy: 4-year results of a pilot study. *Mov Disord* 2000; **15**(2):230–237.

97. Trend P, Kaye J, Gage H, Owen C, Wade D, Short-term effectiveness of intensive multidisciplinary rehabilitation for people with Parkinson's disease and their carers. *Clin Rehabil* 2002; **16**(7):717–725.

98. Wade DT, Gage H, Owen C, Trend P, Grossmith C, Kaye J, Multidisciplinary rehabilitation for people with Parkinson's disease: a randomised controlled study. *J Neurol Neurosurg Psychiat* 2003; **74**(2):158–162.

chapter 14

Coping

Leslie D Frazier and Laura Marsh

Introduction

Once Parkinson's disease (PD) is diagnosed, an individual must begin to cope with the realization that he or she has a chronic, progressive disease that will substantially alter one's life. First, there is the wide range of emotional responses that are common following diagnosis – from anger and denial to despair and sorrow. In addition, studies on the stress of chronic illness find that there is an awareness that life will be different, that goals must be changed, and that managing the illness will become the focus of daily life.[1,2] As a patient with PD begins the adjustment process, the disease pervades the sense of who one is as a person.[3] Some incorporate PD into their identities in positive ways that bode well for adjustment, seeing their symptoms as challenges with which they must find ways to cope, and hoping to make the best of the situation.[4] For example, one person who we saw said that the most important thing for him was to be able to walk in the PD marathon – despite his significant mobility impairments. Others incorporate the illness into their sense of self in negative ways and come to see themselves as victims of the disease; this interferes with their ability to take control and manage the disease in proactive ways. This chapter reviews coping styles in PD and makes some suggestions on positive ways of coping based on research studies as well as clinical experience.

Stress, coping, and adaptation

In order to understand how patients cope with PD, it is necessary to understand the process of coping generally. Whether stress comes from major life events (e.g. the birth of a child, the diagnosis of an illness, a promotion at work, a traffic accident), or daily hassles (e.g., commuter traffic, unpleasant salespeople, bills in the mail), coping is an interactive process between the individual and the environment.[5] According to Lazarus and Folkman,[5] at the moment we become aware of stress, we appraise it to determine if it is threatening or challenging (i.e., primary appraisal) and whether we have the resources to deal with it (i.e., secondary appraisal). An event is stressful when it is perceived as taxing or exceeding one's resources.[5] Adaptation to stressors is affected by coping processes.

There are a number of proposed theories on adaptation to a chronic illness such as PD, but no adaptive process is universal.[6] The phases of adaptation can include periods of shock, anxiety, denial, depression, internalized anger, externalized hostility, acknowledgment, and adjustment. For any given individual, elements may be skipped or reverse, and some individuals stay fixed at one stage (Figure 14.1). A new set of symptoms, such as onset of a depressive episode, or progression of the disease may send a person back to an earlier stage. Importantly, clinicians can facilitate the processes of adaptation, especially the transition from the acknowledgment phase, when patients reconcile the permanency of PD as an aspect of their self-concept, to a final phase of adjustment. The adjusted patient can accept their functional changes and limitations on an emotional level and integrate these changes into their life circumstances. Consequently, the adjusted patient is able to re-establish a positive sense of self-worth, realize new potentials, pursue new goals, and overcome obstacles.

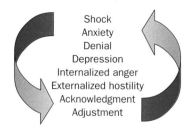

Shock
Anxiety
Denial
Depression
Internalized anger
Externalized hostility
Acknowledgment
Adjustment

Figure 14.1 *Theoretical phases of adaptation to chronic illness.*

Coping is the term used to describe the cognitive and behavioral efforts employed by an individual to manage stressful events,[5] whether they represent specific external circumstances, such as meeting a deadline, or internal experiences, such as the awareness that symptoms of PD accumulate over time.[7] Decades of research on stress have found that a number of personality factors influence adjustment and coping. For example, hardy individuals (those who have a high degree of control over life, a commitment to life, and who see obstacles as challenges and potential avenues for growth) cope better (have better health-related outcomes) than those who are lower in hardiness.[8] Indeed, a great deal of research has focused on the role of perceived control on disease-related stress management. In patients with PD, most studies show that physical aspects of PD and disease severity have a limited role in psychological adaptation to PD and do not correspond directly to subjective well-being.[9,10] However, the strong belief that one is able to control one's adaptation to PD appears to be associated with adaptive coping.[11]

The resources one brings to bear on a situation significantly impact the ability to respond to stressors. Coping resources can range from internal abilities such as creativity and intellect, to external resources such as finances and friends. In particular, social support (both instrumental and emotional) is essential for coping with major stressors such as living with a chronic condition. In general, coping efforts are either directed at changing or ameliorating the stressor (i.e., action-oriented, problem-focused coping), or at managing the emotional impact of the stress (i.e., emotional regulation, emotional or behavioral disengagement, cognitive reframing). More recently, studies have found a beneficial influence of religion and spirituality in relation to coping with illness.[12]

Most people, regardless of the stressor, use a combination of coping strategies and are flexible enough to change or modify strategies that are not working. For coping to be successful, two conditions must be met. First, the coping strategy must be appropriate for the situation. Second, coping strategies must be flexible in order to adjust to the dynamic nature of chronic illness. The importance of developing coping strategies that are tailored to the specific situation cannot be emphasized enough. That is, if one has some degree of control over a situation, then trying to change it may help. However, if the source of stress is something that cannot be controlled, a focus on dealing with the emotional response to the stress may be more adaptive than trying to change the situation. In PD, the belief that one can control the disease itself can be maladaptive if unsuccessful efforts lead to disappointment and anguish.

Research on coping with chronic illness in general,[13] and PD in particular,[4,14] shows that patients who cope best use problem-focused coping for management of symptoms and emotional-focused coping for living with the stress of being a patient with PD. In fact, our research shows that people with PD are extremely creative in managing the wide array of symptoms that may interfere with their functioning, and that those who cope best find new solutions to each change in symptoms. For example, one woman, a former dance instructor, found that as her medications wore off and her walking became difficult she could waltz across the room and get to where she was going easily and gracefully! This person also reported that she turned to gardening and listening to music when she felt discouraged by her illness. Her greatest fear, she said, was that she would become bitter because of her illness. Thus, she was finding action-oriented, problem-focused coping strategies for managing the symptoms and emotional outlets for managing the larger stress of being chronically ill.

Coping with Parkinson's disease

Influence of disease-related stressors on coping strategies

The above anecdote illustrates the general findings from research examining coping in PD.[15] How an individual copes with the specific stressful symptoms of the disease in them has a significant effect on overall function and well-being. Some patterns are more useful and promote better quality of life and adjustment over time.

Based on the idea that different symptoms of PD present different degrees of stress, it seems that the most effective coping occurs when patients are able to tailor coping strategies to the specific types of stressors. In our study,[14] participants were 145 PD patients ranging in age from 48 to 91 (mean age 73). The symptoms of PD were broken down into three groups of disease-related stressors: physical stressors (i.e., bathing/toileting, posture, walking, rigidity, tremor, falling, difficulty with sexual activity, difficulty getting up from a chair, drooling, etc.); cognitive stressors (i.e., forgetfulness, slowed thinking, poor concentration, lack of mental energy, confusion, etc.); and psychosocial stressors (i.e., isolation, dependency on others, feeling of being a burden, feeling misunderstood, depression, loss of self-respect, loss of control, pressure of others' expectations, etc.). For each type of stressor, each participant was asked to pick the "most stressful symptom you are currently coping with." These individuals with PD had been ill for an average of 8 years and most reported that their symptoms (as a whole) were mildly to moderately severe and that their medications (as a whole) were moderately to mostly effective at managing the symptoms. Nonetheless, their symptoms were quite stressful. Table 14.1 shows the percentage of PD patients reporting various types of stressors as their "most stressful symptom."

In the same study,[14] after selecting the "Most stressful symptom" in each category, patients were administered a modified version of the Cope Scale[16] to determine what coping techniques were used to deal with that specific stressor. The coping behaviors were grouped into three distinct coping dimensions (Table 14.2). In this sample, individuals used active coping or emotional regulation most often. There was also an interaction among coping and stressors; that is, patients with PD were indeed using different coping strategies for different types of stressors.

Perhaps more importantly, this study also examined the influence of coping on quality of life. Beyond the influence of PD severity, coping strategies exerted a selective effect on mental and physical health outcomes. Severe symptoms (regardless of type) coupled with the use of distancing

Table 14.1 Types of stressors considered stressful for PD patients[14]

Type of stressor	"Most stressful symptom" (% reporting)
Physical	
Rigidity	17
Tremor	14
Getting up from a chair	11
Falling	11
Cognitive	
Lack of mental energy	26
Difficulty sleeping	14
Forgetfulness	13
Slowed thinking	11
Psychosocial	
Being dependent on others	21
Feeling of being a burden to others	17
Depression	15
Loss of control	14
Feeling misunderstood by others	10

Table 14.2 Types of coping and related behaviors used by patients with PD[14]

Coping dimension	Coping behaviors
Active coping	I take additional action to try to get rid of the problem
	I put aside other activities to concentrate on the problem
	I force myself to wait for the right time to do something about the problem
	I consult others who have had similar problems about what they did
Emotional regulation	I talk to someone about how I feel
	I look for something good in what is happening
	I learn to accept and live with it
	I get upset and let my emotions out
Distancing	I seek God's help
	I refuse to believe it has happened
	I turn to other activities to take my mind off things
	I admit to myself that I can't deal with it, and quit trying

significantly increased stress and lessened quality of life. However, less use of distancing, especially for cognitive stressors, was associated with higher quality of life scores.

In terms of clinical applications of the above data, a key point is that patients with PD report an array of stressful problems with physical and cognitive symptoms as well as psychosocial functioning. More successful coping is evident in those who tailor their coping strategies to specific stressors. Furthermore, there is a greater reliance on emotional regulation across stressors. Because of these results, we believe that successful interventions for PD patients should teach stress appraisal and techniques to match or tailor coping efforts to specific stressful symptoms.

Coping with PD over time

For coping to be successful at relieving distress and promoting quality of life, patients must adapt their strategies to the changing course of their illness. As the illness progresses, new symptoms emerge, old symptoms worsen, functional abilities change, and anxiety and depression fluctuate in response to these changes. Thus, strategies for managing these stressors must change as well.

In order to understand what promotes adaptation to downturns in health within the context of PD, we studied a group of people with PD over a 2-year period.[17] We found that the severity of PD symptoms worsened significantly over time, as did the stress of being ill and quality of life, specifically in the areas of general self-reported health, physical functioning and social functioning. While the symptoms reported as "Most stressful" at baseline did not change, changes in the disease influenced changes in coping. Specifically, when there was greater change in the severity of the illness, patients were more likely to turn to less effective coping strategies, such as distancing. However, positive changes in quality of life over time were related to greater use of effective coping strategies, such as emotional regulation and less distancing.

In this sample of patients, patterns of coping with PD over time generally remained stable, although this predicted poorer quality of life. While the role of cognitive impairments or co-morbid psychiatric disturbances was not examined, patients were more likely to maintain the same coping patterns if they were older, had more severe illness, and experienced greater distress. Yet, there were some patients in the sample with evidence for less stable and more flexible coping patterns. These patients changed their coping approaches, and this pattern was significantly related to optimal outcomes (i.e., better mental and physical health). Thus, among well-adjusted PD patients, being flexible enough to change coping strategies is related to less stress and better quality of life.

The sense of self in coping with PD

Being diagnosed with a chronic illness influences every aspect of a person's life and most deeply affects one's sense of who they are as a person. The process of adaptation that occurs as one begins to manage the illness on a day-to-day basis and cope with the impact it has on one's life, is a process of reorganizing our sense of self. Our work has also examined the extent to which illness becomes embodied in patients' self-representations.[4,17] More specifically, the role of illness in shaping who we are has been of interest as a mechanism for distinguishing among those PD patients who see their illness as a challenge and those who see themselves as victims of their illness. In general, what we have found is that having PD affects all aspects of one's sense of self, and that incorporating the illness into one's sense of self in positive ways promotes better adjustment.

Future directions of research on coping

Psychological research is useful for examining general ways of coping, but it is not able to detail the nuances and unique efforts of individuals in their quest to manage their illness. Also, social support is a whole different arena in which coping occurs and needs to be examined. The studies reported above examine individuals' coping efforts within the context of their illness. However, most of these individuals had spouses, children, caregivers, healthcare professionals, support groups, religious organizations, and other groups of people who help them in their quest to cope with their disease. More research must be done to examine the different types of social support provided to PD patients (i.e., instrumental, emotional, financial, disease-related) in order to determine what social supports are most helpful and how social supports can best facilitate patients' adjustment to illness.[18] Third, coping with PD happens within the context of family and the caregiver is an important influence on the successful adaptation of the patient. Research has also examined coping in caregivers and found that certain patterns lead to better mental and physical well-being in caregivers as well.[19,20] Caregiver stress is discussed in detail in Chapter 19.

Impact of psychiatric disturbances in Parkinson's disease on coping

While coping styles have been examined as predictors of depressive symptoms, the impact of discrete psychiatric disorders or cognitive deficits on coping with PD has not been studied explicitly. In our experience, patients often suggest that their mood disorders are the result of maladaptive coping skills, but the opposite is more likely true. While ineffective coping and poor adjustment can occur in the absence of mood disorders, mood and anxiety disorders undermine some of the most important coping strategies. For example, maintaining a positive attitude is barely an option for an individual with a major depressive disorder and successful coping and adaptation are virtually impossible in the face of an untreated mood disorder. Problem-solving strategies can be difficult to conceive for individuals who feel hopeless or are overwhelmed by anxiety. Memory and executive dysfunction early in the course also affect problem-solving, as discussed in Chapter 5. As PD progresses, the cognitive impairments can affect more domains of functioning and the burden of coping shifts more to the caregiver, whose coping strategies become more relevant and a focus of patient management.[21]

A minority of studies on coping in PD report on the role of depressive symptoms. One study, a postal survey of 136 patients with PD, showed that a positive affect and outlook were related to high self-esteem, instrumental supports (in order to accomplish daily tasks) and positive coping styles (e.g., problem solving and self-reassuring behaviors).[10] By contrast, low self-esteem and negative coping styles such as pessimism, self-criticism, procrastination over practical matters, and eating to take ones mind off things (such as depression) were most predictive of depression. Another study described the patterns or clusters of adaptation among 44 patients with PD.[9] Well-adjusted patients tended to be optimistic and dismiss negative thoughts from their mind. A second group, classified as the "Depressed and worried," constantly struggled with accepting the diagnosis, and this was associated with anxiety, frustration, and depression. Even when there were only mild symptoms, affected patients resented their losses, felt stigmatized, and experienced intrusive anxiety about emotional symptoms. It is possible that at least some of the individuals in the second group had a pervasive mood disorder that limited their successful adaptation and coping. Furthermore, an important component of ongoing psychiatric treatment and relapse prevention should be the facilitation of successful adaptation and coping.

Ways that clinicians can facilitate coping with Parkinson's disease

Coping, by definition, represents the efforts of the individual and it is an integral aspect of disease management. Since most hours in a day are spent apart from medical contact, clinicians must help patients become aware of their role in disease self-management so that they can cope optimally. Clinicians can facilitate self-management by making sure that psychiatric disturbances are identified and treated, distinguishing between psychopathological symptoms and understandable emotional changes, helping patients also appreciate those differences, and analyzing what coping strategies are used. Clinicians should educate patients and their families about PD, including its varied manifestations, the expected outcomes and potential side-effects of different treatments, and interactions between its motor, cognitive, and psychiatric aspects, as described throughout this book. Successful psychoeducational interventions for PD patients should teach stress appraisal and techniques to "match" coping efforts to specific stressful symptoms. Clinicians should also encourage patients to educate themselves independently. To that end, they should be informed about lay PD organizations that are listed in Appendix B and provide invaluable educational resources. On a local level, PD support groups provide a combination of educational programs and social support, both of which are helpful. Advocacy organizations provide similar benefits but strive to increase awareness about PD to the general public and, in particular, government organizations that influence funding for research into and treatment of PD. As described in Chapter 19, involvement in this collective effort has a powerful and favorable impact on how some individuals adjust to PD.

In some patients (or family members), psychotherapy may be needed to help with the process of adaptation. Depending on the circumstances, insight-oriented, supportive and resilience-building, problem-solving oriented, and/or cognitive-behavioral therapies can be appropriate.[22] Different approaches may be needed from day to day. For other patients, it may be necessary to treat a mood disorder before successful adaptation and coping with self-management is possible. Cognitive and physical impairments may also limit problem-solving abilities; this should be acknowledged and incorporated into the treatment plan. However, even patients with advanced PD and dementia benefit from coping strategies that promote emotional self-regulation. One woman with advanced PD and significant cognitive deficits was wheelchair-bound and completely dependent on others for her physical needs. Yet, she could describe her longstanding and ongoing role in the mutual love within her family, and that gave her a positive sense of self-worth.

Practical aspects of coping with Parkinson's disease

Living with PD involves chronic and recurrent physical, emotional, and social stressors on a daily basis and a tendency for increased stress to aggravate motor symptoms.[23] Coping strategies that are most helpful to patients with PD are those that are directed appropriately at either problem-solving or emotional regulation. Table 14.3 shows the top-ten coping strategies used by patients with young-onset PD. It is important to regard obstacles as challenges to be overcome, rather than hopeless barriers. This positive approach allows for a sense of pride, control, hopefulness, and

Table 14.3 Top 10 coping strategies used by patients with young onset Parkinson's disease ($n = 29$) (Gerstenhaber M and Marsh L, unpublished data)

1. Educating self
2. Exercise
3. Being objective about one's various circumstances
4. Taking one step at a time
5. Being aware of one's strengths
6. Advocating for one's self
7. Maintaining a sense of humor
8. Being an active participant
9. Engaging family support
10. Educating others

creativity that, in turn, helps one to cope more effectively. It is often helpful to make a list of the difficulties that are associated with the illness and find practical solutions for each of these. Many times, other individuals with PD will discover creative solutions, so discussing particular problems with others who have the illness can be enlightening. PD support groups are particularly useful for this purpose. Sharing solutions and working together to solve practical problems enhances a collective, as well as an individual, sense of control. For example, some support groups have started "equipment closets" of canes, walkers, and other assistive devices that can be shared as needed by other individuals in the group. In addition, there are many patient-oriented websites (see Appendix B) that provide practical advice. We have also found that the variety of self-help books available may have useful hints and we encourage patients to browse through these books.

Flexibility in coping strategies is extremely important. If one has a strategy that helped in the past but no longer works, try altering the approach. A typical example of this is constipation. An approach that previously worked may not work as well as the illness progresses. There are a variety of strategies available – try the next one. Remember that there are a variety of problems in PD that are physical, cognitive and psychological and may require different approaches. Unwittingly, it is possible to use strategies that aggravate distress, as sometimes happens in response to "off-period" akinetic periods.[24] Try to identify these problems clearly and set reasonable goals.

The importance of social supports in coping with PD cannot be overstated.[23] Do not try to cope alone – work to maintain relationships with your family and friends. As the illness progresses, it can become more difficult to do this, and easier to find reasons to avoid people. In the absence of an untreated psychiatric disturbance, the urge to isolate oneself must be fought. Find practical solutions to the barriers. The sense of community that evolves from participation in PD support groups, community service, volunteer activities, and time with friends is a superb way to cope with the illness. We find that individuals who become involved in advocating for the illness, either through political activity or by volunteering for research projects, find great comfort in their contributions. Be creative in looking for outlets.

Exercise is a wonderful way to cope with many of the physical and psychological problems of this illness. The topic is more fully discussed elsewhere in the book, but mild, regular exercise is crucial. Religion is very helpful to many people trying to cope with this illness. While not everyone comes easily to religion, examine your own life to see if this source of effort may have a role.

Lastly, maintaining hope is crucial for someone coping with PD. A cure for this illness may not be around the next corner, but there have been significant and promising recent advances in PD research. Active involvement in advocacy groups, research, support groups, your religious community, and life in general is the best approach to maintaining hope and coping with this illness.

Acknowledgment

Support for Dr Marsh provided by NIH P50-NS-58366 and NIH RO1-MH069666.

References

1. Dunkel-Schetter C, Feinstein LG, Taylor SE, Falke RL, Patterns of coping with cancer. *Health Psychol* 1992; **11**(2):79–87.
2. Shifren K, Hooker K, Wood P, Nesselroade JR, Structure and variation of mood in individuals with Parkinson's disease: a dynamic factor analysis. *Psychol Aging* 1997; **12**(2):328–339.
3. Frazier LD, Perceptions of control over health: implications for sense of self in healthy and ill older adults. In: Shohov SP (ed.) *Advances in Psychological Research.* Nova Scientific Publishing: New York, 2002; 145–163.

4. Frazier LD, Cotrell V, Hooker K, Possible selves and illness: a comparison of individuals with Parkinson's disease, early stage Alzheimer's disease, and healthy older adults. *Int J Behav Dev* 2003; **27**(1):1–11.

5. Lazarus RS, Folkman S, *Stress, Appraisal, and Coping.* Springer Publishing Co.: New York, 1984.

6. Linveh H, *Psychosocial Adaptation to Chronic Illness and Disability.* Aspen Publishers: Gaithersburg, MD, 1997.

7. Haveman J, *A Life Shaken: My Encounter with Parkinson's Disease.* Johns Hopkins University Press: Baltimore, MD, 2002.

8. Kobasa SC, Stressful life events, personality, and health: an inquiry into hardiness. *J Pers Soc Psychol* 1979; **37**(1):1–11.

9. Dakof GA, Mendelsohn GA, Parkinson's disease: the psychological aspects of a chronic illness. *Psychol Bull* 1986; **99**(3):375–387.

10. MacCarthy B, Brown R, Psychosocial factors in Parkinson's disease. *Br J Clin Psychol* 1989; **28**(Pt 1):41–52.

11. McQuillen AD, Licht MH, Licht BG, Contributions of disease severity and perceptions of primary and secondary control to the prediction of psychosocial adjustment to Parkinson's disease. *Health Psychol* 2003; **22**(5):504–512.

12. Koenig HG, Cohen HJ, *The Link between Religion and Health: Psychoneuroimmunology and the Faith Factor.* Oxford University Press: New York, 2002.

13. Aldwin CM, Brustrom J, Theories of coping with chronic stress: illustrations from the health psychology and aging literatures. In: Gottlieb BH (ed.) *Coping with Chronic Stress.* Plenum Press: New York, 1997; 75–103.

14. Frazier LD, Coping with disease-related stressors in Parkinson's disease. *Gerontologist* 2000; **40**(1):53–63.

15. Brod M, Mendelsohn GA, Roberts B, Patients' experiences of Parkinson's disease. *J Gerontol B Psychol Sci Soc Sci* 1998; **53**(4):213–222.

16. Carver CS, Scheier MF, Weintraub JK, Assessing coping strategies: a theoretically based approach. *J Pers Soc Psychol* 1989; **56**(2):267–283.

17. Frazier LD, Stability and change in patterns of coping with Parkinson's disease. *Int J Aging Hum Dev* 2002; **55**(3):207–231.

18. Monahan DJ, Hooker K, Caregiving and social support in two illness groups. *Soc Work* 1997; **42**(3):278–287.

19. Hooker K, Manoogian-O'Dell M, Monahan DJ, Frazier LD, Shifren K, Does type of disease matter? Gender differences among Alzheimer's and Parkinson's disease spouse caregivers. *Gerontologist* 2000; **40**(5):568–573.

20. Hooker K, Monahan DJ, Bowman SR, Frazier LD, Shifren K, Personality counts for a lot: predictors of mental and physical health of spouse caregivers in two disease groups. *J Gerontol B Psychol Sci Soc Sci* 1998; **53**(2):73–85.

21. Thommessen B, Aarsland D, Braekhus A, Oksengaard AR, Engedal K, Laake K, The psychosocial burden on spouses of the elderly with stroke, dementia and Parkinson's disease. *Int J Geriatr Psychiat* 2002; **17**(1):78–84.

22. Lolak S, Bedside psychotherapy. *Curr Psychiat* 2004; **3**(8):11–20.

23. Backer JH, Stressors, social support, coping, and health dysfunction in individuals with Parkinson's disease. *J Gerontol Nurs* 2000; **26**(11):6–16.

24. Matson N, Made of stone: a view of Parkinson "off" periods. *Psychol Psychother* 2002; **75**(Pt 1):93–99.

chapter 15

Personality issues

Matthew Menza

Introduction

In the first case of Parkinson's disease ever described, James Parkinson commented in 1817 that this was a patient who, "... had industriously followed the business of a gardener, leading a life of remarkable temperance and sobriety."[1] This thought was emphasized in 1913 by Carl Camp, a well known neurologist, writing in *Modern Treatment of Nervous and Mental Diseases* who noted, "It would seem that paralysis agitans affected mostly those persons whose lives had been devoted to hard work. ... The people who take their work to bed with them and who never come under the inhibiting influences of tobacco or alcohol are the kind that are most frequently affected. In this respect, the disease may be almost regarded as a badge of respectable endeavor."[2]

Since that time, many reports have examined the association between personality or behavioral traits and Parkinson's disease (PD). While the concept remains controversial, most of these reports suggest that patients who develop PD generally show a tendency towards a premorbid personality profile of industriousness, inflexibility, punctuality, cautiousness and lack of novelty seeking, and that these traits persist after the onset of the motor illness. Such a proposition, necessarily based on retrospective data and elusive concepts of personality, is, of course, hard to prove. In this chapter, I will review the efforts that have been made to identify personality traits associated with PD, and briefly discuss the importance of these issues for clinical care.

Early studies of personality in Parkinson's disease

Most of the early studies of personality in PD are described in psychoanalytic terms that sound dated to the modern ear. They often suggest that the illness itself is somehow caused by intra-psychic conflicts. While these concepts do not sit well with contemporary psychiatric and neurological theory, the authors of these reports do identify traits that we can recognize today. For example, in 1948, Booth,[3] using the Rorschach and clinical interviews, as well as handwriting from the premorbid period, evaluated 66 PD patients. He found that the personality is characterized by an urge toward action, industriousness, striving for independence, authority and success within a rigid, usually moralistic, behavior pattern. He describes a religious attitude towards success and a loyalty to the mores of their childhood milieu. Prichard et al.[4] evaluated 100 PD patients from private practice and a hospital clinic. They describe the majority of the patients as either submissive, dependent, obsessive and perfectionist, or as worried over their health. In 1960, Mitscherllich,[5] after studying 40 PD patients, notes that the highest values are cleanliness, order, decency and punctuality and that they are usually industrious, very exact and extraordinarily ambitious. Prick, in 1966,[6] comments that, as a group, they were courteous, polite, honest, trustworthy, altruistic, conscientious, punctual. There are many of these early studies that, with fair unanimity, describe these PD patients in similar terms.

Studies in Parkinson's disease patients and control subjects

In the late 1960s, investigators began to apply more sophisticated research methodology to the question of personality in PD. They began to use standardized psychological tests in studying groups of patients with PD and comparing them to other control groups. Hubble et al.[7] in 1993, compared the remote and current personality features in 35 patients with PD and 35 controls. In the premorbid state, patients with PD were viewed as withdrawn and dependent. After disease onset, they were less talkative, less flexible and more generous, even-tempered and cautious than controls. Over the past 30 years there have been many of these studies using assessment instruments such as the California Psychological Inventory,[8] the MMPI,[9] and the NEO-Personality Inventory.[10]

These studies have given somewhat more credibility to the concept of a personality profile common to patients with PD because they attempt to control for various confounds, such as age, gender, and medical illness. These studies reinforced the general description found in the earlier literature; patients with PD, both premorbidly and after the onset of the illness, appear to be more cautious, deferential to authority, driven, and introverted than comparable controls.

Twin studies

In an interesting study, twin pairs discordant for PD were used to look for early differences in personality and behavior. In 1984, Ward et al.[11] interviewed 20 identical twin pairs, discordant for PD, and their relatives and asked a series of questions about their behavior at ages 8 and 16, as well as 10 years before the onset of PD and after the illness began. They report that the twin with PD, at age 8, was less usually the leader and was more self-controlled than the non-affected twin. At age 16 the affected twin was more nervous and more self-controlled. Ten years before the onset of the illness, the affected twin was less usually the leader, was more nervous, less aggressive, more quiet and less confident and lighthearted. This study has obvious methodological limitations but nonetheless suggests that there were differences that greatly predate the motor illness.

Studies of novelty seeking in Parkinson's disease

PD is associated with decreases of at least 80% in nigrostriatal dopamine, and decreases of up to 75% in the dopaminergic neurons that serve the limbic and frontal areas of the brain (A10 neurons).[12,13] Patients with PD are also known to have decreases in dopaminergic function which predate the onset of clinical symptoms.[14] Thus, if there are behavioral traits associated with these dopaminergic systems, PD patients could be expected to show alterations in these behaviors that predate the onset of their motor disease.

The mesolimbic dopaminergic system is generally thought to be the key substrate of pleasure and reward in animals and humans.[15,16] The behavioral traits of novelty seeking and sensation seeking are also thought to be mediated by this dopaminergic system.[17] Novelty seeking has been described as, "a heritable tendency toward intense exhilaration or excitement in response to novel stimuli or cues for potential rewards . . ." Individuals who are high in novelty seeking are described as, "impulsive, fickle, excitable, quick-tempered, extravagant, and disorderly." In contrast, individuals who are lower than average on novelty seeking are described as, "reflective, rigid, loyal, stoic, slow-tempered, frugal, orderly and persistent."[18]

It is easy to see that there is a considerable overlap between these descriptions of novelty seeking, a trait dependent on central dopamine activity, and descriptions of the personality traits that accompany PD. We have suggested that PD patients, because of damage to the mesolimbic dopaminergic system, have an attenuated dopaminergic response to novel stimuli and, therefore, experience these stimuli as less pleasurable. This leads to a less novelty seeking style, i.e., more rigidity, orderliness, etc.[19] However, as discussed in Chapter 12, behavioral disturbances that defy these qualities can occur in patients on dopamine replacement therapy.

Our group has used an instrument, the Tridimensional Personality Questionnaire (TPQ),[18] which measures novelty seeking, in a series of controlled studies of personality in PD. Patients with PD have consistently been shown, when compared to medical controls, to be less novelty seeking before and after the illness began.[20-22] While there continues to be debate over this issue, the connection between dopaminergically mediated pleasure and reward systems in the brain and a personality profile in PD remains intriguing.

Epidemiological finding suggestive of a PD personality

As was seen earlier, Camp[2] suggested in 1913 that PD patients had low premorbid rates of smoking and alcoholism. A host of large epidemiological studies[23-28] has repeatedly demonstrated that PD patients have approximately half the lifetime risk for having smoked as do controls. There are also data indicating that patients who do not drink coffee have an increased risk for PD. The best of these studies followed 8004 Japanese-American men for 30 years and found that non coffee drinkers were more than five times more likely to develop PD than heavy coffee drinkers.[29] While more controversial, most studies have suggested that there is also a decreased lifetime risk for having been a drinker in people who go on to develop PD.[30]

The unifying principle linking the lower rates of use of these substances premorbidly in PD patients again may involve mesolimbic dopaminergic damage. Cigarettes, alcohol, and caffeine (at high doses) are all drugs whose rewarding effects are dopaminergically mediated in the mesolimbic system.[31] Thus, for patients with damage to this dopaminergic system these substances would be expected to be less rewarding. Personality traits such as novelty seeking and sensation seeking are also associated with the use of substances such as cigarettes,[32] presumably through a common mechanism of dopaminergically mediated reward.

Recalling that dopaminergic damage is known to predate the onset of the motor illness, we have explored the relationship between smoking and novelty seeking in PD patients. In 1993 we studied 104 non-demented, idiopathic PD patients and 41 matched medical controls. PD patients were less likely to have been smokers (odds ratio = 0.450) and had significantly less pack-years and years of smoking. Both controls and PD patients who had smoked had higher novelty seeking scores and novelty seeking was significantly correlated with both pack-years and years of smoking in both the controls and in the PD patients.[33]

Other epidemiological evidence that suggests some similar personality profile in PD patients is considerably more conjectural. For instance, stability in both jobs and marriages has been anecdotally suggested but not studied.[3,34]

Impact of these traits on clinical care
There may be important clinical ramifications to the idea that there are a group of personality traits that are common to individuals with PD. The stability that is evident in these patients often leaves them with intact families who are supportive and help to provide an environment that allows for a positive approach to the illness. The careful, detail-oriented personality tends to facilitate adherence to admittedly complex medical regimens, often entailing taking medication six, seven, or more times per day. These individuals often come to the office with detailed lists of their medications and their questions about treatment, which enhances communications with their physicians. Because they often are careful, dedicated patients, we have found that they are very willing to participate in research studies. Their dedication to the greater good is remarkable.

On the other hand, individuals with a tendency towards perfectionism and detail often have great difficulty tolerating the uncertainty of the illness, with motor fluctuations, off periods, and uncertain course. As they generally have functioned throughout their lives by controlling details, they find the lack of control anxiety-provoking. Development of cognitive symptoms, especially the executive function difficulties described in Chapter 5, can hinder the ability to attend to details as closely as usual, causing considerable distress and confusion.

There is, of course, considerable variation from individual to individual. Nonetheless, these patients will generally do best with detailed explanations and thorough answers to their questions. Since they are often hopeful individuals, we find that discussion of the promise of research leading to new treatments is helpful. To engender a sense of control and to allow careful titration of their medication regime, we often give them leeway to adjust their medications, within a range of options. One should allow their strengths to be used in a positive way.

Conclusions

So, are there personality traits or behaviors associated with PD and its premorbid state? The weight of the evidence suggests that there are. Admittedly based on retrospective data and masked by multiple methodical approaches, there do appear to be a group of descriptors including industriousness, punctuality, orderliness, inflexibility, cautiousness, and lack of novelty seeking that are repeatedly used to describe patients with PD. The data suggesting this conclusion come from case-based anecdote studies with standardized personality inventories, studies with control subjects, twin studies, and epidemiological studies suggesting premorbid decreases in smoking, alcohol drinking, and coffee intake.

It is actually surprising that, despite differences in methodology, the use of many different ways of measuring the traits, diffuse concepts of personality and the retrospective nature of the data, the great majority of studies show such similarity in their results. While there does appear to be an association between personality traits and PD, it is important to remember that these differences are not large and that there is considerable variability.

Why is there an association between these behavioral traits and PD? Here we can be much less certain in our conclusions. There is a reasonable case to be made that these traits are the result of the dopaminergic damage that predates the onset of the motor illness, a kind of non-motor manifestation of early damage to the dopaminergic system. The data connecting novelty seeking to mesolimbic dopaminergic damage is compelling, as is the link between this system and the use of cigarettes, alcohol, and caffeine. But the ultimate hypothesis that the underlying dopaminergic damage results in both lower substance abuse rates and the behavioral traits described in PD remains hypothetical.

There are probably important clinical consequences of these findings. The stability that is evident in these patients generally leaves them with intact families who are supportive and help to provide an environment allowing for a positive approach to the illness. The careful, detail-oriented traits allow them to be very adherent to complex medical regimens. On the other hand, they have great difficulty tolerating the uncertainty of the illness, with motor fluctuations, off periods and uncertain course. One needs to take advantage of the positive personality traits in individualizing their treatment.

Acknowledgment

This work was supported by R01NS43144–01A1 from NINDS.

References

1. Parkinson J. *An Essay on the Shaking Palsy*. Sherwood, Neely, and Jones: London, 1817.
2. Camp CD, Paralysis agitans, multiple sclerosis and their treatment. In: White WA, Jelliffe SE, Kimpton H (eds) *Modern Treatment of Nervous and Mental Disease*, Vol 2. Lea and Febiger: Philadelphia, 1913; 651–667.
3. Booth G, Psychodynamics in Parkinsonism. *Psychosom Med* 1948; **10**:1–14.5.
4. Prichard JS, Schwab RS, Tillann WA, The effects of stress and the results of medication in different personalities with Parkinson's disease. *Psychosom Med* 1951; **13**:106–111.
5. Mitscherllich M, The psychic state of patients suffering from Parkinsonism. *Adv Psychosom Med* 1960; **1**:317–324.
6. Prick JJG, Genuine parkinsonism. A psychosomatic, anthropological-psychiatric approach. *Abs World Congress of Psychiatry Madrid*, 1966. Sandorama Special Number IV, 1966.
7. Hubble JP, Benkatesch R, Hassanein RES et al, Personality and depression in Parkinson's disease. *J Nerv Ment Dis* 1993; **181**:657–662.
8. Eatough VM, Kempster PA, Stern GM, Lees JA, Premorbid personality and idiopathic Parkinson's disease. In: *Advances in Neurology*, Vol 53: *Parkinson's Disease: Anatomy, Pathology, and Therapy*. Raven Press: New York, 1990; 335–337.
9. Jimenez-Jimenez FJ, Santos J, Zancada F et al, Premorbid personality of patients with Parkinson's disease. *Acta Neurol (Napoli)* 1992; **14**(3):208–214.
10. Glosser G, Clark C, Freundlich B et al, A controlled investigation of current and premorbid personality: Characteristics of Parkinson's disease patients. *Mov Dis* 1995; **10**(2):201–206.
11. Ward CD, Duvoisin RC, Ince SE, Nutt JD et al, Parkinson's disease in twins. In: Hassler RG and Christ F (eds) *Advances in Neurology*, Vol 40. Raven Press: New York, 1984; 341–344.
12. Hornykiewicz O, Kish SJ, Biochemical pathophysiology of Parkinson's disease. *Adv Neurol* 1986; **45**:19–34.

13. Agid Y, Cervera P, Hirsch E et al, Biochemistry of Parkinson's disease 28 years later: A critical review. *Mov Disord* 1989; **4**(Suppl 1):S126–S144.
14. Bernheimer H, Birkmayer W, Hornykiewicz O et al, Brain dopamine and the syndromes of Parkinson and Huntington: clinical morphological and biochemical correlations. *J Neurol Sci* 1973; **20**:415–455.
15. Liebman JM, Cooper SJ (eds) *The Neuropharmacological Basis of Reward*. Clarendon Press: Oxford, 1989.
16. Iversen SD, Brain dopamine systems and behavior. In: Iversen LL, Iversen SD, Snyder SH (eds) *Handbook of Psychopharmacology*, Vol 8. Plenum Publishing Corp: New York, 1977; 333–374.
17. Bardo MT, Donohew RL, Harrington NG, Psychobiology of novelty seeking and drug seeking behavior. *Behav Brain Res* 1996; **77**:23–43.
18. Cloninger RC, A systematic method for clinical description and classification of personality variants. *Arch Gen Psychiat* 1987; **44**:573–588.
19. Menza MA, Forman NE, Goldstein HS, Golbe LI, Parkinson's disease, personality and dopamine. *J Neuropsychiat Clin Neurosci* 1990; **2**(3):282–287.
20. Menza MA, Forman NE, Goldstein HS, Golbe LI, Parkinson's disease, personality and dopamine. *J Neuropsychiat Clin Neurosci* 1990; **2**(3):282–287.
21. Menza MA, Golbe LI, Cody, RA, Forman NE, Dopamine-related personality traits in Parkinson's disease. *Neurology* 1993; **43**:505–508.
22. Menza MA, Mark M, Burn D, Brooks D, Psychiatric correlates of 18F-dopa striatal uptake: Positron emission tomography results in Parkinson's disease. *J Neuropsychiat Clin Neurosci* 1995; **7**:176–179.
23. Kahn HA, The Dorn study of smoking and mortality among U.S. veterans: Report on eight and one-half years of observation. In: *Epidemiologic Approaches to the Study of Cancer and Other Chronic Disease*. National Cancer Institute Monograph No. 19, Washington, DC: GPO, 1966; 1–125.
24. Hammond CA, Smoking in relation to the death rates of one million men and women. In: *Epidemiologic Approaches to the Study of Cancer and Other Chronic Disease*. National Cancer Institute Monograph No. 19, Washington, DC: GPO, 1966; 127–204.
25. Kessler II, Diamond EL, Epidemiologic studies of Parkinson's disease: I. Smoking and Parkinson's disease: A survey and explanatory hypothesis. *Am J Epidemiol* 1971; **94**:16–25.
26. Marttila RJ, Rinne UK, Smoking and Parkinson's disease. *Acta Neurol Scand* 1980; **62**:322–325.
27. Baumann RJ, Jameson HD, McKean HE et al, Cigarette smoking and Parkinson's disease: I. A comparison of cases with matched neighbors. *Neurology* 1980; **30**:839–843.
28. Gorell JM, Rybicki BA, Johnson CC, Peterson EL, Smoking and Parkinson's disease: a dose-response relationship. *Neurology* 1999; **52**(1):115–119.
29. Ross WG, Abbott RD, Petrovitch H et al, Association of coffee and caffeine intake with the risk of Parkinson disease. *JAMA* 2000; **283**:2674–2679.
30. Jimenez-Jimenez FJ, Mateo D, Ginenez-Rolday S, Premorbid smoking, alcohol consumption, and coffee drinking habits in Parkinson's disease. A case-control study. *Mov Disord* 1992; **4**(4):339–344.
31. Wise RA, Neurobiology of addiction. *Curr Opin Neurobiol* 1996; **6**(2):243–251.
32. Zuckerman M, Ball S, Black J, Influences of sensation seeking, gender, risk appraisal and situational motivation on smoking. *Addict Behav* 1990; **15**:209–220.
33. Menza MA, Forman NE, Sage JI, Parkinson's disease and smoking: the relationship to personality. *Neuropsychiat Neuropsychol Behav Neurol* 1993; **6**:214–218.
34. Paulson GW, Dadmehr N, Is there a premorbid personality typical for Parkinson's disease? *Neurology* 1991; **41**(Suppl 2):73–76.

chapter 16

Rehabilitation

Diane Playford

Introduction

Delivering a comprehensive PD service demands an understanding of the needs of patients at different stages of the disease. MacMahon and Thomas have identified four key stages in the management of a patient with Parkinson's disease.[1] They include a diagnostic stage, a maintenance stage, a stage of complex disability, and finally a period where a palliative approach is required.

Some keys themes underpin the delivery of care at all stages of the disease and these will include the accessibility and expertise of healthcare professionals and the need for education of the patient so they can manage their own disease as exemplified by the "Expert Patient Programme." The Expert Patient Programme (EPP) is a British National Health Service (NHS)-based training program that provides opportunities for people who live with long-term chronic conditions to develop new skills to manage their condition better on a day-to-day basis.[2] It is based on research from the US and UK which shows that people living with chronic illnesses are often in the best position to know what they need in managing their own condition. Provided with the necessary "self-management" skills, which include identifying appropriate sources of support and positive coping styles (e.g., problem-solving and self-reassuring behaviors), they can make an impact both on their disease management and quality of life.

Despite the underlying themes, the needs of patients differ at the varying stages of Parkinson's disease and it is not possible to respond to the range of needs in a single service setting. It is clear from MacMahon's schema that all clinicians have some skills relevant to rehabilitation but the complex disability stage is primarily the domain of the physician who has particular expertise in both the symptomatic management of PD and rehabilitation.

There are a number of different definitions of rehabilitation (see Table 16.1 for alternative definitions of rehabilitation), but one used commonly states "Rehabilitation is a process of active change by which a person who has become disabled acquires the knowledge and skills needed for optimum physical, psychological and social function."[3] This definition recognizes that the disabled person plays an active role in determining the endpoints of the rehabilitation process, and how they may be reached.

Delivery of a comprehensive rehabilitation service demands clear structure and processes. The British Society of Rehabilitation Medicine has proposed clinical standards for in-patient and out-patient specialist rehabilitation services in the UK.[4] These standards relate to both the structures and processes by which rehabilitation is delivered. Rehabilitation includes multidisciplinary assessment and problem definition, treatment planning and delivery, evaluation of effectiveness and reassessment.[5] Even if a coordinated rehabilitation program is not available, clinicians can consider these standards in their management of individual patients with PD.

Table 16.1 Definitions of rehabilitation

A process of active change by which a person who has become disabled acquires the knowledge and skills needed for optimum physical, psychological and social functioning

The application of all measures aimed at reducing the impact of disabling and handicapping conditions, and enabling disabled and handicapped people to achieve social integration

The process of restoration, to the maximum degree possible, of function (physical or mental) or role (within the family, social network, or workforce)

A problem-solving and educational process aimed at reducing the disability and handicap experienced by someone as a result of disease, always within the limitations imposed both by available resources and by the underlying disease

Assessment

A comprehensive rehabilitation assessment is very different from that offered by a physician working independently. At the complex disability stage, the person with PD will have multiple factors affecting functional performance that may present as a single problem.

When a team works together, they need a structure for assessment and description of the difficulties. The World Health Organization (WHO) International Classification of Function (ICF) provides such a structure. It classifies functioning at both the level of body/body part, whole person, and whole person in social context.[6] Disablements are:

1. losses or abnormalities of bodily function and structure (impairments)
2. limitations of activities (disabilities)
3. restrictions in participation (formally called handicaps).

Figure 16.1 shows that disablement and functioning are outcomes of interactions between health conditions and personal and contextual factors. Two sorts of contextual factors are identified: social and physical environmental factors (social attitudes, access to buildings, social attitudes, legal protection, etc.); and personal factors that include gender, age, other health conditions, social background, education, overall behavior pattern, and other factors that influence how disablement is experienced by the individual. They help explain why apparently similar patients have different outcomes. An individual patient may complain of difficulty walking but the reasons for this

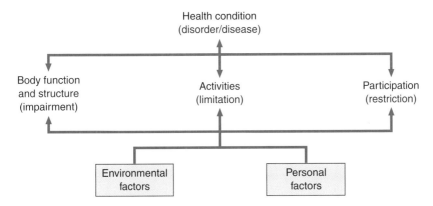

Figure 16.1 *Interaction of concepts from the World Health Organization International Classification of Function 2001.*

may be multiple, as may the social consequences. A typical example of the impairments, activity limitations and participation restrictions associated with PD is shown in Table 16.2.

Treatment planning

Once a patient's problems are clearly elucidated, a management strategy has to be put in place. Multidisciplinary teams may have the best approach to dealing with multiple interacting problems but also have multiple interacting demands. Goal setting is a long-established approach to insuring

Table 16.2 Example of the International Classification of Function (ICF) in PD

Health disorder/disease	Parkinson's disease
Body function and structure (impairment)	Bradykinesia R > L
	Rigidity
	Tremor R > L
	Severe postural instability
	Moderate dysarthria and dysphonia
	Mild dysphagia
	Sialorrhea
	Bladder instability
Activity limitation	Walks with rollator
	Difficulty getting dressed
	Urinary urgency, frequency, and urge incontinence
	Poor intelligibility of speech
	Difficulty feeding himself
Participation restriction	Cannot go out alone because frightened of falling
	Unable to go bowling with friends
	Does not eat in restaurants because "messy"
	Cannot use telephone as cannot be understood
	Unable to work and has lost job
	Financial difficulties due to early retirement
	Can not undertake household tasks, including DIY
Environmental factors	Lives in third floor residence. Lift (elevator) unreliable
Personal factors	Had been Regimental Sergeant Major – valued smart appearance, posture and physical fitness

that everyone on the team knows the expected outcome.[7] A long-term goal can be broken down into short-term goals and action plans.[8] Good goals are specific, measurable, achievable, time limited, and relevant to the patient.[9] Relevance to the patient is crucial, and this often requires that the goals are defined with the patient and are multidisciplinary. Patients, as well as therapists, should have a copy of the goals. Underpinning the achievement of many goals are actions or tasks that have to be undertaken by the multidisciplinary team. Thus, the person with PD may be able to learn over three therapy sessions how to perform a specific task, and thus potentially could change in 3 days. However, if the therapists concerned cannot provide three therapy sessions in 3 days, then the goal must allow for this. Equally, if a patient can learn how to perform a particular task that is dependent on ordering and delivery of a piece of equipment, such as a specialized walker, then that must be recognized, articulated, and allowed for.

Evaluation

Evaluation of the success of any rehabilitation can examine process or outcome. At the simplest level, achieving a specified goal is a measure of outcome. The difficulty of using goals as outcome measures is that they are unique to an individual patient and cannot be used to describe groups or compare outcomes between groups. Where suitable outcome measures exist, i.e., the outcome is appropriate to the intervention, it may be preferable to examine outcome. Clinically, it is important to remember that useful instruments should be easy to administer (e.g., brief, cheap, and easy to analyze), appropriate (that is, measure the outcome relevant to the intervention and relevant to that disease group), and acceptable to patients (being neither intrusive nor upsetting).[10] A number of measures have been developed for use in PD. The simplest clinical scale to assess PD, devised by Hoehn and Yahr,[11] distinguishes between five stages of severity of the disease from (stage 1) unilateral involvement with minimal or no functional impairment to (stage 5) confined to wheelchair or bed. Although this scale is the most widely used rating scale, it is too crude and insensitive to be useful as a measure of outcomes of interventions. The best known is the Unified Parkinson's Disease Rating Scale (UPDRS), which has been thoroughly investigated in terms of its psychometric aspects, however it does not assess the emotional or social impact of PD.[12,13]

Recently, focus has moved from clinician-based scales like the UPDRS to patient-based outcomes that reflect the impact of the disease on health-related quality of life.[14] Some disease-specific measures have been developed for use in PD. These include the Parkinson's Impact Scale (PIMS),[15] Parkinson's Disease Quality of Life Questionnaire (PDQL),[16,17] and the Parkinson's Disease Questionnaire (PDQ-39).[18-20] At present, the PDQ-39 is probably the most appropriate health-related quality of life measure. The PDQ-39 was developed with the patient's perspective central to the method-ology. A series of exploratory open-ended interviews were held with patients with PD who were asked to describe the impact of the disease on their lives. From these interviews, a 65-item questionnaire was developed and sent to patients with PD in the community in England. Statistical analysis of results produced a shorter version (39 items) which was then sent to a further series of respondents along with other questionnaires to examine validity. The resulting questionnaire comprises 39 items contributing to eight scales: mobility, activities of daily living, emotional well-being, stigma, social support, cognitions, communication, and bodily discomfort. Further studies have confirmed its reliability, validity, and responsiveness to change. A sub-sequent community survey of individuals with PD showed that problems of access to services for PD was associated with poorer PDQ-39 scores.[21]

Scales like the PDQ-39 that measure the impact PD has on a patient may be used to identify the impact of a range of interventions, but sometimes evaluating outcome directly is not possible. For example, a PD nurse may spend significant amounts of time with a patient in education, under-standing and adjustment to a specific issue, e.g., bladder management. One approach in this setting is to evaluate the rehabilitation process, rather than try to measure the outcome. This assumes that the outcome is more likely to be satisfactory if the correct interventions are delivered. Evaluation of the rehabilitation process may be performed in a number of ways, including documenting the compliance with a defined care pathway. Given the difficulty in running a seamless service, systems that allow the evaluation of the rehabilitation process are invaluable, particularly when first establishing a service. Evaluating process is facilitated by the devel-opment of an "integrated care pathway" (ICP) (Figure 16.2). An integrated care pathway consists of a document that maps the interventions that should occur during a specific episode of patient care.[22] Typically, the care pathway allows for operationalization of evidence-based practices for a specific setting.

The benefits of ICPs lie in specifying the best possible method for delivering care and in identifying when the pattern of care deviates from that expected, and the reasons for that, known as variance. A variance sheet may be used to record either departures from the pathway "procedural variance" or the reasons for non-achievement of goals. Individual variances are neither good nor bad. They are simply a method of recording what happened to a specific patient and the reasons for it, thus allowing for individualized patient care. The patterns of variances across a group of patients will identify strengths and weaknesses in the processes around particular episodes of care and permit incorporation of new ideas and remediation of problems into the rehabilitation program.[23] When combined with measurement tools it is possible to identify which aspects of care impact positively or adversely on the outcome.

Service development

The barriers to setting up an efficient and effective PD service vary from setting to setting and differ in differing countries. As they are embedded in the historical establishment of services, there is no single approach to a comprehensive service. One major barrier, however, is the paucity of evidence available to support or explain the role of rehabilitation in PD. This is reflected by the recent critical review of the effectiveness of rehabilitation by the British Society of Rehabilitation Medicine,[24] which failed to mention PD. Although the individual elements of the rehabilitation process have little evidence to support their use, there is little doubt in other chronic neurological disorders that rehabilitative approaches are effective. In multiple sclerosis, another chronic progressive condition, randomized controlled trials have provided data to support inpatient rehabilitation[25,26] and physiotherapy.[27] Stroke unit care reduces death, institutionalized care and dependency at 1 year[28] and long term,[29] and there are significant health status gains in the community after head injury.[30]

Anecdotal evidence from patients, health professionals, and the Parkinson's Disease Society of the UK strongly supports the use of paramedical therapies in the comprehensive management of PD in addition to optimal medical and surgical treatment. These paramedical therapies include physiotherapy, occupational therapy, and speech and language therapy. Despite this support for paramedical therapies, several surveys have demonstrated that only 3% to 29% of patients with Parkinson's disease have seen a paramedical therapist.[31-34] This low rate of referral may partly reflect clinicians' beliefs that

	NHNN Neuro Rehabilitation Unit Integrated Care Pathway V. 2.0 November 2002 **WEEKLY FORM**	UCL HOSPITALS

35290

Patient ID

Weeks since admission:			Date:	/	/	

Goal setting	(please tick)	**Date**	**Name**	**Var. Code**
Is this a goal setting week?	☐ Yes ☐ No			
New goals set?	☐ Yes ☐ No ☐ n/a			
Is the list of goals by the patient's bed?	☐ Yes ☐ No			
Length of Stay & Discharge date reviewed?	☐ Yes ☐ No ☐ n/a			
Key worker present at Goal Setting?	☐ Yes ☐ No ☐ n/a			
All team members present at Goal Setting?	☐ Yes ☐ No ☐ n/a			
Discharge Planning	(please tick)	**Date**	**Name**	
External referrals?	☐ Yes ☐ No ☐ n/a			
Neurological Status and drug regime	(please tick)	**Date**	**Name**	
Weekly review completed?	☐ Yes ☐ No ☐ n/a			
Nursing	(please tick)	**Date**	**Name**	
Waterlow score completed?	☐ Yes ☐ No Score:			
Nursing dependency	☐ Yes ☐ No Score:			
Referrals/Assessments	(please tick)	**Date**	**Name**	
Dietician?	☐ Yes ☐ No ☐ n/a			
Hospital visits?	☐ Yes ☐ No			
Hospital code	☐ QS ☐ UCH/Mddx ☐ Other			
Psychologist/counselling	☐ Yes ☐ No			
Social worker?	☐ Yes ☐ No ☐ n/a			
Volunteer agencies (i.e. GBS)?	☐ Yes ☐ No ☐ n/a			
Referrals/Assessments	(please tick)			
Carer contact	☐ Yes ☐ No			

Sessions	PT	OT	SLT	Psych	SW	**Joint Sessions (specify)**
Estimated						
Variance*						
Achieved						
Carer present?	☐ Yes ☐ No	☐ Yes ☐ No	☐ Yes ☐ No	☐ Yes ☐ No	☐ Yes ☐ No	☐ Yes ☐ No

Weekend Leave	(please tick)	**Date**	**Name**
Patient on Weekend Leave?	☐ Yes ☐ No ☐ n/a		

Figure 16.2 *An "integrated care pathway."*

7428

Variance Codes			
Patient/Condition	**Code**	**Internal System**	**Code**
Patient medically deteriorated	05	Date or time of treatment changed	210
Patient cognitive difficulties/memory	10		
Patient cognitive difficulties/other	20	Planned meeting cancelled	220
Patient behavioural problems	30	Awaiting other consultation	230
Patient fatigue	40	Goal timing inappropriate	240
Neurological deterioration	50	Plan of action inappropriate	241
Neurological deterioration due to drug side-effect	51		
UTI	60	Goal considered inappropriate	250
Other infection	70	Goal setting on a day other than Friday	251
MRSA positive	71	Nursing Staff not available but on unit	260
Pressure area concern	80	Medical Staff not available but on unit	261
Tone problems	81	OT not available but on unit	262
Pain	90	PT not available but on unit	263
Patient mood disturbance	91	SW Staff not available but on unit	264
Confidence	100	Psych Staff not available but on unit	265
Neurological improvement	101	SALT Staff not available but on unit	266
Patient/carer	**Code**	Nursing Staff not available/away from unit	270
Patient not available but on unit	110	Medical Staff not available/away from unit	271
Patient on isolation suite	111	OT not available/away from unit	272
Patient at Queen Square	120	PT not available/away from unit	273
Patient at other hospital	130	SW Staff not available/away from unit	274
Patient not on unit (& not at QS)	131	Psych Staff not available/away from unit	275
Patient declines treatment	140	SALT Staff not available/away from unit	276
Patient self-discharge	141	Staff not on shift	279
Patient disagrees with goals	150	Extra therapy sessions given	280
Patient disagrees with plan of action	151	Staff on annual leave	290
		Staff on study leave	295
Carer disagrees with goals	160	Staff on sick leave	300
Carer support level	170	Reduced skill mix (Nursing)	310
Carers unavailable	180	Reduced staffing (Medical)	311
Patient not well motivated	190	Reduced staffing (OT)	312
Patient well motivated	191	Reduced staffing (PT)	313
Safety	200	Reduced staffing (SW)	314
Underestimated patient's cognitive state/conditions	201	Reduced staffing (Psych)	315
Underestimated patient's cognitive state/conditions	201		
External system	**Code**	Reduced staffing (SALT)	316
Alternative accommodation unavailable/adaptions incomplete	400	Equipment not available	320
Home care not yet available	410	Department closed	330
Transfer to other unit/hospital delayed	420	Internal follow-up/treatment delay	340
Transport delay	430	Inadequate information from QS	340
Community care assessment/external assessment delayed	440	Document omission	360
Accommodation not suitable	450	Late admission	370
Unavailability of equipment	460	Early discharge for positive reasons	380
Follow-up therapy not available	470	Early discharge for negative reasons	381
		Extended stay	382
Funding difficulties	480	**Other**	**Code**
Inadequate information from other hospital	490	Other	500
Patient transferred to Queen Square	491	No Carer	501
		Carer at work	502
		Carer too far away	503

Comments & Administration

Please use this space to communicate any message with regard to either the layout or content of the ICP. This information will be treated confidentially unless otherwise requested. Your comments on your ICPs are valued and will be used in further refining the ICPs. Please also mention if you would be interested in seeing a particular aspect of patients' ICPs being reported on. If you are the key worker for this particular ICP and it has been returned to you, an explanation will be documented below. Urgent questions and queries with regard to the ICPs should be addressed to Diane Playford

Date received:
Date returned to Key worker (if necessary):
Date received back from Key worker:
Date data entry completed:

there is little evidence for using such therapy, although the under-provision of such services in the UK may be an additional factor.

Paramedical therapists treating people with PD provide appropriate exercises, aids, education, and advice that aim to help patients to better understand and cope with their disease. All therapies are based upon a number of defined principles. First, the therapy should be patient-centered and tailored to a patient's specific needs and ambitions. The second principle is that teaching patients about management strategies enables them to continue self-management and problem-solving after the intervention by the therapist has been completed. A third principle is that prevention is better than cure. Thus, most therapists believe that they should see people with Parkinson's disease early in order to educate them and to stop the development of preventable complications, such as frequent falls, contractures, pressure sores, and poor posture.[35]

Physiotherapists

Physiotherapists identify and treat the difficulties patients may have with movement and general mobility. They aim to help patients achieve the greatest level of activity using the best quality of movement possible. Physiotherapy (also termed "physical therapy" or PT in the US) is about learning how to move more normally and with less effort. It is not about routine exercise or regular treatment to prevent deterioration, but about learning skills and techniques to make coping with PD easier. For example, PD can make automatic tasks, such as tying a tie or doing up shoe laces, slower. Certain techniques can improve this including learning strategies such as talking through a task while doing it or relying on visual targets to improve performance. These approaches are known as cueing. Sometimes splitting the movement up into a number of steps, or doing the task in a new way can help. Physiotherapists can help teach these techniques.

Parkinson's disease is also associated with stiffness and poor posture. Initially, this is due to the way Parkinson's disease affects movement, but later the posture becomes habitual and muscles and joints become stiffer. Physiotherapists can work to relieve this muscle and joint stiffness.

As movement become more difficult, it is easy to become unfit. Physiotherapists can advise patients about appropriate exercise regimes that will maximize function and minimize physical deterioration, e.g., Alexander technique, swimming.

Occupational therapists (OTs)

Parkinson's disease may impact on daily activity (occupation) so that people with PD develop problems with the practicalities of life, such as washing and dressing, and maintaining family, work, community, and leisure roles. Occupational therapists work with people with PD and their families to identify problems, which are impacting on their life style, and to minimize the effects of these problems. Like physiotherapists, occupational therapists may teach new strategies to use when performing familiar tasks, such as getting dressed. Occupational therapists may provide or suggest simple equipment that makes performing a particular task easier, e.g., using an electric can opener, a kettle tipper, or providing a chair raise. They may also provide advice about adaptations to the home. Examples of simple adaptations include removing loose rugs and floor covers that may cause people with PD to trip, or providing grab rails. Bigger adaptations include shower facilities with a level access or stair lifts.

Many people with PD find day-to-day routines more effortful, and may experience fatigue. OTs will work with the patient to find daily and weekly routines that minimize effort and allow people with PD to continue the activities that are most important to them.

OTs can also provide advice about resources that allow you to continue to work, to use transport, leisure and other community services, so that life within the community remains as active as possible.

Speech and language therapists

Speech and language therapists are involved in the assessment and treatment of people with communication and/or swallowing disorders. About half of people with PD develop some communication difficulties. These include slurred speech, quiet speech, poor expression, and speaking either too quickly or very slowly. Other communication difficulties might include difficulty with writing, limited facial expression, and body language. The speech therapist will work with the person with PD, and where appropriate, with their family or carers to identify where these difficulties impact functioning, e.g., when using the telephone, or when speaking in public at meetings, or in shops. Therapy can include exercises, which work on improving voice loudness, and therefore intelligibility of speech. Some people may find using a voice amplifier helpful.

The types of swallowing problems encountered by people with PD include difficulty controlling saliva, difficulty chewing harder foods, and slowness to swallow. Some people may experience coughing or choking episodes while eating. The speech and language therapist will assess the swallow and provide advice on the easiest food and drink consistencies and the safest approach to eating and drinking.

The therapies listed above are often complementary to one another, as well as to medical and surgical interventions, since they individually work on different components of health and disease, or on similar components in a different way. For example, although both physiotherapists and occupational therapists may work to improve transfers, they will approach this goal in different manners and with differing overall aims. Physiotherapists aim to increase stability and flexibility with specific exercises, and teach better movement strategies, aiming for the patient to get out of the chair as independently as possible. Occupational therapists approach a problem with transfers from a different perspective. "Occupation" is the daily activity that reflects cultural values, provides structure to living and meaning to individuals; these activities meet human needs for self-care, enjoyment and participation in society.[36] Thus, occupational therapists may assess the height and stability of the chair that the person is transferring from, teach movement, cueing, and concentration strategies, and determine why the person needs to get in and out of that chair. Their overall focus will be on the activity, or occupation, that requires them to be able to transfer.

Thus, the management of people with progressive diseases that result in disability demands a team approach with professionals working across organizational boundaries, delivering evidence-based care that is co-ordinated by a "key-worker" or case manager. A key worker role is often essential to balance and co-ordinate care[37] and this person is most commonly a Parkinson's disease nurse specialist, who has additional disease-specific knowledge. In addition, the unique contributions of the patients themselves need to be recognized. Despite a consensus that multidisciplinary effort leads to optimum care for patients, there are no trials of co-ordinated multidisciplinary input.

Recently, six Cochrane systematic reviews have been undertaken to evaluate the efficacy of paramedical therapies for PD, including physiotherapy, occupational therapy, and speech and language therapy for both speech and swallowing problems.[38–43] Eleven trials were identified comparing physiotherapy with placebo or no treatment, and a further seven trials were identified comparing two forms of physiotherapy. Although many of the studies were pioneering, like the study by Marchese,[44] they highlight the difficulties of performing good randomized clinical trials (RCTs) that rigorously evaluate the impact of rehabilitation in progressive neurological disease. All the trials used small numbers of patients, description of the interventions was poor, and placebos were usually inadequate. In addition, randomization was performed in some of the studies but not all, a wide variety of different outcome measures was used, and statistical analysis was less than optimal. This piecemeal approach may in part reflect the low levels of funding available for this type of clinical research. Nonetheless, the principal finding of these reviews is that there is insufficient evidence to support or refute the use of paramedical therapies in PD.

To improve the quality of these studies on the impact of rehabilitative services on PD, a number of changes need to be made. Initially, a consensus is required on what constitutes the "standard" form of each therapy. Large well-designed placebo-controlled randomized trials are needed to demonstrate the efficacy and effectiveness of these paramedical therapies. Outcome measures that are responsive to the chosen intervention and have particular relevance to patients should be selected and the patients monitored for at least 6 months to determine the duration of benefit. The trials should be reported using CONSORT guidelines,[45] which define good practice for clinical trial design and data analysis.

Recommendations for clinical practice can therefore, at present, only be supported by various levels of subjective knowledge. The suggestions below are supported where possible by evidence from trials or formal consensus, on the applicability of each therapy to a person with PD at each stage of the disease.

Physiotherapy

The Physiotherapy Evaluation Project (PEP) examined current physiotherapy practice using a Delphi technique, and developed a consensus approach for physiotherapy in PD.[46] These guidelines are unequivocal in their support of a multidisciplinary approach. They state that physiotherapy should be individually tailored and eclectic in approach, aiming to maximize functional ability in four core areas:

- Gait (upright mobility)
- Transfers (including bed mobility)

- Balance (including instability and falls) and
- Posture (including abnormal limb movements).

Trials of physiotherapy provide limited evidence of efficacy, particularly with specific gait characteristics, such as walking velocity and stride length. Only one study has examined the impact of physiotherapy on "activities of daily living,"[47] this demonstrated an improvement. Similarly, only one study has measured impact of health-related quality of life which did not improve in the one trial in which it was measured.[48]

Early intervention aimed at maintaining posture and flexibility through the prevention of secondary problems such as soft tissue shortening is thought to be helpful.[49] This will involve an education package, and the establishment of an exercise program at diagnosis. This program needs to be incorporated into daily functional or leisure activities. Once a patient becomes more clearly symptomatic, especially with akinesia (e.g., start hesitation or freezing), then visual and auditory cueing techniques, such as white lines on the floor or a ticking metronome, show promise and need further evaluation.[50,51]

At the palliative stage, carers and patients may benefit from teaching effective rolling and lifting techniques.[52]

Occupational therapy

Only two trials of occupational therapy have been performed in PD patients and these produced results of little value, due to problems in the design of the trials that could have led to bias, the small numbers of patients examined, and the marked heterogeneity of the two methods used.[53,54] Both trials examined group occupational therapy, which is unlikely to address an individual's specific occupational aims and needs. However, a Delphi survey to develop a consensus on core occupational therapy practice for Parkinson's disease in the UK demonstrated the following key findings:[55,56]

- Occupational therapists believed that they were generally effective in minimizing limitations and increasing participation, and helping people maintain social roles at all stages of the disease.
- Early and frequent (annual) intervention maximizes potential benefits.

Speech and language therapy

Although the Royal College of Speech and Language Therapists has published consensus guidelines for the therapy of dysarthria, they are not specific for the treatment of PD and do not contain details of style, duration, or intensity of therapy.[57] There are a number of trials that have examined Lee Silverman Voice Therapy® for Parkinson's disease.[58–63] The results are encouraging, suggesting a clinically significant improvement in intelligibility. However, these studies were not placebo-controlled. Again, the lack of firm data suggests that a large multicenter randomized controlled trial is required. Therapy should be provided soon after functional difficulties are noted, and followed up on an annual basis. Speech and language therapy may also be effective in the treatment of dysphagia, but there is very little evidence at any level published in the literature to support the proposition it alters the risk of aspiration, choking, or pneumonia.[63] However, it is important to remember that lack of evidence does not mean lack of efficacy, and there is a strong consensus about the role of speech and language therapies in minimizing the impact of dysphagia.

There are a number of other therapies used in rehabilitation and community settings. These include different forms of exercise including the Alexander technique, yoga, and Pilates and music and art therapy. There is limited evidence to support these approaches, although there are some preliminary studies using the Alexander technique[64] and music therapy[65] that suggest these may have a role.

Music therapy uses music to address physical, emotional, cognitive, and social needs of individuals. Music therapy interventions can be designed to: promote wellness, manage stress, alleviate pain, express feelings, enhance memory, improve communication, and promote physical rehabilitation. Through cueing techniques, there is a clear rationale for the role of music therapy although the evidence is limited.[64]

Art therapy is the use of art materials for self-expression and reflection in the presence of a trained art therapist. Individuals who are referred to an art therapist need not have previous experience or skill in art; the art therapist is not primarily concerned with making an esthetic or diagnostic assessment of the client's image. The overall aim of its practitioners is to enable a client to effect change and growth on a personal level through use of art materials in a safe and facilitating environment. There is no evidence in the literature to support its use as a specific therapy in PD.

In conclusion, the management of PD needs to reflect the different requirements of the patient at different stages of their disease. This demands close liaison between disciplines and services. While there is limited evidence to support rehabilitation interventions, there is a clear consensus about their role and the need for further evaluation of how these services can optimally benefit patients with PD throughout the disease course. The best outcomes for people with PD are likely to occur when there is integrated service provision with co-ordinated care and the individual expertise and needs are clearly recognized.

References

1. MacMahon D, Thomas S, Practical approach to quality of life in Parkinson's disease. *J Neurol* 1998; **245**(Suppl 1): S19–S22.
2. Expert Patient Programme, http://www.expertpatients.nhs.uk/index.shtml.
3. NHS Executive (March 1997) Rehabilitation – A Guide.
4. Turner-Stokes L, Williams H, Abraham R, Duckett S, Clinical standards for inpatient specialist rehabilitation services in the UK. *Clin Rehabil* 2000; **14**: 468–480.
5. Wade DT, *Measurement in Neurological Rehabilitation*. Oxford: Oxford Medical Publications, 1992.
6. International Classification of Functioning, Disability and Health, http://www3.who.int/icf/icftemplate.cfm.
7. Wade DT, Goal planning in rehabilitation: why, what, how? *Top Stroke Rehab* 1999; **6**(2):1–7.
8. Playford ED, Dawson L, Limbert V, Smith M, Ward CD, Wells R, Goal-setting in rehabilitation: report of a workshop to explore Professionals' perceptions of goal-setting. *Clin Rehab* 2000; **14**:491–496.
9. Schut HA, Stam HJ, Goals in rehabilitation teamwork. *Disabil Rehab* 1994; **16**(4):223–226.
10. Hobart J, Rating scales for neurologists. *J Neurol Neurosurg Psychiat* 2003; **74**(Suppl 4):iv22–iv26.
11. Hoehn M, Yahr M, Parkinsonism: onset, progression and mortality. *Neurology* 1967; **17**:427–442.
12. Fahn S, Elton R, Members of the UPDRS Development Committee, The Unified Parkinson's Disease Rating Scale. In: Fahn S, Marsden C, Calne D, Goldstein M (eds) *Recent Developments in Parkinson's Disease*. Florham Park: Macmillan Healthcare Information, 1987; 153–163.
13. van Hilten J, van der Zwan A, Zwinderman A, Roos R, Rating impairment and disability in Parkinson's disease: evaluation of the Unified Parkinson's Disease Rating Scale. *Mov Disord* 1994; **9**:84–88.
14. Hobart J, Measuring disease impact in disabling neurological conditions: are patients' perspectives and scientific rigor compatible? *Curr Opin Neurol* 2002; **15**(6):721–724.
15. Calne S, Schulzer M, Mak E et al, Validating a quality of life rating scale for idiopathic Parkinsonism: Parkinson's Impact Scale (PIMS) *Parkinsonism Relat Disord* 1996; **2**:55–61.
16. de Boer A, Wijker W, Speelman J, de Haes J, Quality of life in patients with

Parkinson's disease: development of a questionnaire. *J Neurol Neurosurg Psychiat* 1996; **61**:70–74.

17. Hobson P, Holden A, Meara J, Measuring the impact of Parkinson's disease with the Parkinson's Disease Quality of Life Questionnaire. *Age Ageing* 1999; **28**(4): 341–346.

18. Fitzpatrick R, Peto V, Jenkinson C, Greenhall R, Hyman N, Health-related quality of life in Parkinson's disease: a study of outpatient clinic attenders. *Mov Disord* 1997; **12**:916–922.

19. Jenkinson C, Peto V, Fitzpatrick R, Greenhall R, Hyman N, The Parkinson's Disease Questionnaire (PDQ-39): development and validation of a Parkinson's disease summary index score. *Age Ageing* 1997; **26**:353–357.

20. Peto V, Jenkinson C, Fitzpatrick R, Greenhall R, The development and validation of a short measure of functioning and well-being for individuals with Parkinson's disease. *Qual Life Res* 1995; **4**:241–248.

21. Peto V, Fitzpatrick R, Jenkinson C, Self-reported health status and access to health services in a community sample with Parkinson's disease. *Disability Rehabil* 1997; **19**:97–103.

22. Playford ED, Rossiter D, Werring DJ, Thompson AJ, Integrated care pathways: evaluating in-patients rehabilitation in stroke. *Br J Therapy Rehab* 1997; **4**:97–102.

23. Riley K, Paving the way. *Health Serv J* 1998; **108**:30–31.

24. Turner-Stokes L (Guest editor) The effectiveness of rehabilitation: a critical review of the evidence. *Clin Rehab* 1999, **13**:1(Suppl).

25. Freeman JA, Langdon DW, Hobart JC, Thompson AJ, The impact of inpatient rehabilitation on progressive multiple sclerosis. *Ann Neurol* 1997; **42**:236–244.

26. Solari A, Filippini G, Gasco P et al, Physical rehabilitation has a positive effect on disability in multiple sclerosis patients. *Neurology* 1999; **52**:57–62.

27. Wiles CM, Newcombe RG, Fuller KJ et al, A controlled randomised crossover trial of the effects of physiotherapy on mobility in chronic multiple sclerosis. *J Neurol Neurosurg Psychiat* 2001; **70**(2):174–179.

28. Stroke Unit Trialists' Collaboration, Organised inpatient (stroke unit) care for stroke. (2003) (Cochrane Review). In: *The Cochrane Library. Issue 2.* Chichester, UK: John Wiley & Sons, Ltd.

29. Indredavik B, Bakke R, Slodahl SA, Rokseth R, Haheim LL, Stroke unit treatment: 10 year follow up. *Stroke* 1999; **8**:1524–1527.

30. Powell J, Heslin J, Greenwood RJ, Community based rehabilitation after severe traumatic brain injury: a randomized controlled trial. *J Neurol Neurosurg Psychiatr* 2002: **72**:197–202.

31. Yarrow S, Members 1998 survey of the Parkinson's Disease Society of the United Kingdom. In: Percival R, Hobson P (eds) *Parkinson's Disease: Studies in Psychological Care.* Leicester: BPS Books, 1999; 79–92.

32. Mutch WJ, Strudwick A, Roy SK, Downie AW. Parkinson's disease: disability, review, and management. *Br J Med* 1986; **293**:675–677.

33. Oxtoby M, *Parkinson's Disease Patients and Their Social Needs.* London: Parkinson's Disease Society, 1982.

34. Clarke CE, Zobkiw RM, Gullaksen E, Quality of life and care in Parkinson's Disease. *Br J Clin Pract* 1995; **49**:288–293.

35. Deane KHO, Playford ED, Non-pharmacological therapies. In: Playford D (ed.) *Neurological Rehabilitation of Parkinson's Disease. Queen Square Neurological Rehabilitation Series.* London: Martin Dunitz, 2003.

36. Crepeau EB, Cohn ES, Boyt Schell BA, *Willard & Spackman's Occupational Therapy,* 10th edn. Philadelphia: Lippincott, Williams and Wilkins, 2003.

37. Dant T, Gearing B, Keyworkers for elderly people in the community: case managers and care co-ordinators. *J Soc Policy* 1990; **19**(3):331–360.
38. Deane KHO, Jones A, Clarke CE, Playford ED, Ben-Shlomo Y, Physiotherapy for patients with Parkinson's disease. *The Cochrane Library*, 2000.
39. Deane KHO, Jones D, Ellis-Hill C, Clarke CE, Playford ED, Ben-Shlomo Y, A comparison of physiotherapy techniques for patients with Parkinson's disease. *The Cochrane Library*, 2000.
40. Deane KHO, Whurr R, Clarke CE, Playford ED and Ben-Shlomo Y, Speech and language therapy for dysphagia in Parkinson's disease. *The Cochrane Library* 2000.
41. Deane KHO, Whurr R, Clarke CE, Playford ED, Ben-Shlomo Y, Speech and language therapy for dysarthria in Parkinson's disease. *The Cochrane Library*, 2000.
42. Deane KHO, Whurr R, Clarke CE, Playford ED, Ben-Shlomo Y, A comparison of speech and language therapy techniques for dysarthria in Parkinson's disease. *The Cochrane Library*, 2000.
43. Deane KHO, Ellis-Hill C, Clarke CE, Playford ED, Ben-Shlomo Y, Occupational therapy for patients with Parkinson's disease.. *The Cochrane Library*, 2000.
44. Marchese R, Diverio M, Zucchi F, Lentino C, Abbruzzese G, The role of sensory cues in the rehabilitation of parkinsonian patients: a comparison of two physical therapy protocols. *Mov Disord* 2000; **15**:879–883.
45. Begg C, Cho M, Eastwood S et al, Improving the quality of reporting of randomized controlled trials. The CONSORT statement. *JAMA* 1996; **276**(8):637–639.
46. Ashburn A, Jones D, Plant R et al, Physiotherapy for people with Parkinson's disease in the UK: an exploration of practice. *Intern J Therapy Rehab* 2004; **11**:160–167.
47. Patti F, Reggio A, Nicoletti F, Sellaroli T, Deinite G, Nicoletti Fr, Effects of rehabilitation therapy on parkinsonian's disability and functional independence. *J Neurol Rehabil* 1996; **10**:223–231.
48. Chandler C, Plant R, A targeted physiotherapy service for people with Parkinson's disease from diagnosis to end stage: a pilot study. In: Percival R, Hobson P (eds) *Parkinson's Disease: Studies in Psychological and Social Care.* Leicester: BPS Books, 1999; 256–269.
49. Schenkman M, Donovan J, Tsubota J, Kluss M, Stebbins P, Butler RB, Management of individuals with Parkinson's disease: rationale and case studies. *Phys Ther* 1989; **69**(11):944–955.
50. Lewis GN, Byblow WD, Walt SE, Stride length regulation in Parkinson's disease: the use of extrinsic, visual cues. *Brain* 2000; **123**(Pt 10):2077–2090.
51. Thaut MH, McIntosh KW, McIntosh GC, Hoemberg V, Auditory rhythmicity enhances movement and speech motor control in patients with Parkinson's disease. *Funct Neurol* 2001; **16**(2):163–172.
52. Ore T, Evaluation of safety training for manual handling of people with disabilities in specialised group homes in Australia. *Aust N Z J Public Health* 2003; **27**(1):64–69.
53. Fiorani C, Mari F, Bartolini M, Ceravolo M, Provinciali L, Occupational therapy increases ADL score and quality of life in Parkinson's disease. *Mov Disord* 1997; **12**(Suppl. 1):135.
54. Gauthier L, Dalziel S, Gauthier S, The benefits of group occupational therapy for patients with Parkinson's disease. *Am J Occ Ther* 1987; **41**(6):360–365.
55. Deane KHO, Ellis-Hill C, Dekker K, Davies P, Clarke CE, A survey of current occupational therapy practice for Parkinson's disease in the United Kingdom. *Br J Occ Ther* 2003; **66**:193–200.
56. Deane KHO, Ellis-Hill C, Dekker K, Davies P, Clarke CE, A Delphi survey of best practice occupational therapy practice for Parkinson's disease in the United Kingdom. *Br J Occ Ther* 2003; **66**:247–254.

57. Taylor-Goh S (ed) *Royal College of Speech and Language Therapy – Clinical Guidelines*. Bicester: Speechmark Publishing 2005.
58. Ramig LO, Countryman S, Thompson LL, Horii Y, Comparison of two forms of intensive speech treatment for Parkinson's disease. *J Speech Hearing Res* 1995; **38**:1232–1251.
59. Ramig LO, Countryman S, O'Brien C, Hoehn M, Thompson L, Intensive speech treatment for patients with Parkinson's disease: Short- and long-term comparison of two techniques. *Neurology* 1996; **47**:1496–1504.
60. Ramig LO, Dromey C, Aerodynamic mechanisms underlying treatment-related changes in vocal intensity in patients with Parkinson's disease. *J Speech Hearing Res* 1996; **39**:798–807.
61. Ramig L, Hoyt P, Seeley E, Sapir S, Voice treatment (LSVT) for IPD: Perceptual findings. *Parkinsonism Relat Disord* 1999; **5**(Suppl.):S42.
62. Ramig LO, Sapir S, Countryman S et al, Intensive voice treatment (LSVT) for individuals with Parkinson's disease: a 2 year follow up. *J Neurol Neurosurg Psychiat* 2001; **71**(4):493–498.
63. Smith ME, Ramig LO, Dromey C, Perez KS, Samandari R, Intensive voice treatment in Parkinson's disease: Laryngostroboscopic findings. *J Voice* 1995; **9**(4):453–459.
64. Stallibrass C, Sissons P, Chalmers C, Randomized controlled trial of the Alexander technique for idiopathic Parkinson's disease. *Clin Rehab* 2002; **16**(7):695–708.
65. Pacchetti C, Mancini F, Aglieri R, Fundaro C, Martignoni E, Nappi G, Active music therapy in Parkinson's disease: an integrative method for motor and emotional rehabilitation. *Psychosom Med* 2000; **62**(3):386–393.

chapter 17

Long-term care and nursing home issues

S Rebecca Dunlop and Melissa Gerstenhaber

Introduction

With advancing disease, many patients with PD need to transition their care to long-term care environments. In such settings, advanced motor disability, ever-changing motor and mental states, and enhanced care needs pose a variety of challenges that can easily strain individual or institutional resources. For clinicians, optimal patient management will minimize or control motor and neuropsychiatric dysfunction and maximize overall function. To achieve this in long-term care settings, clinical care requires working with an interdisciplinary team of physicians, nursing staff, social workers, and rehabilitative therapists in order to best meet the needs of patients and families. This chapter is geared towards nursing staff, medical staff, and informal care givers. It describes the spectrum of long-term care options, identifies the issues in patient management that lead to use of long-term care and the transition from one type of service to the other, and reviews specific disease management problems encountered in long-term care settings. Awareness of these issues provides a basis for clinical interventions that improve quality of life for patients and families and can reduce the impact of neuropsychiatric dysfunction.

Long-term care options

A variety of options are available for the long-term care of individuals with PD. The appropriate intervention depends on the stage of the illness, availability of support, accessibility of services, and the patient's financial ability and eligibility to obtain such services. Figure 17.1 illustrates the continuum of long-term care services that are generally required relative to clinical progression in the later stages of the illness. The stage of PD will influence whether care needs can be met informally or if community or institutionally based long-term care services are needed.

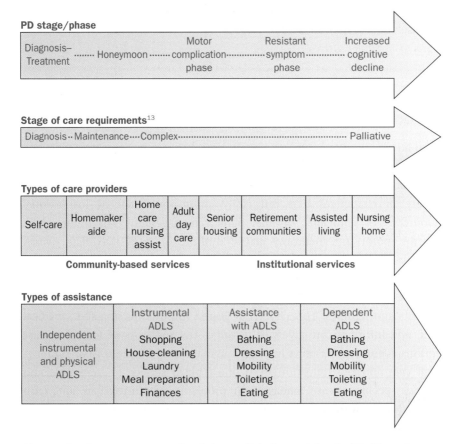

Figure 17.1 *Long-term care needs relative to clinical stage (phase) of Parkinson's disease.*

Informal care

The provision of care by significant others is a component of many chronic illnesses, and most individuals with PD ultimately need some type of care. According to a recent survey, an estimated 44.4 million Americans ages 18 and older provide some type of unpaid care to another adult.[1] The informal caregiver may be the spouse, significant other, adult children, other relatives, close friends, or members of one's faith community. Initially the informal caregiver may simply provide medication reminders, emotional support, or occasionally assist with activities of daily living (ADLs). As the illness progresses, the informal caregiver provides assistance with ADLs as illustrated in Figure 17.1. The caregiver may also bear considerable emotional burden themselves, a topic that is addressed in Chapter 19. Table 17.1 lists common signs of caregiver distress.

As part of the general clinical care, clinicians should inquire regularly, even early in the disease, about a patient's support system. Patients with relatively mild motor or cognitive impairment may feel overwhelmed when they are trying to cope with independent living and management of their PD. For such patients, transition to a more structured and supported living situation frequently leads to a substantial reduction in anxiety, depression, or generalized distress, and may preclude the need to address those symptoms with psychiatric medications.

As illustrated in Figure 17.2, the strength of a patient's support system is inversely proportional to the need for professional supportive services. Individuals without an informal caregiver or with weak support systems will have the greatest need for professional supportive services. Since patients or family members may be reluctant to reveal this vulnerability for any number of reasons (lack of insight, pride/embarrassment, interpersonal issues, etc.), it

Table 17.1 Signs of caregiver distress

Persistent anger, irritability, and resentment
Persistent impatience
Depression
Subjective reports of feeling overwhelmed
Caregiver health problems
Inadequate attention to the patient's physical and mental needs
Inability to provide for the patient's physical and mental needs
Difficulty balancing multiple responsibilities of work and family

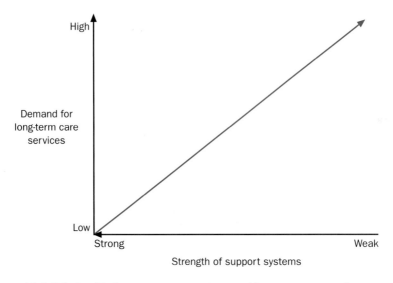

Figure 17.2 *Relationship between support systems and long-term care needs.*

is important for clinicians to observe for signs of an insufficient caregiver/ support system. These signs may include inability to adhere to the medication regimen, missed appointments, frequent calls in crisis from the patient or caregiver, increased falls and injury, slovenly dress or change in hygiene and grooming habits, etc. Identification of an inadequate support system should prompt referral to social workers or community-based nurses.

Community-based services

The addition of community-based services can prolong community living, allowing individuals to remain in the mainstream of life. Such services frequently enhance the quality of life of the person with PD, as well as their caregiver, and may preclude the necessity of nursing home placement. However, since care is provided by individuals who are not family, issues similar to those in nursing home settings may arise. In particular, caregivers provided through community-based services are often unfamiliar with the nuances of PD and will need education in this regard. Table 17.2 lists examples of community-based care providers and their functions. A model for an interdisciplinary home healthcare program for patients with PD that combines skilled assessments by healthcare professionals, case management, and patient and family education has been described.[2]

Table 17.2 Examples of community-based care providers

Homemaker aide	Assists with instrumental ADLs, but no personal care. Usually not certified and has little formal education.
Home health aides/home care nursing assistants	Assists with ADLs and may assist with limited instrumental ADLs. Often certified as a nursing assistant and has limited formal education
Adult medical day services	Provides an array of services during the day within a structured environment. Generally includes transportation as well as meals, activities, therapies, and supervision by licensed nursing professionals. Scope of services varies regionally as does licensing and regulation
Geriatric case managers	Provides assessment of medical needs and financial abilities and develops a personalized plan of care. In most cases, does not provide direct care, but instead supervises implementation of the care plan by other services or informal caregivers. Can be hired privately or may be provided through health insurance or community-based health programs, e.g., local Offices on Aging in the US
Senior housing facilities and group homes	Provides a supervised environment often with varied assistance with instrumental ADLs
Assisted living facilities	Provides a supervised environment 24 hours a day with varied assistance with instrumental ADLs, and periodic assessment by licensed nursing professionals
Continuing care retirement communities (CCRCs)	Provide a continuum of services from independent living facilities to long-term care

Nursing home facilities

A nursing home may serve as a temporary rehabilitative environment after an acute hospitalization or it may be the final home for a patient with advanced PD. Nursing homes are licensed facilities that provide a supervised environment. Licensed staff, including registered nurses, are available around the clock and trained to care for individuals needing partial or total assistance in ADLs. Local health departments establish regulatory operational guidelines and monitor nursing home facilities. These surveys are a matter of public record and are available to individuals considering placement.

Stages of Parkinson's disease and variation in care needs

The slow but progressive and dynamic nature of PD requires different interventions over its course. Likewise, the cumulative needs for assistance along the long-term care continuum will vary from one patient to the next. As suggested by Figure 17.1, care needs are minimal until development of the motor complication period of PD, which may begin anywhere from 3 years to 8 years or more after the point of diagnosis.[3] Resistant symptoms that follow are in some cases accompanied by significant cognitive decline, which generally leads to increased dependencies in daily activities.

Motor complication phase

Motor complications include wearing off, on/off fluctuations, dyskinesias, and dystonias. These complications, which generally require the expertise of a movement disorders specialist, must be optimally managed regardless of the setting in which the patient is living.

Medication timing becomes increasingly important in addressing motor complications since delays in medication administration can contribute to excessive wearing off and more severe fluctuations. Frequently, the importance of timely medication administration needs to be discussed and reinforced with informal and community-based caregivers. This is especially relevant to institutional settings (hospitals or nursing homes), where caregivers change from one shift and one day to the next. Staff may not be familiar with this aspect of PD, and may assume that antiparkinsonian medications, like many other medications, can be administered within an hour or two of the designated administration time.[4] Interventions that may allow for better symptom control are listed in Table 17.3.

Resistant symptom phase

Symptoms beginning during the resistant phase vary greatly from one individual with PD to the next. Almost any of the core or associated symptoms of PD can become resistant to therapy at some point in the illness. These symptoms may include freezing, frequent falls, severe fatigue, sleep cycle

Table 17.3 Interventions to improve on-time administration of antiparkinsonian medications during the motor complication phase

Educate patient and caregiver(s) about motor complications and the role of timely medication administration in symptom control

Medication reminder systems and timers, e.g., pillboxes with alarms

Informal caregiver management of medications

Home safety evaluations to evaluate environmental factors that hinder timely medication administration, e.g., patient keeps medications in another room that is inaccessible when patient is immobile because of "wearing-off"

Personal emergency response systems

Consultation with a dietician to evaluate whether dietary protein interferes with medication response

Consultation with a movement disorder specialist regarding medication regimen

disruption, executive dysfunction, autonomic dysfunction, constipation, urine retention and frequency, speech difficulties, swallowing difficulties, psychiatric complications and behavioral changes, as well as visual complications. The management of these specific problems, which are frequently superimposed on symptoms that arise during the motor complication phase, are discussed elsewhere in this book. During the period of resistant symptoms, the person with PD may also need assistance with instrumental ADLs, including shopping, managing finances, meal preparation, etc.

Involvement of a multidisciplinary healthcare team becomes even more important during this phase of the illness. Disciplines that should be considered when evaluating and treating a PD patient at this stage include movement disorder specialists, psychiatrists, registered nurses, physical therapists, occupational therapists, speech pathologists, dieticians, and family caregivers. These team members will be able to address pharmacological and non-pharmacological approaches, which are discussed further in other chapters in this book. Some specific help may be gathered in the following areas.

Physical therapy evaluation and treatment may include instruction in visual, auditory, and tactile cues to manage freezing, instruction in falling to prevent injury, instruction in a regular exercise regimen, and recommendations to use various assistive devices to prevent injury, e.g., protective hip pads and knee pads, use of a cane, including Step Over Canes® (freezing may decrease by using visual cues, inverting a cane),[5] that assist with management of freezing, rollator walkers (walkers with wheels on all four legs) or devices such as the U-Step Walking Stabilizer® (USWS, a walker with a reverse-braking system and tension-controlled wheels; In-Step Mobility Products Corp., Skokie, IL).[6] Occupational therapy evaluation and treatment may include home safety assessment, characterization of functional abilities including with instruments such as the Assessment of Motor and Processing Skills[7] recommendations to use adaptive devices or strategies to maximize function and safety, and driving assessment.

Speech and language pathology evaluation and treatment may include swallowing and feeding assessments with dietary recommendations to prevent aspiration.[8] Communication augmentation tools such as exercises to increase voice volume and improve communication are available, e.g. the Lee Silverman Voice Treatment Program.[9,10]

Additional specialist consultations, when symptoms cannot be adequately addressed by the movement disorder specialist, might include a urologist for evaluation and management of urine retention, recurrent infections, incontinence,[11] or sexual dysfunction, a gastroenterologist for management of severe constipation, a neuro-ophthamologist for management of double vision, dry eyes, and other ophthalmologic problems and a psychiatrist, if not already involved early in the disease, for management of the psychiatric issues.

Period of cognitive decline

As cognitive function declines, there is a growing dependency on others to provide total assistance with basic ADLs. The caregiver often meets this need along with the assistance of community-based long-term care services. Interventions that improve patient function and management at this stage include: further education of patient and caregiver, proper assessment and treatment of co-morbid psychiatric problems, maintenance of a daily routine to assist with organizational difficulties, orientation exercises, utilization of adult medical day programs, which provide a therapeutic milieu and respite for the caregiver, and consideration of other respite services and home care.[12] If a caregiver is not present, individuals who cannot tend to their basic physical needs may require placement in a long-term care facility.

Making the decision to use a nursing home facility

The decision to move into a nursing home after a 10–20-year disease course is often difficult for both the person with PD and for the caregiver. The progressive physical and cognitive decline contributes to the need for more assistance in ADLs and ultimately dependencies in ADLs as shown in Figure 17.1, limiting the feasibility of community-based care.[13] Multiple variables including psychosis,[14] older age, lack of a caregiver, immobility, falls, and cognitive decline[15] contribute to nursing home placement. European studies suggest that 5–10% of nursing home residents have PD.[16] Two American studies report prevalence rates of 5.2%[17] and 6.8%.[16] In both studies, the PD patients in nursing homes had severe dependencies in ADLs. Depression, polypharmacy, impairment of balance, communication and swallowing problems, bowel and bladder incontinence, and restraint use were all associated with the diagnosis of PD.[16] While the decision to place a patient in a nursing home is frequently difficult for patients and families, it is often the best option for meeting the complex needs of the patient with advanced PD.

Factors discouraging nursing home placement

Caregiver expectations and an unwillingness to relinquish control of a patient's care often argue against a decision to seek the assistance of nursing home professionals. Caregivers may feel considerable guilt or feel that they have failed the patient when they make this decision.[13] Concerns about finances, proper medication management, and general PD management may also deter the decision. Healthcare professionals can be instrumental in helping the patient and the caregivers to develop insight into their own feelings and recognize the value of using community-based or nursing home services. Anticipating these responses from the caregiver will enable healthcare professionals to assist the caregiver toward acceptance of the realities of long-term care services.

Role of the informal caregiver in the nursing home setting

After deciding to place a loved one in a nursing home, the caregiver quickly learns that his or her role has changed. Healthcare professionals with an established relationship with the caregiver may be able to educate the caregiver regarding the new realities of the nursing home setting. It is often a tremendous challenge for caregivers to accept that nursing homes cannot deliver one-on-one care. Caregivers may need to be encouraged to assume instead the role of supportive spouse or informal caregiver, an educator to staff about the PD-related care needs of the patient. The most important positive outcome from nursing home placement is the time and energy that the informal caregiver gains, which allows the caregiver to be a supportive spouse, devoted to their relationship with the person with PD. This additional time spent enjoying the company of their loved one is one of the benefits of nursing home placement. As an advocate and educator, caregivers should be encouraged to work proactively with the staff and develop a positive collaborative relationship. A first step towards a positive relationship with the staff of a nursing facility is to enlist the assistance of the nurse manager. Nurse managers are usually team leaders, who facilitate interactions of the multidisciplinary team and help solve identified problems. By contrast, direct criticism of the staff often sets the stage for a hostile relationship.

Specific care issues that arise in nursing home settings

Nursing home issues for patients with PD vary as much as the disease itself. Many of the issues that require increased physician attention are discussed in the chapters on dementia, psychosis and disinhibition. Table 17.4 provides a guide for other staff and family as to the possible approaches to common PD-related issues that often arise in the nursing home setting. Issues that arise commonly and are of particular concern are discussed below.

Timely administration of antiparkinsonian medications

Although PD patients comprise at least 5% of nursing home residents, parkinsonism tends to be underrecognized[18] suggesting that education about PD and parkinsonism is needed in this setting. At least via consultation, movement disorder specialists should be actively involved in clinical management of patients at this most fragile stage. Timely administration of antiparkinsonian medications is a major concern for most patients and caregivers when they enter any institutionalized setting. Since at least half of patients with PD experience motor fluctuations about 3–5 years into the illness,[3] medication use in PD patients will have been monitored carefully by most caregivers and a patient's neurologist for several years. At the time of entry into the nursing home, the most effective medication schedule has often been reached after months, even years, of fine-tuning. Depending on the severity of motor fluctuations, the medication regimen may be so regimented that doses of antiparkinsonian medications are administered at precise times to avoid disabling on-off fluctuations. Nursing home staff who are unfamiliar with advanced PD often need to be educated about motor

Table 17.4 Nursing home care plan guide for patients with Parkinson's disease

System	Problem	Suggested approaches
Cardiac	Hypotension	1. Monitor orthostatic blood pressure 2. Encourage to get up slowly 3. Consider a fall risk 4. Consider medication side effects 5. Liberalize salt if not contra-indicated 6. Encourage fluid intake 7. Consider medications to increase blood pressure 8. Assess for confusion
Gastro-intestinal	Constipation and potential impaction	1. Increase hydration 2. Increase fiber 3. Increase exercise 4. Laxatives 5. Monitor and record BMs 6. Assess bowel sounds 7. Assess for distention
Genito-urinary	Incontinence	1. Schedule toileting 2. Assess frequency and urgency 3. Urologic consult 4. Assess urine color, odor, and signs and symptoms of infection 5. Consider use of incontinence products, adult briefs, condom catheters, etc.
Integument	Potential skin breakdown	1. Turn and reposition every 2 hours 2. Encourage appropriate exercise 3. Assess skin regularly 4. Maintain adequate nutrition and hydration

continued

Table 17.4 continued

System	Problem	Suggested approaches
Neurologic	Decreased mobility and fall prevention	1. Develop maintenance exercise program 2. Consider medication timing relative to activity 3. Provide assist with ambulation as needed 4. Educate staff and enlist their assistance to assess on/off fluctuations, dyskinesias, and wearing off 5. Encourage use of walker or cane 6. Consider shoes, obstacles, room configuration, and nightlight 7. Maintain call light in close proximity 8. Physical therapy consult
Ophthalmologic	Double vision, dry eyes	1. Consider neuro-ophthalmologic consult 2. Glasses with prisms 3. Artificial tears 4. Talking books 5. Activities that don't require visual acuity
Psychosocial	Depression, psychosis, anxiety, and apathy	1. Psychiatric consult 2. Consider psychiatric medications 3. Consider timing of PD medication relative to mood changes 4. Assess activity interests 5. Engage in activity program 6. Recreation therapy and music therapy 7. Create structured environment and routine schedule
	Caregiver distress	1. Engage in care plan process 2. Maintain open communication 3. Encourage to articulate concerns 4. Validate appreciation for 10–20 years of informal caregiving 5. Encourage to share knowledge of PD

Table 17.4 continued

System	Problem	Suggested approaches
Speech and swallowing	Low voice volume and dysarthria	1. Speech language pathology (SLP) consult
		2. Encourage to speak slowly
		3. Encourage to speak loudly
		4. Follow SLP recommended exercises
		5. Communication augmentation devices
	Altered nutrition	1. Monitor weight
		2. Monitor intake of nutrition
		3. Dietician consult
		4. Assess calorie count
		5. Provide supplements
		6. Assess for dehydration
		7. Feed as needed
		8. Consider gastrostomy tube or PEG
	Aspiration potential	1. Assess for frequent coughing and choking at meals or with intake
		2. SLP evaluation and swallowing study
		3. Provide feeding assistance
		4. Encourage to tuck chin and swallow twice
		5. Select food of appropriate consistency

complications of PD and associated non-motor features, the importance of timely medication administration, and that the patient may suffer physically or psychiatrically if a dose is delayed or missed.

The very real need of the patient to have medication on time can become a major source of tension between families and staff if adequate steps are not taken to prevent or resolve problems. In some cases, patients become terrified that they will not receive their medications on time, and the associated anxiety or distress can be misinterpreted by staff. Likewise, family caregivers become concerned and then complain about having to stress the need to have medication administered on time when patients are hospitalized or in a nursing home setting. A particular obstacle in nursing homes is that medications are often administered two, three, or four times daily, and these regimens generally fall outside the range required by the patient with PD. While healthcare regulations may permit nurses to administer medications up to

2 hours before or after a prescribed time to give a medication, this is often inadequate for PD patients with motor fluctuations. Such patients may need to take antiparkinsonian medications every hour or every 2 hours, sometimes around the clock, and this regimen can be very difficult, if not impossible, for the staff of a long-term care facility to follow given staff:patient ratios and the competing demands of other patients. We strongly encourage family members and patients to address strategies to accommodate this unique need of the PD patient individually with the nursing facility staff. Importantly, nursing home staff often benefit from developing care plans that enable patients to complete tasks such as eating, brushing teeth, showering, and other therapies while in the "on" state with increased mobility and dexterity.[4]

Mobility

The management of mobility problems is a primary safety concern, but also a significant factor in the prevention of problems associated with immobility, such as contractures, incontinence, and skin breakdown. The goal of maintaining safe mobility is paramount when managing the individual with advanced PD. Physical therapy will help identify the most appropriate assistive device for each individual. Patients may need a cane, rollator walker, wheelchair, or scooter in order to retain safe mobilization. Regular exercise and strengthening regimens help maintain mobility. Nursing facilities should develop walking maintenance programs for this population.

The mobility problems of PD patients place them at risk for falls and fractures. Nursing home staff need to be aware of the potential development of postural hypotension and impairment of postural reflexes which contributes to greater fall risk.[19] When assessing the fall risk, nightrails, bathroom lights, and the location of the call bell must be considered. Some facilities may insist upon personal protective restraints that will limit mobility, but may prevent a catastrophic fall.

Feeding/nutrition

Mealtime for patients with advanced PD can be difficult for families. Drooling, choking, and food on the patient or floor can be unattractive and distressing for patients who have cognitive awareness or family members who are visiting. Consultation with dieticians and speech/language therapists may be helpful. To preserve dignity as much as possible, dietary staff may consider cutting food before it is placed at the table, serving softer food, and using utensils that will hold food during tremors. An occupational therapy assessment may also identify assistive devices or strategies that maximize function in this setting. Perhaps a patient needs softer food, as chewing may be difficult. Calorie counts and evaluation of the patient's ability to self-feed will guide interventions. Supplemental nutrition may be needed to provide adequate calories. Since silent aspiration can occur, the warning signs of coughing or choking during meals may not be present. A swallowing study will determine if the patient is aspirating. Physicians and/or dieticians may request weekly or more frequent weighing. Feeding tubes may be an option to discuss with the family.[19]

Speech/communication

Communication difficulties often arise and hinder patient care. In particular, patients can have difficulty communicating their needs or interacting socially with staff, other patients, and families. This can be the case in groups or in one-on-one interactions. Simple strategies need to be adopted, such as moving closer to the patient when speaking with them. Reminders to speak louder and more slowly may help as well.[19,20] PD patients may be able to utilize other forms of communication depending upon their motor ability. Consultation with a speech language therapist will assist the patient, family, and the team to identify other appropriate interventions for communication deficits.[19]

Bowel and bladder function

Autonomic dysfunction occurs in PD and contributes to disturbances in bowel and bladder function that are often a management issue for the patient and the staff. Encouraging patients to use the bathroom regularly may help decrease accidents. Toileting schedules as frequently as every 1–2 hours may be utilized. Use of pads, diapers or condom catheters for men may help ward off isolation. A urology consult for further suggestions, including surgery depending on how difficult this problem is to manage, may be necessary.

Sleep

Disturbances in the sleep–wake cycle may have contributed to nursing home placement. Sleep disturbances and their management are discussed further in Chapter 11. In nursing homes, common problems are that patients may nap often during the day and then experience nocturnal awakenings. There may be vivid dreams or REM behavior disorder (RBD) with agitation while sleeping.[21] Night-time staff need to be aware of these phenomena. Nocturnal enuresis and/or nocturnal immobility may contribute to disrupted sleep as well as skin breakdown and discomfort.[21]

Sweating

Many PD patients complain of sweating, especially in the "off" state or during periods of dyskinesia.[22] Sweating may be embarrassing as well as uncomfortable. Quality of life has been affected by sweating.[22] Suggestions to decrease sweating include: wearing lightweight clothes, keeping the temperature low, avoiding environments that are too hot, and considering medication regulation to decrease "off" periods and dyskinesias.[22]

Psychiatric symptoms

The prevalence of mood disorders in nursing home patients with PD is 20.3% or one in five residents.[23] Mood changes in PD patients are important to recognize, evaluate, and treat as appropriate since they frequently have adverse effects on overall functioning and impact caregivers as well as other aspects of the disease. In nursing homes, mood disorders can present significant challenges since they often accompany changes in sleep and appetite, as well as agitation and distress. These issues are addressed in Chapter 8.

As discussed further in Chapters 10 and 12, psychosis, agitated behavior and disinhibition can present as substantial management problems in nursing home settings. Hallucinations and delusions that are disruptive may contribute to aggressive behavior. As the severity of dementia increases, the frequency of behavior problems in PD patients in nursing homes increases.[24]

The physicians and nursing staff should be attuned to the prospect of behavioral disturbances in PD patients in nursing homes and establish procedures for alerting the physician and acute treatment. The management of these problems is discussed in Chapters 6, 10, and 12. Careful assessment and management of psychosis and other behavioral disturbances can achieve good symptom control without a significant decline in motor function.

Paranoia and/or disorientation and confusion may make patients combative when attempting to interact with them, such as when care is provided for ADLs. Patients may misinterpret their interactions with staff and may act aggressively.

Dementia in PD generally occurs in later stages and may contribute to nursing home placement. Dementia needs to be evaluated and treated by a specialist as discussed in Chapter 6. Additional options that may help orient and reassure patients include: keeping a calendar available to review dates and times every day or frequently during the day, placing a picture of the patient outside their bedroom door with their name so it can be seen as they enter, having pictures of significant family members and friends within their sight and labeled as to who they are and their relationship to the patient. Symptoms may be worse in the evening as with other nursing home patients ("sun-downing syndrome"), so routines should be kept consistent and simple. It may also be beneficial to complete as much as possible of the individual's care during the day and have the evening be very quiet with decreased stimulation.

End of life care

End of life care is frequently an issue in nursing homes because it is often the final residence for a patient. The patient who requires palliative care may not be able to tolerate dopaminergic therapy, may be unsuitable for surgery, and often has other illnesses occurring simultaneously.[25] In one study, the 3-year mortality rate of PD patients in long-term care was 50%, with aspiration pneumonia the primary cause of death.[26] Optimal care of the patients at the end stages of a neurodegenerative condition requires different types of inter-ventions by physicians and staff. Palliative care perspectives and approaches used for advanced cancer patients can also apply to patients with PD when curative treatment is no longer an option.[27] Ideally, clinicians will have had conversations about the end-stages of PD with the patient and family members well in advance of any significant demise. Discussions regarding comfort and supportive measures for pain, palliative care, and life support provide an understanding of the patient's values and encourage advanced care planning and decision-making. In the absence of such earlier conversa-tions, clinicians should be prepared to meet with families to discuss the patient's status and modify decisions as appropriate. Patients and families often need to decide whether the patient should have a feeding tube placed, be treated for recurrent medical problems, or be resuscitated. Referral to hospice may be an appropriate intervention. However, end of life does not mean end of care, so ongoing clinical assessment should aim to reduce troubling symptoms, including depression, pain, anxiety, or delirium. Families should be supported in their end of life decisions.

Nursing home staff have a unique opportunity to provide support during an emotional and often traumatic time for patients and their families. The need for families to discuss the issues surrounding the pending death of a loved one may come and go. The staff needs to be available to listen during set meetings and impromptu meetings with the family. The needs of family members may be very basic and concrete, such as "how to plan a funeral," or more abstract, including questions about religious beliefs related to death and dying.

Nursing home staff who make themselves available for discussions with the families about death and dying need to be comfortable with the topic and related issues. Staff need the opportunity to discuss these issues among themselves, as often PD patients may have been in the nursing home for a few years and staff may have developed a relationship with the patient and family. Death is a part of life, and is not a failure of the function of the staff.[19]

Conclusions

The long-term care of individuals with PD poses many challenges for clinicians, staff and caregivers. We need, though, to provide comprehensive care to the patient with PD throughout the course of the illness. As is the case with many chronic illnesses, the slow progressive debilitation requires multiple disciplines, as well as the patient and family, engaged in a constructive dialogue about the patient's health, both physical and mental. This dialogue must be dynamic in nature as clinical exigencies will change. The input of all interested parties will allow for the successful management of the individual with advancing PD.

Acknowledgments

Support for Ms Dunlop provided by the National Parkinson's Foundation (NPF) to the Johns Hopkins NPF Center of Excellence and for Ms Gerstenhaber by NIH (P50-NS-58366) for the Johns Hopkins Morris K. Udall Parkinson's Disease Research Center of Excellence.

References

1. *National Survey of Caregivers funded by MetLife Foundation.* AARP, July/Aug 2004.
2. Vickers LF, O'Neill CM, An interdisciplinary home healthcare program for patients with Parkinson's disease. *Rehabil Nurs* 1998; **23**(6):286–289, 299.

3. *Parkinson's Disease: The Life Cycle of the Dopamine Neuron.* Proceeds of meeting by NY Acad Sci, Fall 2003.

4. Rosto L, Promise for Parkinson's. *Advance for Providers of Post-Acute Care* 2004; **7**(3):44–47.

5. Dunne JW, Hankey GJ, Edis RH, Parkinsonism: upturned walking stick as an aid to locomotion. *Arch Phys Med Rehabil* 1987; **68**(6):380–381.

6. Harris-Love MO, Siegel KL, Paul SM, Benson K, Rehabilitation management of Friedreich ataxia: lower extremity force-control variability and gait performance. *Neurorehabil Neural Repair* 2004; **18**(2):117–124.

7. Pan AW, Fisher AG, The assessment of motor and process skills of persons with psychiatric disorders. *Am J Occup Ther* 1994; **48**(9):775–780.

8. McAndrews W, Making mobility manageable. *Advance for Providers of Post-Acute Care* 2004; **7**(3):48–49.

9. Ramig LO, Fox C, Sapir S, Parkinson's disease: speech and voice disorders and their treatment with the Lee Silverman Voice Treatment. *Semin Speech Lang* 2004; **25**(2):169–180.

10. Ramig LO, Sapir S, Countryman S et al, Intensive voice treatment (LSVT) for patients with Parkinson's disease: a 2 year follow up. *J Neurol Neurosurg Psychiat* 2001; **71**(4):493–498.

11. Rigby D, Whelan L, Parkinson's disease – continence management. *Nurs Times* 2001; **97**(30):65–66.

12. Belsky J, Disease, disability, and health care. In: Brace-Thompson J (ed.) *The Psychology of Aging Theory, Research, and Interventions*. Pacific Grove: Brooks/Cole Publishing Company, 1999; 131–163.

13. MacMahon T, Managing Parkinson's disease in long-term care. *Nursing Older People* 2002; **14**(9):23.

14. Goetz CG, Stebbins GT, Risk factors for nursing home placement in advanced Parkinson's disease. *Neurology* 1993; **43**(11):2227–2229.

15. Aarsland D, Larsen JP, Tandberg E, Laake K, Predictors of nursing home placement in Parkinson's disease: a population-based, prospective study. *J Am Geriatr Soc* 2000; **48**(8):938–942.

16. Mitchell SL, Kiely DK, Kiel DP, Lipsitz LA, The epidemiology, clinical characteristics, and natural history of older nursing home residents with a diagnosis of Parkinson's disease. *J Am Geriatr Soc* 1996; **44**(4):394–399.

17. Lapane KL, Fernandez HH, Friedman JH, Prevalence, clinical characteristics, and pharmacologic treatment of Parkinson's disease in residents in long-term care facilities. SAGE Study Group. *Pharmacotherapy* 1999; **19**(11):1321–1327.

18. Friedman JH, Fernandez HH, Trieschmann MM, Parkinsonism in a nursing home: underrecognition. *J Geriatr Psychiat Neurol* 2004; **17**(1):39–41.

19. Calne SM, Kumar A, Nursing care of patients with late-stage Parkinson's disease. *J Neurosci Nurs* 2003; **35**(5):242–251.

20. Coumarassamy M, Saravanan B, Nursing care of patients with Parkinson's disease – a rehabilitative view. *Nurs J India* 2002; **93**(11):253–254.

21. Crabb L, Sleep disorders in Parkinson's disease: the nursing role. *Br J Nurs* 2001; **10**(1):42–47.

22. Swinn L, Schrag A, Viswanathan R, Bloem BR, Lees A, Quinn N, Sweating dysfunction in Parkinson's disease. *Mov Disord* 2003; **18**(12):1459–1463.

23. Jones RN, Marcantonio ER, Rabinowitz T, Prevalence and correlates of recognized depression in U.S. nursing homes. *J Am Geriatr Soc* 2003; **51**(10):1404–1409.

24. Fernandez HH, Lapane KL, Ott BR, Friedman JH, Gender differences in the frequency and treatment of behavior problems in Parkinson's disease. SAGE Study

Group. Systematic Assessment and Geriatric drug use via Epidemiology. *Mov Disord* 2000; **15**(3):490–496.

25. Thomas S, MacMahon D, Parkinson's disease, palliative care and older people: Part 1. *Nurs Older People* 2004; **16**(1):22–26.

26. Fernandez HH, Lapane KL, Predictors of mortality among nursing home residents with a diagnosis of Parkinson's disease. *Med Sci Monit* 2002; **8**(4):CR241–CR246.

27. Low JA, Pang WS, Chan DK, Chye R, A palliative care approach to end-stage neurodegenerative conditions. *Ann Acad Med Singapore* 2003; **32**(6):778–784.

chapter 18

Advocacy and the Parkinson's disease community: a true triumph of the spirit

Laura Jane Cohen, Amy L Comstock and Benjamin J Kirby

"Advocacy means I put away self and serve others by standing up and educating, whether from public speaking, or published writings. Activism is about showing others how to become proactive instead of reactive . . . Advocacy to me is leaving the cause in better shape than when it was first found."

Terry Bowers, PAN Texas State Co-Coordinator and
young-onset Parkinson's disease patient

Though no scientific evidence exists to measure the impact of advocacy on individuals with chronic diseases and specifically Parkinson's disease, we believe that advocacy is one way for Parkinson's patients and their loved ones to recapture a sense of power over their lives. We have seen first hand the life-altering effects of successful advocacy efforts. In a sense, many patients feel as if they have gotten their voice back. As Joan Samuelson, the founder of the Parkinson's Action Network (PAN) has said, "The day you got your Parkinson's diagnosis, you joined a very empowered group of people."

As you will read in other chapters of this book, Parkinson's disease is an equal opportunity debilitative disease. It strikes young and old, rich and poor, male and female, with no regard for one's ability to handle the diagnosis, physically or mentally.

This disease strikes at the heart of all of our innate fears, "will I be able to ... take care of my family, take care of myself, keep my job, walk my daughter down the aisle, hold my grandchildren, enjoy my retirement, keep my independence, contribute to my marriage?" All of these questions are frightening and few can be answered in the moments after you are diagnosed. These questions are made all the more frustrating by the fact that the answer will be different for virtually everyone with Parkinson's disease.

What appears to be universal, however, in Parkinson's patients and their families, are the feelings that come with a diagnosis of Parkinson's disease. These feelings include helplessness, hopelessness, anger, sadness, fear, and denial among others. Some of our advocates have expressed their feelings after a Parkinson's diagnosis in the following ways:

"The idea of knowing there is a problem with your body and seeing it get worse over time can deteriorate one's well being. The walls of your home are a place that nobody sees on a day-to-day basis; walls that you can hide behind; walls that shut out the world ...

So, as this was happening to me, I began to hide. I did not want to go anywhere; I liked the walls of my home to hide behind. Not only did I hide behind the walls of my home, but also I began to build walls around me to hide behind in public, walls that I would eventually call the 'steel curtain.' I began to live on the computer, not going anywhere for days on end. I began to shut off my outside world and hide behind my curtain.

The steel curtain I hid behind began to strengthen, and I did anything I could to hide, like walking with my hands in my pockets. I would actually concentrate on everything I did to make myself look 'normal.' I found it very tiring to keep up my outer image, sometimes to the point of literal exhaustion. When I walked I had to think and concentrate on every step."

Michael Vest, PAN West Virginia State Coordinator and
young-onset Parkinson's disease patient

"When first diagnosed with Parkinson's, the Parkinson's brain takes us to a safe-haven ... a place called denial.

I remember going to Arizona in 1996 for a Parkinson's symposium. I taped every speaker that day on my cassette recorder. I figured that when I got back home to Las Vegas I would listen to the tapes. I never would have believed that it would be the year 2003 before I had the courage to listen to the tapes for the first time. All I did that day at the symposium was look around the room at all the people with Parkinson's. It was so depressing. I just kept thinking that I was going to look like those folks sooner than I cared to. I decided then that I didn't want to go to any support groups or anything that resembled what I had just seen. What I saw that day was ugly, scary, and unbelievably depressing. I needed to stay in my little safe haven in order to survive.

There was a problem though with that type of survival. How would I get better? If I stayed in denial, 'in a closet,' so to speak, how would anyone know that I existed? Back then I thought that everyone knew about Parkinson's disease and that it was just new to me. I thought that all the doctors, scientists, researchers, and politicians knew the cause, the cure, and all the idiosyncrasies of Parkinson's disease. So I was silent like almost everyone else with the disease. However, there were several people there that day at the symposium who were making a difference. One lady in particular, Joan Samuelson, founder and president of Parkinson's Action Network PAN, said, 'We will be invisible no more!'

Gale Lauer, PAN Nevada State Coordinator and
young-onset Parkinson's disease patient

The advocacy work that PAN does continues to empower patients and their loved ones by giving them back a sense of ownership over their disease and their lives. That sense comes from the feeling that they have some measure of control over their disease, that they, not just the scientists with beakers and Bunsen burners, have the ability to affect positive change in Parkinson's disease. We see that patients who advocate for what they need and deserve feel they are making a difference, not only for themselves, but for future generations who may be diagnosed with Parkinson's disease.

We have also found that the positive feelings patients get from advocacy are typically not diminished whether or not they believe that their advocacy will directly impact their own disease. Many examples of this are evident at our annual Research and Education Forum & Public Policy Forum. At the Forum, patients and their loved ones from around the country come to Washington, DC, to learn about the latest research in Parkinson's disease and learn the tools to become a Parkinson's advocate. The Forum concludes with all the participants attending meetings on Capitol Hill to speak with their Members of Congress about Parkinson's disease and what the Members can do to help.

One example from a recent Forum involved a long-time Parkinson's patient in his seventies who went to meet with his Member of Congress with a group of other Parkinson's patients. At the meeting, the gentleman turned to his Member of Congress and said "It's too late for you to help me, but I am here because it is not too late to help her." At this, he pointed to his friend, a 35-year-old Parkinson's patient with three young children at home. At the end of the day, he told us that the Forum was one of the most uplifting experiences he had had since being diagnosed.

The Forum has become so much more than a conference for our advocates. For many, it has become a pivotal event in how they view themselves and the disease.

> "As many people with Parkinson's spoke out for the first time, and lobbied their senators and representatives, they learned that they could indeed make a difference. As we became more visible, vocal and empowered as individuals, so did the Parkinson's community as a whole."
>
> Linda Herman, PAN New York State Coordinator and
> young-onset Parkinson's disease patient

"My introduction to PAN came from my dear friend Jaye. In a few short weeks of planning, I found myself at the 9th Annual Public Policy Forum for PAN.

After many people commented that I was not showing symptoms for some time, I decided to let my guard down and began to let some of my symptoms show. It was a true relief for me and it felt good to relax. When information began to flow at the PAN forum, I could concentrate on the speaker and not so much as to how I looked.

I fit in with a group that knew exactly how I felt. I feel thankful for those who said those words to me that led me to put down my guard. A special bond took place talking with those people who understood. A few times the best conversations were not focused on Parkinson's disease but just things we enjoy as people.

The kindness of people and the helpfulness I experienced will carry me on a journey that has been started by so many wonderful people. Their work will continue but now has the added support of many more getting involved. I have been shown a path and this path will give me a chance to talk with Parkinson's disease patients in my state and how they view topics of research and of government issues. I feel I should do my duty and be a voice for those who have lost their own. I want to extend my thanks to those who have helped me find my way in this Parkinson's community. My personal steel curtain has fallen, and I believe I am going to continue to let this curtain fall. Thank you to those who helped me at PAN."

Michael Vest, PAN West Virginia State Coordinator and
young-onset Parkinson's disease patient

"I have become an advocate to help get the funding necessary to find the cure for Parkinson's disease. I am obligated to myself and everyone else who has Parkinson's disease, Alzheimer's, movement disorders, and spinal cord injuries. I am obligated to get the message out. Once the cure for Parkinson's is found, the cure for other neurological disorders will follow.

I became an advocate to get people to understand what it is like to have Parkinson's. You wouldn't know it by looking at me or spending a few days with me, but I am in the later stages (the fourth of five stages) of Parkinson's.

I became an advocate because I believe we are so close to finding the cure for Parkinson's. We are so close. If we weren't so close, I wouldn't care as much, but I am truly in a race against time. The fact is that the brain cells I need are dead and I am dying.

I am determined to make advocacy a big part of my life. After all, suffering with Parkinson's has been a big part of it. Now I want to be a part of getting Parkinson's disease eradicated. I am invisible no more. Hear me rrrroar!"

Gale Lauer, PAN Nevada State Coordinator and
young-onset Parkinson's disease patient

"To me though, the best thing about the Forum was the people who attended. Since my diagnosis, I have met some great people, who know and understand what life is like with Parkinson's disease. I have never been together with so many of them at one time. I was very touched by what a close-knit family we are, and if anyone ever feels like they are alone with this disease, all they have to do is attend a function like the Forum, and they will know that they will never be alone."

Michael O'Leary, PAN Arizona State Coordinator and
young-onset Parkinson's disease patient

PAN has established a State and Congressional Advocacy Coordinator Program. This program began with five State Advocacy Coordinators and in just 1 year has grown to 59 Coordinators in 39 states and the District of Columbia. PAN aims to have coordinators in all states and will add more in certain key Congressional districts. This program is a critical component of the work that PAN does. Our "unified voice" is the voice of many people in the Parkinson's community working with us towards a cure.

In fact, PAN's "unified voice" not only speaks for the advocates in the Parkinson's community. PAN is proud to be supported by other major national Parkinson's organizations; the National Parkinson Foundation, The Michael J. Fox Foundation for Parkinson's Research, the Parkinson's Disease Foundation, the Parkinson Alliance and Unity Walk, and the American Parkinson Disease Foundation. These organizations not only provide financial assistance to PAN, but are also in regular communication with PAN about our legislative agenda. We all share the same ultimate goal: finding a cure for Parkinson's disease and easing the burden. Never has the community come together in such a way as they have through PAN and we are very pleased to be able to be a conduit for increased collaboration.

> "We all study civics in high school, but most of us have forgotten everything except perhaps the rudimentaries. Somewhere between the Declaration of Independence and the Gettysburg Address we seem to recall that we the People are the government, we are responsible for our own governance. To discharge our duty we must participate in the process. Granted, for most people that means being an informed voter. But we are thrust into a unique situation when we become ill with Parkinson's disease.
>
> We have the opportunity to become patient advocates, able to represent thousands of similarly afflicted people to ensure that we get the public funding necessary for effective research into the cause and cure of Parkinson's disease. Our voices carry an authority beyond any others. This is our disease, this is our life and this will be our death if we are not cured. That is our message and that is what we must shout through the halls of Congress and the White House until we are not only heard but ultimately cured and, thus, freed."
>
> Ann Campbell Wasson, PAN Northern California State Co-Coordinator
> and young-onset Parkinson's disease patient

Joan Samuelson began the Parkinson's Action Network (PAN) in 1991 because she correctly believed that Parkinson's disease was not receiving enough funding or attention from the federal government. We have made great progress since 1991, but there is still a lot for PAN and PAN advocates to do. We do not yet have a cure, and better treatments for Parkinson's disease still need to be found. Because of this, PAN will continue to increase awareness about Parkinson's disease, and will continue to advocate for increased federal funding for many other federal programs.

Although we will continue to fight until a cure is found, PAN has a track record of success. For example, PAN successfully urged Congress to direct the National Institutes of Health to develop a first-of-its-kind Parkinson's Disease Research Agenda – a 5-year plan that called for a $1 billion investment in Parkinson's research. PAN played – and will continue to play – a key role in supporting the Department of Veterans Affairs "Parkinson's Disease Research, Education and Clinical Centers." PAN led the effort to enact the Morris K. Udall Parkinson's Disease Research Act of 1997 – the first law to focus entirely on the need to expand the Parkinson's disease research program administered by the NIH. PAN was the principal advocate for congressional language supporting NIH Director Elias Zerhouni's "Road Map" initiatives. The language, adopted by the House of Representatives, authorized substantial funding for these initiatives and urged the Director to emphasize "translational research," expediting the delivery of new treatments and cures from the laboratory to the bedside. PAN has increased our partnerships on Capitol Hill. In February 2004, PAN was a leader in creating the first Bi-Cameral Parkinson's Disease Working Group/Caucus. There are 70 Members of the House and Senate participating in this important Caucus, and the numbers will continue to grow.

"The amount of money spent on research into the cause and treatment of Parkinson's disease is directly effected by the political process and our participation, or lack of participation, in it.

We are at a crossroads. We can sit on our rumps and complain about our aches and pains and wait to die. Or we can believe in our own power to affect our future and change our own prognosis."

Greg Wasson, PAN Northern California State Co-Coordinator and young-onset Parkinson's disease patient

Another unique phenomenon in this community is the presence of individuals at the Forum and other advocates involved with PAN who have lost their loved one with Parkinson's disease. Many of our State and Congressional Coordinators are the children, siblings, and spouses of Parkinson's patients who have passed away. This really speaks to the overarching feeling that advocacy gives to all people. It is truly the sense that you are having a part in changing the world – and not just your world. At PAN, we have a unique opportunity to get to know Parkinson's patients before they become involved with advocacy and after they become advocates. The change in them is tremendous. Even as their symptoms eventually worsen, their spirits remain unmoved.

In the words of one of our advocates:

"There is no limit to what we can accomplish if we empower people with Parkinson's disease."

Perry Cohen, PAN Washington, DC,
Coordinator and Parkinson's disease patient

We urge you to get involved. The benefits to you, your loved ones, and others who have this illness, are great. Appendix B lists contacts for various organizations involved in advocacy for PD. You can also check with your neurologist for organizations in your area.

chapter 19

Caregiving

Geoffrey W Lane, Lee Hyer and Gerald Leventhal

Introduction

The vast majority of care for people with PD is provided by family members rather than paid or professional caregivers.[1] While this help is willingly given, it often comes at a cost; sleepless nights, emotional exhaustion, and financial sacrifice. Caregiving cannot be successful over a sustained period unless the caregiver's health, daily functioning, and quality of life are protected. Effective help for caregivers is that which holds caregiver stress at an acceptable level, buttresses the caregiver's psychological adjustment and health, and at the same time fosters effective caregiving behaviors. Helping PD caregivers learn better ways to emotionally and practically cope with the severe physical decline, unique to PD, needs to go hand-in-hand with treating the medical problems specific to PD patients themselves.

Additionally, the economic costs of PD are substantial,[2] but cost estimates may not consider the economic impact of informal caregiving by family members or forced changes in their outside employment. For example, family members often serve as unpaid caregivers; the occurrence of PD may force changes in family members' job activities, e.g., a wife who had never worked must now become the breadwinner due to her husband's illness.[3]

Most research on caregiving has focused on Alzheimer's dementia (AD), with Parkinson's disease (PD) receiving relatively little attention.[4,5] Nonetheless, this chapter will review what is known about caregiving in PD and will show that the problems faced by PD caregivers are distinct from those faced by caregivers who tend to the needs of family members that suffer from other neurodegenerative illnesses. In addition, we will make recommendations on how to reduce stress in caregivers and maximize both the function of the patient with PD and the relationship with the caregiver.

Who are the caregivers and what are their roles?

A caregiver is one who helps a patient manage tasks of daily living, including the management of symptoms and the integration of the patient's treatment regimen into his or her patterns of daily life. Most caregiving for persons with PD is provided by family members rather than paid or professional caregivers.[1] The roster of caregivers includes family members of all types, but their efforts are often supplemented by nurses' aides who reside in or work in the PD patient's place of residence, whether at home or in a long-term care setting.[1]

Family caregivers are one of three clusters of supports that are crucial for the PD patient's care and well-being. A second cluster involves the team of medical practitioners, e.g., neurologist, primary care geriatrician, psychiatrist, geropsychologist, physical therapist, etc. This team's task is to diagnose problems, conduct ongoing assessment, and monitor disease progression, and prescribe and evaluate the effectiveness of treatment regimens. Family caregivers interface with the medical team in various ways that are crucial to the PD patient's medical care and quality of life. For example, caregivers may transport a PD patient to medical appointments, provide information to medical team members about the patient or the patient's home environment, and accept guidance and follow instructions from medical team members with respect to the PD patient's care. The third cluster of care support comes from the patient himself whose personal health beliefs and behaviors are critical for effective PD disease management, particularly for the patient's daily interactions with family caregivers. By definition, family caregivers interface frequently and intensively with their family member with PD. It is important that caregivers and the PD patient share a common frame of reference and agree on major aspects of what is necessary and helpful. Without such agreement, the quality of caregiving will be compromised.

Symptoms most relevant to the PD caregiving situation

Our discussion of PD caregiving is based on the assumption that every debilitating chronic disease generates a specific profile of caregiving demands and burdens, a profile that is unique to that illness.[6] However, we further recognize that there are many similarities across chronic diseases in the challenges posed for caregivers. Though the profile of demands and burdens may differ from one disease entity to the next, there is much overlap.[7,8] For example, regardless of disease entity, the onset and progression of debilitating chronic illness in a family member are likely to force changes in the family division of labor, impose limitations on caregivers' pursuit of other life goals, and generate anxiety, frustration, and strained relationships. Regardless of the disease entity, and of whether the caregiver is a spouse or an adult child, the caregiver is likely to experience high psychological cost, and the caregiver's patience, tolerance for stress, and problem-solving skills will surely be tested.[9–12]

That said, an important guiding assumption here is an emphasis on primary stressors, i.e., the activities that PD caregivers must perform as a direct result of the current state of the patient's illness, the treatments, and the patient's reactions to the illness.[12,13] While caregivers may differ greatly in how they adapt to the stresses of caregiving, it is the properties of the disease and its treatment that drive the PD patient's behavior and care needs, and in turn, drive the care demands to which the caregiver must respond. Table 19.1 lists aspects of the disease that impact caregiver tasks. The table also includes aspects of the patient's health behaviors, personality, and psychiatric status that impact the pattern of care demands and caregiver burden.

With a diagnosis of PD comes a number of disabling symptoms specific to the disorder that can be highly distressing for the patient and caregiver. The most salient ones related to the caregiver include movement and neuromuscular control problems, severe functional and physical problems, cognitive decline, problems with sleep, and emotional problems.

Movement and neuromuscular control problems

Mobility and physical safety are pre-eminent concerns for the PD patient and PD caregiver.[14–16] Problems with moving safely and performing motor tasks central to daily living, e.g., dressing, getting out of bed, avoiding falls, etc., are a direct consequence of the symptomatic features of PD. Though

> **Table 19.1** Characteristics of patient's disease status, health behavior, personality, and emotional and cognitive behavior that impact caregiver's tasks and role
>
> 1. *Disease status*
>   Rate of progression (highly variable)
>   Complexity of symptom pattern; idiopathic PD as primary vs PD plus other Parkinsonian co-morbidities
>   Level of physical impairment, e.g., risk of falls, ability for self-care, general medical co-morbidities
>   Cognitive and neurological status
>
> 2. *Health behavior and beliefs*
>   Self-regulation concepts that the patient brings to the task of disease management
>   Self-monitoring of current biological and psychological function
>
> 3. *Personal and emotional qualities that affect collaboration with caregiver*
>   Emotional reactions and psychiatric status; depressed mood, anxiety, etc.
>   Independence–dependence; comfort with/resistance to accepting help; overreliance on others' assistance
>   Sense of entitlement; interpersonal demandingness

dramatic behavioral dyscontrol problems are rare in the earlier stages of PD, problems such as freezing, "on-off" periods, and gait difficulties, are sources of strain for caregivers.

Cognitive decline

Dementia is not a central feature of PD,[17] but memory and cognitive problems generally develop.[18,19] In fact, as discussed in Chapters 5, 6, and 7, there exists a spectrum of cognitive deficits in PD that includes mild cognitive impairment, presenting with problems in multiple cognitive domains,[20] as well as dementia, with a profile of unique features involving a dysexecutive syndrome and visuospatial and behavioral symptoms[19] and co-morbid with features of other dementias.[21] While the exact neuropsychological profile differs for any individual, symptoms generally include difficulty with apathy, judgment, impulsivity, and memory.[22]

There are many cases in which core PD symptoms are accompanied by both cognitive and physical co-morbidities. From the perspective of PD caregiving issues, these co-morbidities can be viewed as additional burdens. For example, in many cases, dementia evolves later in the course of PD and may even represent the co-occurrence of Alzheimer's disease (AD) pathology superimposed on PD.[11] In cases of dementia with Lewy bodies, some form of dementia or cognitive dysfunction is present when parkinsonian symptoms are first noted.[23] It is in these cases that the role of the PD caregiver is less distinct from that of the typical AD family caregiver. When PD and dementia converge,[24] the role of the PD caregiver and AD caregiver also converge and become more similar with respect to the profile of care demands. However, the physical burdens of care may be greater for the PD caregiver, especially when the dementia is in its earlier stages but motor symptoms are relatively more advanced.

Sleep problems

Disordered sleep is a common co-occurring problem in PD; patients may suffer from a variety of difficulties, which are reviewed in Chapter 11. These sleep difficulties have profound implications for the health and well-being of the PD caregiver.[25,26] Insomnia, the most common sleep disorder seen in PD often leads to sleep deprivation in the caregiver, resulting in exhaustion during the day. Bed partners may also be at risk for injury as many of the sleep disorders include abnormal behavior during sleep, from restlessness to wild thrashing. Comella et al.[27] looked at a small sample of PD patients and their caregivers and found that 5% of the patients reported that they had injured their sleeping partner, a result replicated in other studies.[28]

Other potentially troublesome sleep problems that PD patients (and their caregivers) may encounter include excessive daytime sleepiness and "sleep attacks",[25] which are potentially disabling.

Procedures that reduce PD patients' sleep problems are an important target area for improving their quality of life and also for decreasing caregiver burden. We urge caregivers to discuss these problems with the appropriate medical professions. A thorough discussion of the treatment of sleep disorders can be found in Chapter 11.

Psychiatric difficulties

Depression and anxiety are found in approximately 50% of those with PD.[29,30] The loss of mental energy, initiative, self-esteem, as well as the dysphoric mood and feelings of worthlessness, that accompany depression may have profound implications for caregivers.[31] The loss of vitality and enjoyment can make the caregiving relationship less satisfying, and so reduce his or her motivation and personal investment in the caregiving process. Again, caregivers should bring these problems to the attention of the appropriate medical professional. Advice on how to manage these problems is found in other chapters in this book.

Patients with PD frequently experience psychotic symptoms, including hallucinations and delusions (fixed, false beliefs) which result in significant stress and challenge for the family caregivers in the home.[32-34] Delusions and hallucinations are particularly burdensome as they are resistant to reasoning and may be persecutory. That is, the patients may develop the belief that their spouse is being unfaithful or that the spouse intends to harm them. Placed in the context of caregiving, in which the spouse may have sacrificed considerably to continue to care for the individual with PD, one can easily see the distress that would ensue. In fact, in a Norwegian sample studied by Aarsland et al.[32] the presence of hallucinations was the strongest predictor of placement in institutions such as nursing homes. Furthermore, hallucinations were found to be a major burden for PD caregivers, and thereby are likely to lead to institutionalization (Goetz as cited in reference 35).

The problems with sleep, depression, hallucinations, and psychotic symptoms may be important targets for medical as well as psychosocial intervention in order to improve the well-being of PD caregivers and care recipients.[36] The treatment of these disorders is specifically addressed in other chapters in this book.

Stress and social support in the patient–caregiver dyad

Stress management for PD caregivers is important because it affects the patient's clinical status and quality of life, but also because stress can have serious adverse physical health consequences for the caregiver.[37,38] Managing stress must be based on a recognition that caregiving involves an ongoing interaction between two participants, the patient and the caregiver. Each party is coping with stress from his or her own perspective, and so the process cannot be understood unless that perspective is considered.[39]

Caregivers and patients also form an interactive pair, and the stress of one party can quickly become the stress of the other. Interventions that reduce the patient's stress then are likely to reduce the caregiver's stress. Conversely, interventions that are effective for the caregiver and result in more effective caregiving are likely to reduce the patient's stress. Caregivers who fail to adequately adjust to demands of the caregiving situation are more likely to trigger problem behaviors in the patient. Schulz et al.[40] report that dementia caregivers who are depressed trigger higher levels of patient problem behaviors, e.g., wandering and agitation. Additionally, when caregivers adopt a more personal, supportive style of relating, the patients display better adjustment.[4] From the PD patient's perspective, it is difficult to over-state the importance of a stable, emotionally supportive caregiving environment as shown in the poignant comments of one PD sufferer.[16]

> My disabilities become distinctly greater at the time of some break in the habits of daily living to which I have become accustomed. Even babysitting for our grandchildren for a weekend, in our own home, can produce repercussions: exaggerated tremor, more fatigue and nighttime insomnia, . . . more difficulty in moving about. All are no doubt related to feelings of insecurity – fear of being unable to avert some impending accident. I can't even imagine the effect of a serious emotional clash with one of my loved ones. I fear that in my present semi-dependent situation, such a confrontation would devastate me. Constant reassurance that my loved ones are supportive, patient, caring, understanding, and loving is, I believe, my greatest asset and most secure source of happiness.
>
> (p. 74)

From the PD caregiver's perspective, providing effective, supportive care-giving yields benefits to the caregiver as well as the PD patient. The patient's improved response fosters a positive feedback loop resulting in greater social support for the PD caregiver and so has a stress-protective effect on the care-giver. However, there are situations in which, despite the caregiver's best efforts, a negative feedback loop exists between PD patient and PD caregiver that increases caregiver stress and diminishes the caregiver's personal satisfaction as shown in the pained comments of one PD caregiver cited by Greenberg[41] (p. 19).

> My mother has always been domineering and now my brother and I know what my father went through. She has had home-health aides, but none was good enough for her. She complained about each one. This one left a dish in the sink; that one didn't like her, etc. . . . She tells me if I were a "good daughter" I would come over and do the things an aide

does. I have always been a good daughter; in fact, I was never able to say no to her, but now I don't know what to do. I have a career which I love and need, two teenage children who need me, and a husband who is furious with me, because at the end of the day I have nothing left for him and the kids. All I do is talk about my mother, to my friends, to my relatives; she has become an obsession. If my mother falls and there is no one there to help her she'll fall again, maybe hurt herself more seriously this time, and it will be my fault.

Approaches at ameliorating caregiver stress are best that take account of several clusters of variables involved in the stress process. The first cluster has already been outlined in Table 19.1 and consists of primary stressors, e.g., the specific stresses associated with caring for a relative who has problems of gait, dysphagia, "freezing," etc. The second cluster consists of mediators of stress, e.g., the individual caregiver's personal appraisals of events, coping resources and skills, and relevant personality characteristics. The third cluster consists of situational and background factors related to stress, e.g., the immediate physical environment in which caregiving takes place, the availability and effective utilization of social supports, etc.

Table 19.2 lists some personal resources that can mediate caregiver stress and effectiveness, e.g., knowledge of the illness, caregiving skills, stress tolerance, patience, stamina, and comfort and satisfaction with the caregiving role. The table also outlines other factors that mediate caregiver stress and effectiveness, including the quality of the caregiver's past relationship with the patient, the availability of material resources and social supports from other helpers, and other life demands on the PD caregiver. It is likely that these other factors that affect PD caregivers are similar to those that affect caregivers for other degenerative disorders. Thus, PD caregiver characteristics, such as age (elderly versus middle-aged) or gender (women on average being better prepared for and more comfortable with caregiving roles), are likely to affect PD caregivers' motivation, stamina, and satisfaction with caregiving in the same way they affect other varieties of caregiver.[42,43] Finally, as memory and cognitive abilities decline, caregiving problems become more severe and more formal care services are required, especially for patients with PD.[44]

Table 19.2 Caregiver personal resources and contextual factors that mediate caregiver stress

1. *Personal resources*
   Health knowledge and beliefs related to PD, PD treatments, and PD course
   Mastery of knowledge and skills relevant to caregiving tasks; problem solving ability; past experience and training in caregiving roles
   Stress tolerance and stress coping skills; patience; resilience against burnout; physical and emotional stamina
   Motivation, commitment, and satisfaction with caregiving roles and activities; altruistic orientation

2. *Quality of past and current personal relationship with PD patient*
   Marital satisfaction
   Adult child's relationship to parent

3. *Availability of material resources and social support*
   Quality of physical environment in which caregiving takes place
   Assistance from other family members
   Assistance from home health aids, friends, and other non-family helpers
   Financial factors that affect ability to hire personnel, acquire special equipment, etc.

4. *Other life demands on caregiver*
   Outside job/occupation
   Young children in the home

Intervention

While there is little formal research in this area, several therapeutic approaches have been employed to alleviate PD caregiver stress and maximize caregiver effectiveness. The following is a discussion of several aspects of the caregiving process that may be useful to caregivers.

Problem-focused and psychoeducational intervention

Caring for a spouse or loved one who is not cognitively impaired, but is significantly impaired in both instrumental and primary activities of living (e.g., talking, eating, moving) is a common problem for the PD caregiver. Qualitative research on the experience of PD caregivers indicates they are greatly disturbed by their loved one's loss of motor skills and loss of function.[45,46] Wallaghen and Brod (as cited in reference 4) report that the best predictor of caregiver burden in PD caregivers is the feeling of control over the patient's symptoms, a finding consistent with the idea that PD caregivers are likely to favor problem-focused coping methods.[39] In this view, the caregivers' efforts should be directed at the specific nature of the stress-producing problems that confront them.[5] In the case of PD, this involves attending to the PD patient's motor control problems. The PD patient finds it increasingly difficult to perform tasks of daily living such as buttoning one's clothes, putting on socks, using a knife to cut food, getting out of bed, and so forth. Such deficits are sources of stress the PD patient and PD caregiver must deal with. For example, a retired heart surgeon with PD described his problem with tying shoelaces and his wife's assistance as follows.[16]

> Consider the technical challenge of tying my shoelaces – a skill that had, over the past few years … virtually vanished. My fingers had become strangers to the task. They just didn't know what to do, even after many trials. More and more frequently, my wife had to come tie the laces – how humiliating for a once dexterous surgeon! … So I set out to give myself lessons in shoelace tying …
>
> (p. 141)

In this instance, the patient, himself, a highly resourceful, intelligent man, was able to initiate a trial-and-error learning process that involved analysis of the movements in knot tying and weeks of intensive practice. Through careful observation and persistence, he was able to recover some portion of a lost skill he had first learned as a child – only a temporary victory in the face of PD's unrelenting progression, to be sure, but a victory nonetheless.

From the caregiver's perspective, the daughter of an elderly PD patient described the difficulties of coping with the problem of her mother's slow, poorly coordinated movements when they went shopping.[41]

> With her halting gait and poor balance, it would take us almost 5 minutes to maneuver the 30 yards, replete with seven steps, to my car. This slow pace would remain unchanged throughout the day. Further restraint and patience would be required of me in the shopping process itself. Respecting my mother's strong wish to be independent, I would merely stand by as she painstakingly got in and out of her garments to try on clothes, not allowing me to assist her with anything, save perhaps a difficult button on the sleeve.

Although I would grit my teeth in exasperation and anger, I could not help but admire her courage and tenacity. That I love my mother and her company were not enough to stave off the complete exhaustion I would experience at the end of our sojourn together. The strain of constant vigilance combined with the slowing down of my normal rhythm to remain in sync with hers would wipe me out.

(p. 46)

This caring daughter would benefit from problem-focused intervention that would reduce stress and help her continue her caregiving tasks with renewed energy and a sense of inner calm.

Hooker et al.[42] provide empirical support for the view that PD caregivers frequently focus on problems generated by the PD patient's motor dysfunctions. They studied 175 spouse caregivers of PD and AD patients and found that, compared with AD caregivers, PD caregivers were more likely to respond to their stressful situation by engaging in coping strategies that were largely problem-focused. Other data indicate that PD caregivers are likely to favor and accept prescriptive therapeutic interventions[47,48] that emphasize education, practical problem solving, and externally focused therapeutic content[42,49] as opposed to inwardly, emotionally focused interventions and therapy content.

Educational interventions are a fruitful area to target for the caregiver. In Table 19.3, we outline four general areas an educational program should address. They include assuring that the caregiver has: (1) a valid biomedical understanding of PD disease process and treatment; (2) an ability to accurately evaluate the PD patient's current physical and emotional states and cognitive capacity; (3) a broad range of effective caregiving responses from which the caregiver can select; (4) an enhanced ability to monitor his own stress and utilize appropriate self-care and stress-coping procedures to manage stress.

Family therapy intervention

There is evidence from qualitative and survey-based data that the spouses of patients with PD experience considerable stress on family relationships, and on key family issues such as maintaining privacy and independence.[45] Greene and Griffin[50] found that marital quality significantly influenced symptoms, a finding that suggests that the quality of at least some parkinsonian symptoms may be influenced by the quality of the caregiver–care

Table 19.3 Potential areas to cover in effective PD caregiver educational interventions

1. *Assure biomedical validity of caregiver understanding of PD disease process and treatment*
   Provide realistic expectations re the course and progression of PD
   Increase understanding of potential medication side-effects that increase patient and caregiver stress

2. *Enhance caregiver ability to correctly assess PD patient's current biological and emotional states, and level of cognitive functioning*
   Enhance ability to correctly interpret changes in patient's state, especially short-term fluctuations associated with L-dopa therapy as the patient moves through on/off phases
   Enhance ability to recognize how patient's deficits/impairment are linked to patient's emotional reactions (e.g., anxiety/depressed mood) and how these emotional reactions in turn affect patient functioning

3. *Expand caregiver's array of effective alternative caregiving responses from which caregiver can select those that best fit the PD patient's current need*
   Provide tips and guidance for managing the patient's problems of movement and neuromuscular dyscontrol, and for insuring patient safety
   Provide tips and guidance re steps to encourage patient compliance with treatment, and maximize patient self-reliance

4. *Enhance caregiver's ability to recognize and effectively manage his own stress*
   Educate in personal stress recognition, basic self-care, and stress coping methods
   Educate re available community resources and in methods for mobilizing support from other family members

recipient relationship. This impact of the spousal relationship on the management of the disease is further supported by research showing that the level of expressed (negative) emotion between AD caregivers and AD care recipients predicts poorer outcomes.[51]

These findings imply that couples therapy may be a valuable treatment for caregivers. Indeed, there is already a manualized "relationship enhancement therapy" that has been successfully piloted with patient–caregiver couples.[45] There appears to be considerable promise for further application of family therapy approaches to managing stress and improving caregiver effectiveness in the PD caregiving situation.[6,8,52] Certainly, it is reasonable to direct couples to marital therapy if there is difficulty in their relationship.

Intensiveness of therapeutic intervention

Research suggests that caring for a patient with PD who is not cognitively impaired is less stressful overall than caring for a loved one who is significantly cognitively impaired.[42] Consequently, an intervention to reduce stress for the average PD caregiver may require less intensive intervention than for the average AD caregiver. For example, fewer sessions may be necessary to achieve significant change in the life of a stressed PD caregiver, and there may be less need for antidepressant or anxiolytic medication.[53] That said, issues related to personality or meaning may become prepotent and deserve attention.

Patient participation in interventions to manage caregiver stress

We have emphasized the caregiver side of the issue but efforts to manage caregiver stress must also consider the patient's potential to serve as an active participant in stress management interventions. The design of PD caregiver interventions then should allow for significant involvement and input from the PD care recipients themselves,[49,54] as this would maximize the chances of significant therapeutic change. Several coping strategies, including relaxation, skills training, and communication may be helpful. But, as we noted above, the patient's level of cognitive impairment has special significance for crafting stress management interventions for caregivers.[53]

Cognitive functions in PD tend to be preserved in PD to a much greater degree than in AD, and so it is feasible to directly involve the patient in interventions that will benefit the caregiver. As implied above, cognitive impairment becomes a more notable problem at later stages of PD, at which time patients may then have reduced capacity to participate in voluntary planned actions to ameliorate caregiver stress.

Outcome assessment in PD caregiving

Because caregiving is a two-sided process, it is necessary to have criteria for assessing the impact of therapeutic intervention on both the PD caregiver and the patient. From the caregiver's side, caregiving cannot be successful over a sustained period unless the caregiver's health, daily functioning, and quality of life are protected. Effective caregiver interventions are those that hold caregiver stress at an acceptable level, buttress the caregiver's psychological adjustment and health, and at the same time foster effective caregiving behaviors. The first section of Table 19.2 presented a partial list of criteria that can be used to evaluate the PD caregiver's success in adapting to demands of the caregiving process. The caregiver's personal resources must be sufficient to meet the demands of the caregiving situation, including sustained effectiveness in problem-solving, stress-coping, stamina, motivation for caregiving, satisfaction with the caregiving role, and mastery of skills and knowledge necessary for performing caregiving tasks.

With respect to criteria for assessing the PD patient's outcomes, the criteria must be based on whether the goals of caregiving are achieved, i.e., whether the caregiving process succeeds in maximizing the PD patient's health, daily functioning, and quality of life. Table 19.4 presents a caregiver-centered approach to assessing the success of caregiving by using outcome assessment measures that reflect the effectiveness of the PD caregiver's actions. As shown in Table 19.4, the PD caregiver's effectiveness is measured by successful interaction with the patient's medical team, accurate assessment of the PD patient's symptoms and response to treatments, success in encouraging treatment compliance and patient self-reliance, and ability to assure a safe, supportive environment. Other indicators of caregiver

Table 19.4 Criteria for evaluating effectiveness of PD caregiving

1. *Interaction with medical providers*
   Exchanges information with medical team about disease management, i.e., on patient functioning, treatment effectiveness, and side effects
   Makes effective use of information/recommendations provided by health providers

2. *Interaction with PD patient*
   Accurate assessment of changes in patient symptoms and functioning over the course of a single day as well as from day to day
   Accurate monitoring of patient's response to treatment regimens; ability to encourage patient compliance
   Assures safe, supportive environment for PD patient
   Fosters self-reliance and independent functioning by the patient; regulates type and degree of assistance in accord with patient's current capabilities and symptoms

3. *Interaction with other caregivers and relevant parties*
   Communicates with other family members, home health aides, attorneys, etc.
   Mobilizes and collaborates with other helpers

effectiveness assess the caregiver's ability to mobilize and collaborate with other sources of help and support.

Conclusion

Much of the care of people with PD is provided by family members and this care is crucial in determining how well the illness is managed. Clinicians, patients, and caregivers themselves need to consider stress levels in the caregiver when dealing with PD; caregiving cannot be successful over a sustained period unless the caregiver's health, daily functioning, and quality of life are protected.

Much of the stress of caregiving is determined by the symptoms, and the severity of the patient's illness. The core motor manifestations of the illness, as well as cognition, sleep, and psychiatric problems need, therefore, to be maximally managed to reduce stress on the caregiver. Beyond these measures, one must consider the interaction between the caregiver and the patient, with attention given to their relationship. Strategies directed at the caregiver may include education and stress management of various types. Social support systems are crucial to avoiding a sense of isolation and are to be encouraged. Helping PD caregivers learn better ways to emotionally and practically cope with the severe physical decline unique to PD needs to go hand-in-hand with treating the medical problems specific to PD patients themselves.

References

1. Lieberman AN, Williams FL, *Parkinson's Disease: A Complete Guide for Patients and Caregivers*. New York: Simon & Schuster, 1993.
2. Jarman B, Hurwitz B, Cook A, Madhavi B, Lee A, Effects of community based nurses specializing in Parkinson's disease on health outcome and costs: randomized controlled trial. *BMJ* 2002; **324**:1–8.
3. Whetten-Goldstein K, Sloan F, Kulas E, Cutson T, Schenkman M, The burden of Parkinson's disease on society, family, and the individual. *J Am Geriatr Soc* 1997; **45**:844–849.
4. Haynie DA, Risk factors associated with caregiving for relatives with Parkinson's disease: Assessment and comparison. *Dissert Abstract Intern* 1998; **59**(08): 4447B.
5. Lane G, Coping as a mediator of caregiver distress. *Dissert Abstract Intern* 2004; **64**(11):5789B.
6. McDaniel SH, Hepworth J, Doherty WJ, *Medical Family Therapy*. New York: Basic Books, 1992.
7. Rolland JS, Toward a psychosocial typology of chronic and life-threatening illness. *Family Systems Med* 1984; **2**:245–262.

8. Rolland JS, Chronic illness and the life cycle: A conceptual framework. *Family Proc* 1987; **26**:203–221.
9. Cavanaugh JC, Caregiving to adults: A life event challenge. In: Nordhus IH, VandenBos GR, Berg S, Fromholt P (eds) *Clinical Geropsychology*. Washington, DC, American Psychological Association, 1998; 131–140.
10. Kurylo M, Elliott TR, DeVivo L, Dreer LE, Caregiver social problem solving abilities and family member adjustment following congestive heart failure. *J Clin Psychol Med Sett* 2004; **11**:151–157.
11. Shewchuk RM, Rivera PA, Elliott TR, Adams AM, Using cognitive mapping to understand problems experienced by family caregivers of persons with severe physical disabilities. *J Clin Psychol Med Sett* 2004; **11**:141–150.
12. Zarit SH, Johansson L, Jarrott SE, In: Nordhus IH, VandenBos GR, Berg S, Fromholt P (eds) *Clinical Geropsychology*. Washington, DC, American Psychological Association, 1998; 345–360
13. Zarit SH, Interventions with family caregivers. In: Zarit SH, Knight BG (eds) *A Guide to Psychotherapy and Aging*. Washington, DC, American Psychological Association, 1996; 139–159.
14. Clapcich J, Goldberg MA, Walsh E, *Be independent! (revised)*. New York: American Parkinson Disease Association, 1999.
15. Duvoisin RC, Golbe LI, Mark MH, Sage JI, Walters AS, *Parkinson's Disease Handbook (revised)*. New York: American Parkinson Disease Association, 2004.
16. McGoon DC, *The Parkinson's Handbook*. New York: Norton, 1990.
17. Samii A, Nutt JG, Ransom BR, Parkinson's disease. *The Lancet* 2004; **363**:1783–1793.
18. Aarsland D, Litvan I, Salmon D, Galasko D, Performance on the dementia rating scale in Parkinson's disease with dementia and dementia with Lewy bodies: Comparison with progressive supranuclear palsy and Alzheimer's disease. *J Neurol Neurosurg Psychiat* 2003; **74**:1215–1223.
19. Emre M, What causes mental dysfunction in Parkinson's disease? *Mov Disord* 2003; **18**:63–71.
20. Fernandez H, Crucian G, Okun M, Price C, Bowers D, Mild cognitive impairment in Parkinson's disease: The challenge and the prodrome. *Neuropsychiat Dis Treat* 2004; **1**:37–50.
21. Ridenour T, Dean R, Parkinson's disease and neuropsychological assessment. *Intern J Neurosci* 1999; **99**:1–18.
22. Zgaljardic D, Borod J, Foldi N, Mattis P, A review of the cognitive and behavioral sequelae of Parkinson's disease: Relationship to frontostriatal circuitry. *Cognitive Behav Neurol* 2003; **16**:2003.
23. Ballard CG, Definition and diagnosis of dementia with Lewy bodies. *Dementia Geriatr Cognit Disord* 2004; **17**:15–24.
24. Aarsland D, Andersen K, Larsen JP, Lolk K, Kragh-Sørenson P, Prevalence and characteristics of dementia in Parkinson's disease: An 8-year, prospective study. *Arch Neurol* 2003; **60**:287–302.
25. Stacy M, Sleep disorders in Parkinson's disease: Epidemiology and management. *Drugs Aging* 2002; **19**:733–739.
26. Happe S, Berger K, FAQT investigators, The association between caregiver burden and sleep disturbances in partners of patient's with Parkinson's disease. *Age Aging* 2002; **31**:349–354.
27. Comella C, Nardine TM, Diederich NJ, Stebbins GT, Sleep-related violence, injury, and REM sleep behavior disorder in Parkinson's disease. *Neurology* **51**:526–529.
28. Bernath O, Guilleminault C, Sleep-related violence, injury, and REM sleep behavior disorder in PD. *Neurology* 1999; **52**:1924–1925.

29. Brown R, Disorders of intention in Parkinsonian syndromes. In: Bedard MA (ed.) *Mental and Behavioral Dysfunction in Movement Disorders.* Humana Press: Totowa, NJ, 2003; 101–112.

30. Menza MA, Psychiatric aspects of Parkinson's disease. *Psychiatr Ann* 2002; **32:**99–104.

31. Hodgson JH, Garcia K, Tyndall L, Parkinson's disease and the couple relationship: A qualitative analysis. *Families, Systems Health* 2004; **22:**101–118.

32. Aarsland D, Larsen JP, Tandberg E, Laake K, Predictors of nursing home placement in Parkinson's disease: A population-based, prospective study. *J Am Geriatr Soc* 2000; **48:**938–942.

33. Henderson MJ, Mellers JDC, Psychosis in Parkinson's disease: "Between a rock and a hard place." *Intern J Psychiatr* 2000; **12:**319–334.

34. Naimark D, Jackson E, Rockwell E, Jeste DV, Psychotic symptoms in Parkinson's disease patients with dementia. *Am J Geriat Psychiat* 1996; **44:**296–299.

35. Ismail MS, Richard IH, A reality test: How well do we understand psychosis in Parkinson's disease? *J Neuropsychiat Clin Neurosci* 2004; **16:**8–18.

36. Hely MA, Morris JGI, Traficante R, Reid WGJ, O'Sullivan DJ, Williamson PM, The Sydney multicentre study of Parkinson's disease: progression and mortality at 10 years. *J Neurol Neurosurg Psychiatr* 1999; **67:**300–307.

37. Pearlin LI, Mullan JT, Semple SJ, Skaff MM, Caregiving and the stress process: An overview of concepts and their measures. *The Gerontologist* 1990; **30:**583–594.

38. Schulz R, Beach SR, Caregiving as a risk factor for mortality: The caregiver health effects study. *JAMA* 1999; **282:**2215–2219.

39. Lazarus RS, Folkman S, *Stress, Appraisal and Coping.* New York: Springer Publishing Company, 1984.

40. Schulz R, O'Brien AT, Bookwala JF, Psychiatric and physical morbidity effects of dementia caregiving: Prevalence, correlates, and causes. *The Gerontologist* 1995; **35:**771–789.

41. Greenberg VE, *Respecting Your Limits when Caring for Aging Parents.* San Francisco: Jossey-Bass, 1998.

42. Hooker K, Manoogian-O'Dell M, Monahan DJ, Frazier LD, Shifren K, Does type of disease matter? Gender differences among Alzheimer's and Parkinson's disease spouse caregivers. *The Gerontologist* 2000; **40:**568–573.

43. Beutler LE, Moos R, Lane G, Coping, treatment planning, and treatment outcome: Discussion. *J Clin Psychol* 2003; **59:**1151–1167.

44. Murman DI, Chen Q, Colucci PM, Colenda CG, Gelb DJ, Liang J, Comparison of healthcare utilization and direct costs in three degenerative dementias. *Am J Geriat Psychiat* 2002; **10:**328–336.

45. McRae C, Sherry P, Roper K, Stress and family functioning among caregivers of person's with Parkinson's disease. *Parkinsonism Relat Disord* 1999; **5:**69–75.

46. Haberman B, Spousal perspective of Parkinson's disease in middle life. *J Advan Nurs* 2000; **31:**1409–1415.

47. Beutler LE, Clarkin JF, Bongar B, *Guidelines for the Systematic Treatment of the Depressed Patient.* New York: Oxford University Press, 2001.

48. Beutler LE, Harwood TM, *Prescriptive Psychotherapy.* New York: Oxford University Press, 2000.

49. Oertel WH, Ellgring H, Parkinson's disease – medical education and psychosocial aspects. *Patient Edu Counsel* 1995; **26:**71–19.

50. Greene S, Griffin WA, The influence of marital satisfaction on symptom expression in Parkinson's disease. *Psychiatry* 1998; **61:**35–45.

51. Vitaliano PP, Young HM, Russo J, Romano J, Magana-Amato A, Does expressed emotion in spouses predict problems among care recipients with Alzheimer's disease? *J Gerontol* 1993; **4:**202–209.

52. Doherty WJ, Rigidity in the family: A case of Parkinson's disease. In: McDaniel SH, Hepworth J, Doherty WJ (eds) *The Shared Experience of Illness*. New York: Basic Books, 1997; 351–357.
53. Sörenson S, Pinquart M, Habil D, Duberstein P, How effective are interventions with caregivers? An updated meta-analysis. *The Gerontologist* 2002; **42**:356–372.
54. Kowal J, Johnson SM, Lee A, Chronic illness in couples: A case for emotionally-focused therapy. *J Marit Fam Ther* 2003; **29**:299–310.

Appendix A

Table A.1 Antipsychotics used in Parkinson's disease

Generic name	Tradename	Doses (mg)	Indications/special considerations
Typical antipsychotics			
None indicated			Do not use – poorly tolerated
Atypical antipsychotics			
Aripiprazole	Abilify	5–30	Psychosis (variable tolerability)
Clozapine	Clozaril	6.25–150	Psychosis, behavioral disturbances (agranulocytosis)
Olanzapine	Zyprexa	2.5–15	Psychosis, behavioral disturbances (not well-tolerated)
Quetiapine	Seroquel	12.5–150	Psychosis, behavioral disturbances
Risperidone	Risperdal	0.5–6	Psychosis (poorly tolerated)
Ziprasidone	Geodon	10–60	Psychosis (variable tolerability)

Table A.2 Antidepressant medications used in Parkinson's disease

Generic name	Tradename	Dose (mg)	Indications
Tricyclic antidepressants			
Clomipramine	Anafranil	25–150	Depression
Desipramine	Norpramin	25–150	Depression
Doxepin	Sinequan	25–200	Depression
Imipramine	Tofranil	25–200	Depression
Maprotiline	Ludiomil	10–150	Depression
Nortriptyline	Pamelor	10–75	Depression
Protriptyline	Vivactil	5–30	Depression
Trimipramine	Surmontil	25–150	Depression
Serotonin-selective reuptake inhibitors (SSRIs)			
Citalopram	Celexa	10–60	Depression
Escitalopram	Lexapro	5–30	Depression, anxiety disorders
Fluoxetine	Prozac	5–60	Depression, anxiety disorders
Fluvoxamine	Luvox	25–200	Depression, OCD
Paroxetine	Paxil	10–50	Depression, anxiety disorders
Paroxetine	Paxil CR	12.5–50	Depression, anxiety disorders
Sertraline	Zoloft	25–200	Depression, anxiety disorders
Others			
Atomoxetine	Strattera	40–100	ADHD-type symptoms
Bupropion	Wellbutrin	50–300	Depression
Bupropion	Wellbutrin–SR	50–300	Depression
Bupropion	Wellbutrin–XL	50–300	Depression
Duloxetine	Cymbalta	20–60	Depression, diabetic pain
Mirtazepine	Remeron	15–45	Depression
Nefazodone	Serzone	25–200	Depression (caution liver failure)
Trazodone	Desyrel	25–300	Hypnotic
Venlafaxine	Effexor XR	37.5–300?	Depression, anxiety disorders
Venlafaxine	Effexor	37.5–300?	Depression, anxiety disorders

Table A.3 Medications used for insomnia in Parkinson's disease

Generic name	Tradename	Dose	Indications
Non-benzodiazepine hypnotics			
Eszopiclone	Estorra		Approval expected in 2005
Zaleplon	Sonata	5–10	Insomnia
Zolpidem	Ambien	5–10	Insomnia
Benzodiazepines			
Alprazolam	Xanax	0.25–6	Anxiety
Chlordiazepoxide	Librium	5–60	Anxiety
Clonazepam	Klonopin	0.5–3.0	Anxiety, used for insomnia, REM behavior disorder (RBD), periodic leg movements of sleep (PLMS)
Clorazepate	Tranxene	7.5–30	Anxiety, used for insomnia
Diazepam	Valium	2–30	Anxiety, used for insomnia
Estazolam	ProSom	0.5–2	Insomnia
Flurazepam	Dalmane	15–30	Insomnia
Lorazepam	Ativan	0.5–6	Anxiety, used for insomnia
Antidepressants			
Amitriptyline	Elavil	10–75	Depression, used for insomnia
Doxepin	Sinequan	10–75	Depression, used for insomnia
Imipramine	Tofranil	10–75	Depression, used for insomnia
Trazodone	Desyrel	12.5–150	Depression, widely used for insomnia

Appendix B

A listing of web-based resources and contact information for clinician education, patient and caregiver education and support, research funding, and advocacy.

General information

Doctors Guide – Personal Edition
www.docguide.com

A source for peer-reviewed literature, case studies, webcasts, continuing medical education courses, news updates and patient education. Available in multiple languages.

WE MOVE™
Worldwide Education and Awareness for Movement Disorders
1-800-437-MOV2
www.wemove.org

WE MOVE™ is an internet-based resource that provides information on movement disorders to patients, healthcare workers, and the public. Its focus is on research and treatments along with links to support groups and the news updates on research results. WE MOVE™ also designs and provides professional and patient internet-based learning modules, teaching slide sets, office tools, moderated patient/family Web chats, E-MOVE news features (www.imakenews.com/wemove), and post-chat print newsletters.

Massachusetts General Hospital Neurology Web Page

neuro-www.mgh.harvard.edu:16080/forum/ParkinsonsDiseaseMenu.html

This is a webforum to discuss and comment on Parkinson's disease. It is used by many individuals with PD.

The Parkinson's Web

pdweb.mgh.harvard.edu

For clinicians, this web-based resource links to national PD organizations, medical centers and other sites offering clinical care of PD patients, private institutes and foundations, government resources, and professional organizations. Separate links for families and patients are also provided.

Caregiver information

Family Caregiver Alliance (FCA)

(800) 445.8106 (San Francisco, CA)

www.caregiver.org

Founded in 1977, the FCA was the first community-based non-profit organization in the USA to address the needs of families and friends providing long-term care at home. FCA provides programs at national, state and local levels to support and sustain caregivers. It also operates the National Center on Caregiving to promote public awareness, policy and research to develop high-quality, cost-effective support programs for family caregivers across the nation.

National Family Caregivers Association (NFCA)

1-800-896-3650 (Kensington, MD)

www.thefamilycaregiver.org/

The NFCA conducts advocacy efforts and provides support and education to individuals who care for a chronically ill, aged, or disabled loved one. The NFCA is dedicated to address caregiving issues that extend beyond individual diagnoses and different life stages.

Parkinson's disease organizations

American Parkinson's Disease Association (APDA)
1-800-223-2732 (Staten Island, NY)
1-800-908-2732 (Los Angeles, CA)
888-400-2732 (Contact for Local Information and Referral Center)
www.apdaparkinson.org

The APDA has many local chapters and affiliated support groups. The organization provides education and support to patients. It also provides annual grants to researchers and takes part in public education about PD through events and fund-raisers.

American Parkinson's Disease Association
Young Parkinson's Information and Referral Center
800.223.9776 or 847.657.5787 (Glenview, Illinois)
www.youngparkinson.org

The APDA has a website targeted to the issues and concerns of the younger patient population (ages 21–50). It provides information and resources for living well with PD. The site also includes a photo gallery of young people with Parkinson's and their stories, the opportunity to be connected one-to-one to other young people with PD and a library of downloadable APDA educational materials.

European Parkinson's Disease Association (EPDA)
++44 (0) 1732 457 683 (Kent, UK)
www.epda.eu.com

The EPDA is a non-profit organization that includes memberships from over 30 Parkinson's patient organizations in Europe. It is devoted to increasing international understanding about PD and providing information and education to patients and their families about PD. The site provides links to PD organizations throughout the world.

Michael J. Fox Foundation for Parkinson's Research
1-800-708-7644 (New York, NY)
www.michaeljfox.org

Michael J. Fox started this non-profit organization to teach patients and caregivers about living with PD and to raise funds to support aggressive research towards finding a cure. The website and newsletter provide news updates on PD research, news, and events.

National Parkinson Foundation, Inc (NPF)
1-800-327-4545 (Miami, Florida)
www.parkinson.org

The NPF is the largest organization in the United States for individuals with PD and their families. The website provides information about new research, events, and support groups as well as grant funding opportunities for researchers. The NPF site provides extensive links to caregiver resources.

Parkinson's Action Network (PAN)
1-800-850-4726 (Washington, DC)
www.parkinsonaction.org

PAN is the unified education and advocacy voice of the Parkinson's community in the USA. PAN provides individuals with PD and other advocates opportunities for education and interaction with the Parkinson's community, scientists, policy and opinion leaders, as well as the public at large. PAN promotes its advocacy efforts via an informed grassroots network that focuses on an increased and accelerated investment of public resources for PD research and care.

Parkinson's Disease Foundation (PDF)
1-800-457-6676 (New York, NY)
www.pdf.org

The PDF is a national non-profit organization in the United States that is devoted to education, advocacy, and the funding of research.

Parkinson's Disease Society (PDS)
020 7931 8080 (London)
www.parkinsons.org.uk

A charitable organization, the PDS provides support, advice, and information to people with Parkinson's, their carers, families and friends, and to health and social services professionals involved in management and care. It has many branches and support groups throughout the UK. The PDS engages in advocacy and fundraising for research and has developed models of good practice in service provision, such as Parkinson's Disease Nurse Specialists and respite care.

People Living With Parkinson's

www.plwp.org

This website is supported by patients. It provides chat rooms, message boards, and facts on PD.

Parkinson's Information Exchange Network's Online (PIENO)

parkinsons-information-exchange-network-online.com

PIENO provides an international e-mail list and website about Parkinson's that includes patients, caregivers, family members, medical professionals, and healthcare industry representatives. The language is English.

The Parkinson's Alliance (PA)

1-800-579-8440
www.parkinsonalliance.net/home.html

This is a United States-based non-profit organization dedicated to raising funds to help finance the research to find the cause and cure for Parkinson's disease.

World Parkinson's Disease Association

(39) 02 66713111 (Italy)
www.wpda.org

A non-profit organization, fostered by APDA and the Italian Parkinson Association (AIP), that serves the world Parkinson community through education and promotes greater cooperation and exchange of communications among the various national patients' organizations.

Research programs and opportunities

ClinicalTrials.org

www.clinicaltrials.gov

Proves regularly updated information about federally and privately supported clinical research in human volunteers.

Parkinson's Disease Research Web
National Institutes of Health: National Institute of Neurological Disorders and Stroke
www.ninds.nih.gov/parkinsonsweb

This NIH disease-specific website was developed to facilitate research efforts on Parkinson's disease, track the progress of the PD Research agenda and Matrix activities, and provide both the research and lay community with information and resources. The Parkinson's disease research portfolio is managed by the NINDS Neurodegeneration Group.

PDTrials.org
www.PDtrials.org

This site provides information on Parkinson's clinical research and clinical trials that are currently looking for participants. The website was recently developed as part of a national public awareness campaign, *Advancing Parkinson's Therapies* (APT), coordinated by the Parkinson's Disease Foundation with leadership from American Parkinson Disease Association, The Michael J. Fox Foundation for Parkinson's Research, the National Parkinson Foundation, the Parkinson's Action Network, the Parkinson Alliance, and WE MOVE.

Center Watch: Clinical Trials Listing Service
617-856-5900 (Boston, MA)
www.centerwatch.org

This site is maintained by a Boston-based publishing and information services company and is a business of The Thomson Corporation. It provides information about clinical research, including listings of more than 41 000 active industry protocols and government-sponsored clinical trials, as well as new drug therapies in research for patients interested in participating in clinical trials and for research professionals in pharmaceutical, biotechnology, and medical device companies, CROs, and research centers involved in clinical research around the world.

Index

Numbers in bold type indicate figures, italics indicate tables.